Infectious Diseases, Microbiology and Virology

Infectious Diseases, Microbiology and Virology

A Q&A Approach for Specialist
Medical Trainees

Luke S. P. Moore
Consultant in Infectious Diseases, Microbiology & Virology, Chelsea & Westminster NHS Foundation Trust, Imperial College London

James C. Hatcher
Consultant in Infectious Diseases and Microbiology, Great Ormond Street Hospital for Children

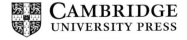
CAMBRIDGE
UNIVERSITY PRESS

CAMBRIDGE
UNIVERSITY PRESS

University Printing House, Cambridge CB2 8BS, United Kingdom

One Liberty Plaza, 20th Floor, New York, NY 10006, USA

477 Williamstown Road, Port Melbourne, VIC 3207, Australia

314–321, 3rd Floor, Plot 3, Splendor Forum, Jasola District Centre, New Delhi – 110025, India

79 Anson Road, #06–04/06, Singapore, 079906

Cambridge University Press is part of the University of Cambridge.

It furthers the University's mission by disseminating knowledge in the pursuit of education, learning and research at the highest international levels of excellence.

www.cambridge.org
Information on this title: www.cambridge.org/9781316609712
DOI: 10.1017/9781316659373

© Luke S. P. Moore and James C. Hatcher 2020

First published 2020

Printed in the United Kingdom by TJ International Ltd, Padstow Cornwall

A catalogue record for this publication is available from the British Library.

Library of Congress Cataloging-in-Publication Data
Names: Moore, Luke S.P. author. | Hatcher, James C., author.
Title: Infectious diseases, microbiology and virology : a Q & A approach for specialist medical trainees / Luke S.P. Moore, James C. Hatcher.
Description: Cambridge ; New York, NY : Cambridge University Press, 2019. | Includes bibliographical references.
Identifiers: LCCN 2019019458 | ISBN 9781316609712 (pbk.)
Subjects: | MESH: Communicable Diseases | Microbiology | Virology | Problems and Exercises
Classification: LCC RC111 | NLM WC 18.2 | DDC 616.9–dc23
LC record available at https://lccn.loc.gov/2019019458

ISBN 978-1-316-60971-2 Paperback

....

Contents

Preface

Training in infection-related specialities in the United Kingdom has undergone substantial changes over the past years. Combination of specialities (microbiology, virology, tropical medicine and infectious diseases) and the desire for infection specialists to increase clinical activities and reduce laboratory-based practice have led to a fundamental change in examination methodology. Our aim was to produce a book that mapped to the current infection training curriculum in line with the examination style of 'best of five' answers.

We have designed this book to test the knowledge of candidates preparing for examinations in infection specialities, but it is also our aim to have a broader appeal to other specialities with infection as a core component of their training. The book has 300 'best of five' questions; along with the answers, there are detailed explanations and background to the answers, including suggestions for further reading around the subject. Readers who through this book identify curriculum areas where their understanding may be sub-optimal can then focus their revision to optimise their learning.

We are both practising infection consultants supervising current infection trainees preparing for examinations during busy clinical placements and have a deep understanding of the stress that assessments can cause. We hope you enjoy the book and it provides knowledge and guidance that will serve you beyond the examinations.

Reference Ranges

Haematology

Hb	Male	130–180 g/L
	Female	115–165 g/L
WCC	Total	$4\text{--}11 \times 10^9$/L
	Neutrophils	$1.5\text{--}7 \times 10^9$/L
	Lymphocytes	$1.5\text{--}4 \times 10^9$/L
	Monocytes	$0\text{--}0.8 \times 10^9$/L
	Eosinophils	$0.04\text{--}0.4 \times 10^9$/L
	Basophils	$0\text{--}0.1 \times 10^9$/L
Platelets		$150\text{--}400 \times 10^9$/L
Reticulocyte count		0.5–2.5%
ESR	Male	0–20 mm/first hour
	Female	0–30 mm/first hour

Clotting

Fibrinogen	1.8–5.4 g/L
INR	<1.4

Biochemistry

ALT	5–35 U/L
Albumin	37–49 g/L
ALP	45–105 U/L
Amylase	60–180 U/L
AST	1–31 U/L
B_{12}	115–1000 pmol/L
Bicarbonate	22–30 mmol/L
Bilirubin	
Total	1–22 mmol/L
Conjugated	0–3.4 mmol/L
C-reactive protein	<10 mg/L

Creatine kinase

    Male   25–195 U/L

    Female   35–170 U/L

Folate   2–20 ng/mL

Creatinine   20–70 μmol/L

Glucose (fasting plasma)   3.0–6.0 mmol/L

Immunoglobulin

    IgA   0.8–3.0 g/L

    IgG   6.0–13.0 g/L

    IgM   0.4–2.5 g/L

    IgE   <120 kU/L

Lactate (plasma)   0.6–1.8 mmol/L

Protein   60–76 g/L

Urea   2.5–7.5 mmol/L

Potassium   3.5–5 mmol/L

Sodium   135–145 mmol/L

Blood Gases

H^+ 35–45 nmol/L

pH   7.35–7.45

$PaCO_2$ 4.7–6.0 kPa

PaO_2 11.3–12.6 kPa

Base excess   +/− 2 mmol/L

CSF

Cell count

    Neutrophils   None

    Lymphocytes   60–70%

    Monocytes   30–50%

    Red cells   None

Protein   0.15–0.45 g/L

IgG   5–10 mg/L

Glucose   3.3–4.4 mmol/L

Opening Pressure   5–18 cmH_2O

Abbreviations

ABG	Arterial blood gas
BCG	Bacillus Calmette-Guerin
BTS	British Thoracic Society
CAP	Community-acquired pneumonia
CRP	C-reactive protein
ELISA	Enzyme-linked immunosorbent assay
ESBL	Extended-spectrum beta-lactamase
GCS	Glasgow Coma Scale
HAP	Healthcare-associated pneumonia
HAV	Hepatitis A virus
Hb	Haemoglobin
HBV	Hepatitis B virus
HCAI	Healthcare-associated infection
HCV	Hepatitis C virus
HDV	Hepatitis D virus
HEV	Hepatitis E virus
HIV	Human immunodeficiency virus
HPV	Human papilloma virus
HTLV	Human T-lymphocyte virus
INR	International normalised ratio
MC&S	Microscopy, culture and susceptibility
Neut	Neutrophil count
NICE	National Institute for Health and Care Excellence
NTM	Non-tuberculous *Mycobacterium* spp.
OCP	Ova, cysts and parasites
PCR	Polymerase chain reaction
PHE	Public Health England
RCC	Red cell count
TPHA	*Treponema pallidum* haemagglutination
VAP	Ventilator-associated pneumonia
VDRL	Venereal disease reference laboratory
WCC	White cell count
WHO	World Health Organization

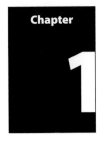

Biology of Bacteria, Viruses, Fungi and Parasites and the Host–Pathogen Interactions

Microbial and host cellular biology and interactions dictate the breadth of clinical infection practice, from colonisation to invasion to infection. Understanding the classifications used for bacteria, viruses, fungi and parasites aids clinical and laboratory diagnosis and ultimately patient management. Understanding the common host responses to infective agents at the cellular level enables appropriate clinical management both with direct acting anti-infectives and other supportive therapy.

Questions

Q1.1 A 21-year-old female presents with a fever, and a novel viral infection is suspected. Electron microscopy is performed. Which of the following might be present in a virus?
A. Nucleus
B. An envelope
C. Metabolic pathways
D. Ribosomes
E. A cell wall

Q1.2 A 46-year-old male presents with a fever of unknown origin, and a whole blood sample is sent to the virology laboratory for polymerase chain reaction testing. The test identifies a DNA virus. Which of the following class of viruses contain DNA?
A. Rhabdoviridae
B. Orthmyxoviridae
C. Enteroviridae
D. Flaviviridae
E. Parvoviridae

Q1.3 A 1-year-old male awaiting repair of a ventricular septal defect is being considered for palivizumab prophylactic therapy for respiratory syncytial virus (RSV). What type of virus is RSV?
A. Single-stranded (−) RNA
B. Single-stranded (+) RNA
C. Double-stranded RNA

D. Single-stranded DNA

E. Double-stranded DNA

Q1.4   A 21-year-old female presents with a fever and leucopaenia, and a viral infection is suspected. Which of the following is a paramyxovirus?

A. Rubella virus

B. Influenza B virus

C. Polio virus

D. Nipah virus

E. Parvovirus B19

Q1.5   A 25-year-old female is recalled after cervical screening. Which of the following is true regarding human papillomavirus (HPV)-associated malignancy?

A. HPV-6 and HPV-11 are associated with genital cancers

B. HPV-16 and HPV-18 are associated with genital cancers

C. HPV late viral proteins inhibit tumour suppressor genes

D. HPV-6 and HPV-11 are associated with anal in-situ neoplasia

E. HPV late viral proteins are products of proto-oncogenes

Q1.6   A 27-year-old female with sickle cell anaemia presents in aplastic crisis with a fever. Her blood results demonstrate:

Haemoglobin 50 g/L

Reticulocyte count 0.1%

White cell count 12.3×10^9/L

Lymphocytes 8.6×10^9/L

CRP 34

Which genus is the most likely causative virus from?

A. Dependovirus

B. Henipahvirus

C. Pneumovirus

D. Parvovirus

E. Erythrovirus

Q1.7   A 31-year-old female is referred from occupational health. A chronic infective carrier state may occur in which viral infection?

A. Hanta virus

B. Hepatitis A virus

C. Hepatitis E virus

D. Hepatitis C virus

E. Nipah virus

Q1.8 A 54-year-old male presents with fever, tachycardia and hypotension. A blood culture is taken and becomes positive in 12 hours. The Gram stain is shown in Figure 1.1.

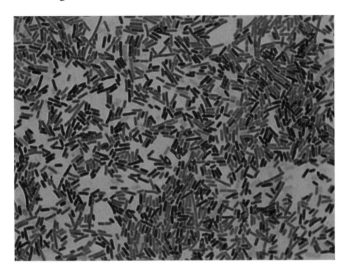

Figure 1.1 Gram stain from a positive blood culture. (A black and white version of this figure will appear in some formats. For the colour version, please refer to the plate section.)

Which of the components of the Gram stain is a fixative?
A. Safranin
B. Carbol fuchsin
C. Acetone
D. Crystal violet
E. Iodide

Q1.9 A 54-year-old male presents with fever, tachycardia and hypotension. A blood culture is taken and becomes positive in 12 hours, and *Escherichia coli* is identified. It is demonstrated to have in vitro resistance to many penicillins and cephalosporins. Through what mechanism is an extended-spectrum beta-lactamase gene most likely to be present in this *E. coli*?
A. Transduction
B. Transformation
C. Conjugation
D. Constitutively
E. De novo mutation

Q1.10 A 28-year-old male presents with diarrhoea. A non-lactose fermenting coliform is isolated from faeces, and serological investigation of the isolate is performed. The "O" antigen is positive, but the "H" antigen is negative. What is the most likely explanation for this?
A. The isolate is non-motile
B. The isolate needs boiling prior to agglutination
C. The presence of a "Vi" antigen is masking the "H" antigen
D. The isolate is in a non-specific phase
E. The isolate is not a *Salmonella* species

Q1.11 A 35-week pregnant female recalled a flu-like illness 2 days prior to delivery. She was treated for peri-partum sepsis, and her new-born child was born in poor condition and admitted to the neonatal intensive care department. Blood cultures (and subsequently cerebrospinal fluid) grew the organism depicted in Figure 1.2.

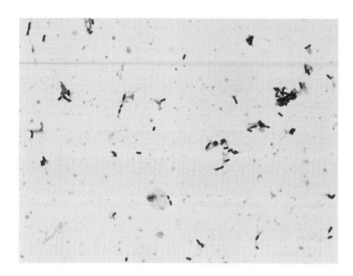

Figure 1.2 Gram stain of cerebrospinal fluid. (A black and white version of this figure will appear in some formats. For the colour version, please refer to the plate section.)

Which laboratory test would be the most useful to confirm identification?
A. Coagulase
B. Catalase
C. Oxidase
D. Haemolysis on blood agar
E. Tumbling motility

Q1.12 A 34-year-old man presents with a fever, and an aerobic blood culture bottle grows a Gram-negative rod. Which one of the following organisms is a strict aerobe?
A. *Bacteroides fragilis*
B. *Kluyvera* spp.
C. *Proteus vulgaris*
D. *Prevotella melaninogenica*
E. *Pseudomonas aeruginosa*

Q1.13 A 42-year-old patient presents with septic shock and is found to have a soft tissue infection. Which component of the cell wall of Gram-positive bacteria may contribute to the development of septic shock in Gram-positive infections?
A. Capsular protein
B. Endotoxin
C. Peptidoglycan
D. Phospholipid
E. Teichoic acid

Q1.14 A 23-year-old female presents with a urinary tract infection. Which of the following is true about urease producing bacteria?
A. Urease acidifies the urine rendering neutrophils inactive
B. *Escherichia coli* is urease positive
C. Acidifying the urine can lead to precipitation of struvite calculi
D. *Morganella morganii* is potentially a urea-splitting bacteria
E. Are commensal organisms that prevent hepatic encephalopathy

Q1.15 A 63-year-old female is diagnosed with urosepsis. She is profoundly hypotensive. What is the most important endotoxin component leading to septic shock from Gram-negative bacteria?
A. Lipopolysaccharide core oligosaccharides
B. Outer membrane vesicles
C. Lipid A
D. O antigens
E. Capsule

Q1.16 A 21-year-old female presents with necrotising fasciitis. Which of the following is not a virulence factor of *Staphylococcus aureus*?
A. Lecthinase
B. Toxic shock syndrome toxin-1
C. Panton-Valentine leukocidin
D. Enterotoxin A
E. DNase

Q1.17 A 31-year-old male returns from Ethiopia and presents with a recurrent febrile illness. What is the cause of the relapsing nature of fever in *Borrelia recurrentis* infection?
A. Antigenic drift
B. Antigenic shift
C. Rapidly developing antibody resistance
D. Antigenic variation
E. Encapsulation

Q1.18 A 16-year-old male presents with respiratory distress. Which organism produces a toxin similar in action to that of *Corynebacterium diphtheriae*?
A. *Bordetella pertussis*
B. *Pseudomonas aeruginosa*
C. *Serratia marcescens*
D. *Haemophilius influenzae*
E. *Clostridium tetani*

Q1.19 An 18-year-old female presents with difficulty swallowing. A throat swab demonstrates club-shaped organisms with differential staining. *Corynebacterium diphtheriae* is suspected. What are *Corynebacterium diphtheriae* volutin granules made of?
A. Carbohydrate
B. Protein
C. Lipid
D. Phosphate
E. Collagen

Q1.20 A 45-year-old female presents with a heart block following a minor dog bite to the palm of her hand (Figure 1.3).

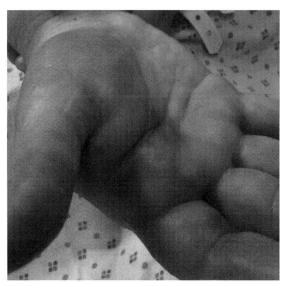

Figure 1.3 Clinical appearance of the right hand following a minor dog bite.

Corynebacterium ulcerans is isolated from the wound, and an Elek test is positive. How does diphtheria toxin act?
A. ADP ribosylation of EF2
B. Ergosterol synthesis inhibition
C. Peptidoglycan disruption
D. Protein synthesis inhibition at the ribosome
E. Acetyl choline esterase inhibition

Q1.21 A 50-year-old male who underwent traumatic splenectomy two years ago presents with tachypnoea, tachycardia and hypoxia. A mucoid *Streptococcus pneumoniae* is subsequently grown (Figure 1.4).

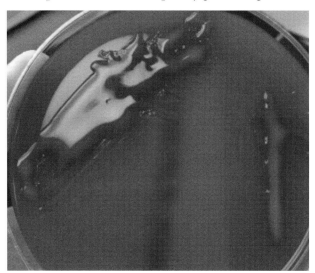

Figure 1.4 Growth on blood agar incubated in an aerobic environment at 37°C for 24 hours. (A black and white version of this figure will appear in some formats. For the colour version, please refer to the plate section.)

An avirulent, non-capsulate strain of pneumococcus can change to virulent capsulate strains through which mechanism?

A. Plasmid transfer
B. Bacteriophage
C. Naked DNA transformation
D. Homogenous recombination
E. Slipped strand mispairing

Q1.22 A 56-year-old male is diagnosed with native valve endocarditis. A blood culture grows a Gram-positive cocci on both blood agar and MacConkey agar, which is ampicillin resistant. What is the likely identification of this organism?

A. *Enterococcus faecalis*
B. *Enterococcus faecium*
C. *Streptococcus pneumoniae*
D. *Streptococcus bovis*
E. *Streptococcus anginosus*

Q1.23 A 14-month-old child is admitted with a two-week history of coughing and is admitted with severe paroxysms of coughing leading to hypoxia. Pertussis is suspected. Which of the following is true about *Bordetella pertussis*?

A. Polymorphonuclear leucocytosis seen during infection
B. Can be clinically diagnosed initially within days of onset
C. Organism is isolated from the throat for several days following infection
D. Vaccine gives lifelong immunity
E. Tetracycline is effective in the paroxysmal stage

Q1.24 A 56-year-old female with urosepsis is not improving despite treatment with an intravenous third-generation cephalosporin. Which bacteria are most likely to harbour an extended-spectrum beta-lactamase gene?

A. *Klebsiella pneumoniae*
B. *Enterobacter cloacae*
C. *Citrobacter freundii*
D. *Morganella morganii*
E. *Proteus mirabilis*

Q1.25 A 49-year-old homeless patient attends the emergency department complaining of itching and fever. He describes the onset of fever approximately 7 days ago. On examination, he has a widespread rash and excoriation marks. What is the most likely vector for this illness?

A. *Aedes aegypti*
B. *Anopheles gambiae*
C. *Pediculus humanus humanus*
D. *Glossina* spp.
E. *Culex* spp.

Q1.26 A 54-year-old male presents with a flitting rash and an eosinophilia eight weeks after return from the tropics. Which of the following infections require an intermediate snail host?
A. Diphylobothriasis
B. Schistosomiasis
C. Echinococcosis
D. Paragonamiasis
E. Strongyloidiasis

Q1.27 A 31-year-old male presents with diarrhoea several days after return from Nigeria. *Entamoeba* is seen on stool microscopy. Which of the following is a non-pathogenic variant of *Entamoeba histolytica*?
A. *Entamoeba dispar*
B. *Escherichia coli*
C. *Entamoeba hartmanni*
D. *Endolimax nana*
E. *Enterobacter cloacae*

Q1.28 A 21-year-old female presents with a fever, adenopathy and a rash. Blood tests demonstrate a lymphocytosis. Serological diagnosis of a primary viral infection may be made by detection of which viral-specific immunoglobulin?
A. IgA
B. IgD
C. IgE
D. IgM
E. IgG

Q1.29 A 23-year-old male student has been recently admitted with invasive meningococcal disease. He has made a good recovery but gives a history of a previous episode of meningococcal septicaemia when he was 15 years old. There is no history of other recurrent infections. Which immunodeficiency is most likely in this patient?
A. Adenosine deaminase deficiency
B. C7 deficiency
C. Job's syndrome
D. Myeloperoxidase deficiency
E. Selective IgM deficiency

Q1.30 An 18-year-old male with chronic granulomatous disease (CGD) has recurrent staphylococcal infection. What is the mechanism behind this?
A. Chemotaxis inhibition
B. Defect in phagocyte oxidase
C. Lack of C3d receptor
D. Failure of phago-lysosome fusion
E. IgM deficiency

Q1.31 A 63-year-old female is diagnosed with urosepsis. She is profoundly hypotensive. The lipopolysaccharide of Gram-negative bacteria is the principle ligand for which specific toll-like receptor (TLR)?
A. TLR3
B. TLR4
C. TLR5
D. TLR7
E. TLR10

Q1.32 A 31-year-old male presents with acute hepatitis. He is found to have hepatitis C, but subsequently clears this infection. Which pattern of cytokines is produced by TH1 lymphocytes?
A. IL4 and IL10
B. TNF-β and IL1
C. IL2 and IFN-γ
D. IL1 and IL12
E. IL4, IL5, IL6 and IL13

Answers

A1.1 **Answer B: An envelope**
Viruses (Latin for toxin) contain DNA or RNA but not both. The central ribonucleic core is surrounded by a protective shell (not a cell wall) of repeating protein units called capsomeres. This has a symmetry which is either helical or icosahedral. Viral particles contain polymerases and integrases but no true metabolic pathways. As completed virions move from the host cell nucleus to the cytoplasm or from the cytoplasm to the extracellular space, an external lipid-containing envelope may be added to the nucleocapsid.

Further Reading

Abrescia NGA, Bamford DH, Grimes JM, Stuart DI. Structure unifies the viral universe. *Ann Rev Biochem.* 2012;81:795–782.

A1.2 **Answer E: Parvoviridae**
There are several methods of classifying viruses, but perhaps the most widely used is the Baltimore system developed in 1971, which designates viruses into one of seven groups depending on the nature of the nucleic acid within the virus. Four aspects are considered: (i) whether the nucleic acid is DNA or RNA, (ii) whether it is single stranded or double stranded, (iii) whether it is positive or negative sense, and (iv) the method of replication.

Table 1 Classification of viruses.

I	II	III	IV	V	VI	VII
Double-stranded DNA	Single-stranded DNA	Double-stranded RNA	Single-stranded (+) RNA	Single-stranded (−) RNA	Single-stranded (+) reverse transcriptase RNA	Double-stranded reverse transcriptase DNA
Adeno	Parvo	Reo	Picorna	Orthomyxo	Retro	Hepadna
Herpes			Toga	Paramyxo		
Pox			Flavi	Rhabdo		
Papilloma			Corona	Filo		
			Calici	Arena		
			Hepe	Bunya		

Data from Baltimore (1971).

Further Reading

Baltimore D. Expression of animal virus genomes. *Bacteriol Rev.* 1971;35(3):235–241.

A1.3 Answer A: Single-stranded (−) RNA

RSV is a single-stranded (−) RNA virus of the family Paramyxoviridae. Infection with this virus usually produces only mild symptoms, often indistinguishable from common cold and minor illnesses. It is, however, also the most common cause of bronchiolitis and pneumonia in children less than 1 year of age and can also cause croup. These syndromes are more likely to occur in patients that are immunocompromised or infants born prematurely. No antivirals are effective – the mainstay of therapy is oxygen. Palivizumab (a monoclonal antibody against RSV surface fusion protein) can be given as monthly injections begun just prior to the RSV season (usually for five months) as RSV prophylaxis for infants that are premature or have either cardiac or lung disease.

Further Reading

Andabaka T, Nickerson JW, Rojas-Reyes MX, Rueda JD, Bacic Vrca V, Barsic B. Monoclonal antibody for reducing the risk of respiratory syncytial virus infection in children. *Cochrane Database Syst Rev.* 2013;4:CD006602.

A1.4 Answer D: Nipah virus

The paramyxoviridae (ss(−)RNA) family includes viruses causing many common infections. However, it has a complex taxonomy:

Subfamily Paramyxovirinae

  Genus Henipavirus (Hendra virus and Nipah virus)
  Genus Morbillivirus (Measles virus)

Genus Respirovirus (Human parainfluenza viruses 1 and 3)

Genus Rubulavirus (Mumps virus and Human parainfluenza viruses 2 and 4)

Subfamily Pneumovirinae

Genus Pneumovirus (Human respiratory syncytial virus)

Genus Metapneumovirus (Human metapneumovirus)

Rubella virus is of the genus Rubivirus from the Togaviridae family (ss(+)RNA). Influenza B virus is a genus of the Orthomyxoviridae family (ss(−)RNA). Polio virus is of the genus Enterovirus from the Picornaviridae family (ss(+)RNA). Parvovirus B19 is of the genus Erythrovirus from the Parvoviridae family.

Further Reading

Virtue ER, Marsh GA, Wang LF. Paramyxoviruses infecting humans: the old, the new and the unknown. *Future Microbiol.* 2009;4(5):537–554.

A1.5 Answer B: HPV-16 and HPV-18 are associated with genital cancers

HPV is a DNA virus from the papillomavirus family, of which there are numerous serotypes. Serotypes 6 and 11 most frequently cause ano-genital warts, while serotypes 16 and 18 are linked with ano-genital cancers. The E6 and E7 early viral proteins are considered oncogenic, inhibiting tumour suppression genes: E6 inhibits p53, while E7 inhibits p53, p21 and RB. Diagnosis is through PCR on sample obtained during colposcopy.

Further Reading

Cutts FT, Franceschi S, Goldie S, Castellsague X, de Sanjose S, Garnett G, Edmunds WJ, Claeys P, Goldenthal KL, Harper DM, Markowitz L. Human papillomavirus and HPV vaccines: a review. *Bull World Health Organ.* 2007;85(9):719–726.

A1.6 Answer E: Erythrovirus

Humans can be infected by viruses from three genera from the Parvoviridae family, but no members of the genus Parvovirus are currently known to infect humans. This creates a confusion of terms because the human parvoviruses are not in genus Parvovirus. They are from the genera: Dependoviruses (e.g. Adeno-Associated Virus), Erythroviruses (e.g. Parvovirus B19) and Bocaviruses. In healthy individuals, the major presentation of B19 infection is erythema infectiosum, but in patients with underlying haematological disorders, infection can lead to aplastic crisis. In immunosuppressed patients, persistent infection may develop that presents as pure red cell aplasia and subsequent chronic anaemia. In utero infection may result in hydrops fetalis, miscarriage or congenital anaemia.

Further Reading

Rogo LD, Mokhtari-Azad T, Kabir MH, Rezaei F. Human parvovirus B19: a review. *Acta Virol.* 2014;58(3):199–213.

A1.7 Answer D: Hepatitis C virus

Viruses typically have one of three natural histories; acute infection (e.g. influenza, hepatitis A, Hanta, Nipah, hepatitis E), latent infection (e.g. herpes simplex, varicella zoster, cytomegalovirus) or chronic infection (e.g. hepatitis B, hepatitis C, HIV).

The global annual incidence of hepatitis C is estimated at four million, of whom 18–34% will spontaneously clear the virus. Acute infection with hepatitis C is clinically mild and may even be unrecognised or undiagnosed; acute resolution is not associated with any long-term sequelae. The remainder of the patients are deemed to have chronic hepatitis C, which is now the leading cause of end-stage liver diseases and liver-related deaths in much of the world. Progression of liver fibrosis in chronic hepatitis C is extremely variable, and is influenced by viral, host and environmental factors.

Further Reading
Westbrook RH, Dusheiko G. Natural history of hepatitis C. *J Hepatol.* 2014;61(S1):S58–S68.

A1.8 Answer E: Iodide
Clinical samples requiring a Gram stain, such as sterile fluids and positive blood cultures, must be heat fixed to a slide. A Gram stain can then be undertaken to determine the presence of Gram-positive or Gram-negative bacteria and to enable morphological characterisation. The slide should be flooded with crystal violet for 1 minute, which penetrates through cells and cell membrane. This is then followed by addition of iodide for a further minute, which also enters the cell wall and then binds with the crystal violet, forming larger molecules which are insoluble in water and are therefore fixed in place. A decolouriser is then washed over the slide for a few seconds, in the form of either acetone or alcohol, and the slide is then rinsed with water. This dehydrates and therefore tightens the cell wall of Gram-positive organisms, stopping the large crystal violate-iodine complexes from exiting the cells. Contemporaneously the decolouriser degrades the outer membrane of Gram-negative organisms and the thin cell wall cannot retain the crystal violet-iodine solution. A counterstain is then applied for 1 minute, usually safranin or carbol fuchsin, which cannot stain the dehydrated Gram-positive organisms, but does adhere to Gram-negative organisms.

Gram-positive organisms have a single cell membrane, around which is a thick peptidoglycan cell wall. Gram-negative organisms have a thin peptidoglycan cell wall, but have two cell membranes, one on either side of the cell wall. Cell wall deficient bacteria cannot be readily characterised by the Gram stain.

Further Reading
Public Health England. UK Standards for Microbiology Investigations TP39: Staining procedures. 2015. Available at: www.gov.uk/government/publications/smi-tp-39-staining-procedures

A1.9 Answer C: Conjugation
Bacteria can demonstrate resistance to antimicrobials through a number of mechanisms, including target alteration, enzymatic destruction, porin loss and efflux pumps. The different genes which dictate these cellular mechanisms can be constitutively present in some genera and species of bacteria, or, more rarely may arise through de novo mutations in those organisms which did not previously harbour them. More usually however, genetic material encoding antimicrobial resistance mechanisms is transferred between organisms, either of the same species, of different species in the same genera, or less frequently between genera. This transfer of genetic material can occur through three main mechanisms: transduction, transformation and conjugation (Figure 1.5).

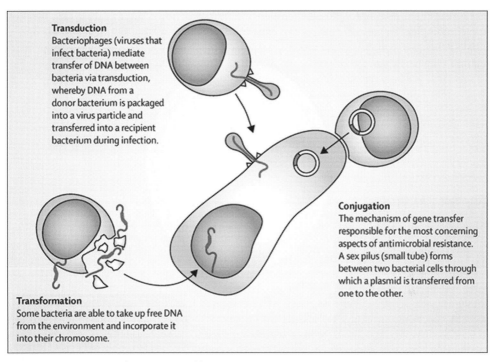

Figure 1.5 Transmission of genetic material between microorganisms.

In this case, *Escherichia coli* does not constitutively harbour an extended-spectrum beta-lactamase (ESBL) gene in their chromosomal genetic material, and the development of a de novo ESBL gene would be rare. Similarly, in the context of both this organism (*E. coli*) and this family of resistance genes (ESBL), transduction and transformation is unlikely. Instead, it is conjugation, and the transmission of plasmids with their additional genetic material, which will bring to the host *E. coli* lineage the ability to produce ESBL proteins and confer resistance to many penicillins and cephalosporins.

Further Reading

Holmes AH, Moore LSP, Sundsfjord A, Steinbakk M, Regmi S, Karkey A, Guerin PJ, Piddock LJ. Understanding the mechanisms and drivers of antimicrobial resistance. *Lancet.* 2016;387 (10014):176–187.

A1.10 **Answer A: The isolate is non-motile**
Salmonella species are non-lactose fermenting (with the exception of *Salmonella* Arizonae and *Salmonella* Indiana) coliforms which produce hydrogen sulphide (with the exception of some isolates of *Salmonella* Paratyphi *A* and *Salmonella* Typhi) when sub-cultured in the presence of sulphur-containing amino acids (on agar plates such as xylose-lysine-desoxycholate agar (XLD) or desoxycholate citrate (DCA)).

Two antigens are examined when identifying serovars of clinical *Salmonella* isolates; somatic (oligosaccharide) "O" antigens and flagella "H" antigens. Variations in these antigens aid identification for clinical and epidemiological purposes; however, laboratory identification can be complex. *Salmonella* isolates can exist in two "H" phases; phase I being motile and phase II being non-motile (the latter as in this case). Isolates that are non-motile on primary culture may be switched to a motile phase using a Cragie tube or the Jameson plate.

Somatic "O" antigens are heat stable and alcohol-resistant, but flagellar "H" antigens are heat-labile. Some surface antigens in *Salmonella* may mask somatic antigens, meaning bacteria will not agglutinate with somatic "O" antisera – one specific surface antigen is the "Vi" antigen. The "Vi" antigen may only occur in three *Salmonella* serovars (out of over 2000): Typhi, Paratyphi C and Dublin, but is variably detected. Other non-lactose fermenting coliforms can cause diarrhoea, including *Shigella* species, but as a rule these do not produce hydrogen sulphide.

Further Reading

Public Health England. UK Standards for Microbiology Investigations B30: Investigation of faecal specimens for enteric pathogens. 2014. Available at: https://assets.publishing.service.gov.uk/government/uploads/system/uploads/attachment_data/file/343955/B_30i8.1.pdf

A1.11 **Answer E: Tumbling motility**
Neonates are at a greater risk of sepsis and meningitis than other age groups due to deficiencies in humoral and cellular immunity and in phagocytic function. Infants younger than 32 weeks' gestation receive little maternal immunoglobulin. Inefficiency in the neonates' alternative complement pathway compromises their defence against encapsulated bacteria and poor migration and phagocytic function of neutrophils is apparent. Group B *Streptococcus* is the most commonly identified organism, implicated in roughly 50% of cases, with *Escherichia coli* accounting for a further 20%, meaning identification and treatment of maternal genitourinary infections is an important prevention strategy. *Listeria monocytogenes* is the third most common pathogen, causing 5–10% of cases. Patients exposed to *L. monocytogenes* in pregnancy often describe a mild flu-like illness but the organism exhibits transplacental transmission leading to sepsis in both mother and neonate. Listeria is a catalase-positive, haemolytic Gram-positive rod that exhibits tumbling motility at 25°C but not at 37°C. Tumbling motility is specific to *Listeria* and identified by the hanging drop test. The cerebrospinal fluid response usually reflects the intracellular nature of *Listeria* with a predominant mononuclear pleocytosis.

Further Reading

National Institute for Health and Care Excellence. Neonatal infection: antibiotics for prevention and treatment NICE guidance. 2012. Available at: www.nice.org.uk/guidance/cg149

A1.12 **Answer E: *Pseudomonas aeruginosa***
P. aeruginosa is an obligate aerobe. It is a Gram-negative, non-lactose fermenting organism which is oxidase positive. It is a common commensal in wounds, but can become an opportunistic pathogen.

Bacteroides spp. (Gram negative) and *Clostridium* spp. (Gram positive) are examples of non-spore-forming and spore-forming strict anaerobes, respectively. Other obligate anaerobes include *Peptostreptococcus* spp. and *Veillonella* spp. *Bacteroides melaninogenicus* has recently been reclassified as *Prevotella melaninogenica* while *Porphyromonas gingivalis* (commonly found in the oral cavity) were originally classified in the *Bacteroides* genus. *Kluyvera* spp. has been put forward as a new member of the Enterobacteriales and as such is only a facultative anaerobe. *P. aeruginosa* is an obligate aerobe.

Further Reading
Moore LSP, Cunningham J, Donaldson H. A clinical approach to managing *Pseudomonas aeruginosa* infections. *Br J Hosp Med (Lond)*. 2016;77(4):C50C54.

A1.13   Answer E: Teichoic acid
The outside of a Gram-positive cell wall is covered with a thick layer consisting of peptidoglycan (PGN) and lipoteichoic acid (LTA), which resembles Gram-negative lipopolysaccharide (LPS). LTA and PGN are able to induce the release of nitric oxide, IL-1, IL-6 and TNF-α by monocytes and macrophages and to activate the oxidative burst in vitro. Furthermore, the effects of LTA and PGNs may be synergistic. Lipoteichoic acid can bind to CD14 and to TLR – binding to TLR-2 has shown to induce NF-kB expression (a central transcription factor), elevating expression of both pro- and anti-apoptotic genes. Its activation also induces mitogen-activated protein kinases (MAPK) activation. LTA bound to targets can interact with circulating antibodies and activate the complement cascade to induce a passive immune kill phenomenon. It also triggers the release from neutrophils and macrophages of reactive oxygen and nitrogen species and cytotoxic cytokines. Therefore, LTA shares many pathogenic similarities with endotoxins.

Further Reading
Ginsburg I. Role of lipoteichoic acid in infection and inflammation. *Lancet Infect Dis.* 2002;2(3):171–179.

A1.14   Answer D: *Morganella morganii* is potentially a urea-splitting bacteria
Bacterial urease alkalinises urine, and urease-producing bacteria play a prominent role in the formation of infection-induced urinary stones. Struvite stone formation occurs when ammonia production increases and urine pH elevates to decrease the solubility of phosphate. *Proteus* spp., *M. morganii* and *Klebsiella pneumoniae* are all potentially urea-splitting bacteria, whereas while *E. coli* is the most common cause of lower urinary tract infections, it is not associated with significant alkalinisation, nor is infection with *Pseudomonas aeruginosa*. Hyperammonaemia can result from the production of excessive amounts of ammonia due to bacterial urease, and its subsequent re-absorption into the systemic circulation, which is implicated in hepatic encephalopathy.

Further Reading
Clericetti CM, Milani GP, Lava SAG, Bianchetti MG, Simonetti GD, Giannini O. Hyper-ammonaemia associated with distal renal tubular acidosis or urinary tract infection: a systematic review. *Pediatr Nephrol*. 2018;33(3):485–491.

A1.15   Answer C: Lipid A
Endotoxins are part of the outer membrane of the cell wall of Gram-negative bacteria. Lipopolysaccharide (LPS) is a major component of the outer membrane, contributing greatly to the structural integrity and protecting the membrane from chemical attack. LPS

comprises three parts: O antigen, core oligosaccharide and Lipid A. Lipid A is associated with the toxicity of Gram-negative bacteria. It is the innermost of the three regions of the lipopolysaccharide molecule, and its hydrophobic nature allows it to anchor the LPS to the outer membrane. Lipid A (and LPS) is believed to activate cells via the Toll-like receptor system. The polysaccharide components produce immunogenicity.

Further Reading

Van Amersfoort ES, Van Berkel TJC, Kuiper J. Receptors, mediators, and mechanisms involved in bacterial sepsis and septic shock. *Clin Microbiol Rev.* 2003;16(3):379–414.

A1.16   Answer A: Lecthinase

S. aureus is a common skin commensal, but can cause skin and skin structure infections, including cellulitis and necrotising fasciitis. Different strains of *S. aureus* produce various different exotoxins, some of which are associated with differing disease presentations and differing severity.

Panton-Valentine leukocidin (PVL) is a cytotoxin produced by *S. aureus* which destroys neutrophils and causes tissue necrosis, recurrent skin and soft tissue infections and necrotising pneumonia. Toxic shock syndrome toxin-1 (TSST-1) is a superantigen produced by *S. aureus* which stimulates IL1, IL2 and tumour necrosis factor leading to toxic shock syndrome. Enterotoxin A can result in the emetic response seen in *S. aureus* food poisoning, but in addition staphylococcal enterotoxins A, B and C are also associated with toxic-shock syndrome presentations. DNase (deoxyribonuclease) production is often used in microbiology laboratories to differentiate *S. aureus* from other species of staphylococci (which can hydrolyse DNA for a source of carbon).

Several bacteria produce phospholipases including *Listeria monocytogenes* but not *S. aureus*. Lecithinase is a type of phospholipase produced by *Clostridium perfringens* causing myonecrosis and haemolysis.

Further Reading

Spaulding AR, Salgado-Pabón W, Kohler PL, Horswill AR, Leung DYM, Schlievert PM. Staphylococcal and Streptococcal superantigen exotoxins. *Clin Microbiol Rev.* 2013;26(3):422–447.

Tong SY, Davis JS, Eichenberger E et al. *Staphylococcus aureus* infections: epidemiology, pathophysiology, clinical manifestations, and management. *Clin Microbiol Rev.* 2015;28 (3):603–661

A1.17   Answer D: Antigenic variation

Borrelia recurrentis (louse-borne relapsing fever) are spirochaetes. A single spirochaete can lead to infection and multiply every 6–12 hours in the blood. The organism can invade the brain, eye, liver, heart and other organs. Each febrile episode is characterised by marked spirochaete-aemia following which there is clearance of the circulating microbes and a development of antibodies against the antigens displayed during the episode. Later episodes will involve spirochaetes displaying a different antigen, similar to trypanosomes, enabling reappearance in the blood. This is accomplished through a process of antigenic variation – specifically site-specific recombination.

Antigenic shift and antigenic drift are the mechanisms through which influenza changes its genetic structure and epitopes over time. Slipped strand mispairing can function as mechanism for phase variation in *Escherichia coli*. Transposons have varied roles in infectious diseases, but perhaps of most clinical relevance are responsible for transfer of anti-microbial resistance genes.

Further Reading

Elbir H, Raoult D, Drancourt M. Relapsing fever borreliae in Africa. *Am J Trop Med Hyg.* 2013;89(2):288–292.

Boutellis A, Mediannikov O, Bilcha KD, Ali J, Campelo D, Barker SC, Raoult D. *Borrelia recurrentis* in head lice. *Ethiopia. Emerg Infect Dis.* 2013;19(5):796–798.

A1.18   Answer B: *Pseudomonas aeruginosa*
Diphtheria toxin is an exotoxin which is encoded by a bacteriophage. It catalyses the ADP-ribosylation of eukaryotic elongation factor-2 (eEF2), inactivating this protein. In this way, it acts as a RNA translational inhibitor. The exotoxin A of *P. aeruginosa* uses a similar mechanism of action. It is an extremely potent exotoxin with only a single toxin molecule required to kill a human cell.

Further Reading

van 't Wout EF, van Schadewijk A, van Boxtel R, Dalton LE, Clarke HJ, Tommassen J, Marciniak SJ, Hiemstra PS. Virulence factors of *Pseudomonas aeruginosa* induce both the unfolded protein and integrated stress responses in airway epithelial cells. *PLoS Pathog.* 2015;11(6):e1004946.

A1.19   Answer D: Phosphate
Corynebacterium is named from the Greek word 'Coryne' which refers to the club shape of bacteria. Volutin, or metachromatic granules, are cytoplasmic granules located in bacterial cytoplasm. These contain polymerised metaphosphate and represents a storage form for inorganic phosphate and energy. These metachromatic granules stain red with methylene blue dye and forms the basis of Albert's stain for the microbiological identification of *C. diphtheria*.

Further Reading

Pallerla SR, Knebel S, Polen T, Klauth P, Hollender J, Wendisch VF, Schoberth SM. Formation of volutin granules in *Corynebacterium glutamicum*. *FEMS Microbiol Lett.* 2005;243(1):133–140.

A1.20   Answer A: ADP ribosylation of EF2
Diphtheria toxin is an exotoxin which is encoded by a bacteriophage. It catalyses the ADP-ribosylation of eukaryotic elongation factor-2 (eEF2), inactivating this protein.
Toxin-mediated systemic sequelae occur in up to 15% of cases, predominantly in respiratory diphtheria but also in those with cutaneous diphtheria where disease is extensive. These manifest in two ways; myocarditis or peripheral neuropathy. Myocarditis can lead to complete heart block and cardiomyopathies. Toxin-mediated neuropathies can manifest as bulbar dysfunction, limb weakness or respiratory failure. Symptoms can be protracted – one series found symptoms persisted for a median of 49 days.

Further Reading

Moore LSP, Leslie A, Meltzer M, Sandison A, Efstratiou A, Sriskandan S. *Corynebacterium ulcerans* cutaneous diphtheria. *Lancet Infect Dis.* 2015;15(9):1100–1107.

A1.21 Answer C: Naked DNA transformation

S. pneumoniae is a Gram-positive cocci which is a common upper respiratory tract commensal. It has the ability to become pathogenic however, and has several virulence factors to aid this. One such virulence factor is the extracellular capsule, which resists phagocytosis by host immune cells. *S. pneumoniae* can alter its production of such capsules through phase variation; a switch between all or none protein expression which is usually reversible. This system can be used to adapt to more than one environment and provides mechanisms to evade the host immune system. Across different genera, phase variation occurs through several mechanisms: slip strand mispairing (e.g. meningococcal capsule formation), homologous recombination, site-specific recombination (e.g. DNA inversion in type 1 fimbrial variation in *Escherichia coli*), epigenic regulation (e.g. altered methylation of regulatory DNA regions in *E. coli* outer membrane protein formation) or transformation of exogenous DNA (e.g. pneumococcal opacity, as in this case).

Further Reading

Engholm DH, Kilian M, Goodsell DS, Andersen ES, Kjærgaard RS. A visual review of the human pathogen *Streptococcus pneumoniae*. *FEMS Microbiol Rev.* 2017;41(6):854–879.

A1.22 Answer B: *Enterococcus faecium*

Enterococci grow well on MacConkey agar unlike streptococci. *E. faecalis* are generally sensitive to ampicillin and resistant to quinupristin/dalfopristin (synercid®). *E. faecium* are resistant to ampicillin and sensitive to quinupristin/dalfopristin. These characteristics are useful in laboratory identification of enterococci, however quinupristin/dalfopristin is difficult to obtain for clinical use and is not universally tested in laboratory practice.

Further Reading

Public Health England. Standards for Microbiological Investigation ID 4: identification of Streptococcus species, Enterococcus species and morphologically similar organisms. 2014. Available at: www.gov.uk/government/publications/smi-id-4-identification-of-streptococcus-species-enterococcus-species-and-morphologically-similar-organisms

A1.23 Answer C: Organism is isolated from throat for several days following infection

Bordetella spp. are small Gram-negative coccobacilli of the phylum proteobacteria and are highly fastidious obligate aerobes. *Bordetella pertussis* is an exclusive human pathogen. Transmission occurs by direct contact or respiratory aerosol droplets. It is highly contagious with over 90% of household contacts developing disease. The incubation period averages 7–10 days (range 5–21 days). Activity tends to peak at the ages of 3–4 years. Bacteria initially adhere to ciliated epithelial cells in the nasopharynx causing an initial catarrhal phase, which lasts for 1–2 weeks during which large numbers of bacteria can be recovered from the pharynx. Paroxysms of cough increase in frequency and severity as illness progresses for 2–6 weeks. During this stage toxins cause ciliostasis and facilitate the entry of bacteria to tracheal/bronchial ciliated cells. *B. pertussis* also produces a lymphocytosis-promoting factor, which causes a decrease in the entry of lymphocytes into lymph nodes and leads to a marked lymphocytosis. Complications include pneumonia, seizures and encephalitis.

Diagnosis can be made via culture of the organism, serology or molecular detection. A nasopharyngeal swab can be cultured on Bordet-Gengou agar to select for the organism, which shows mercury-drop colonies. Culture lacks sensitivity, decreasing with age and specimen quality. It is unlikely to culture positive after 2 weeks of illness. Serology testing detects anti-pertussis toxin IgG antibody levels using ELISA. This is used in older children and adults at least 14 days after onset of cough. Serology is not recommended within a year of vaccination. Genomic detection by PCR improves sensitivity. This can be performed on nasopharyngeal swabs or aspirates and is recommended on any acutely unwell child <12 months of age.

Macrolide antibiotics are first line treatment. Antibiotic therapy has limited effect on improving the clinical course but prevents secondary transmission. In 2007, a Cochrane review showed short course are as effective. Clarithromycin is recommended for neonates, erythromycin in pregnancy and azithromycin for infants, older children and adults. Neither vaccination nor natural disease confers complete or lifelong protective immunity against pertussis with immunity waning after 5–10 years. In 2012, a national UK outbreak was declared due to increase case detection. In response the Department of Health introduced an immunisation programme for pregnant women between 28 and 38 weeks gestation. Boosting maternal antibodies would thus lead to higher neonatal antibody levels.

Further Reading

Public Health England. Standards for Microbiological Investigation B 6: Culture of specimens for *Bordetella pertussis* and *Bordetella parapertussis*. 2014. Available at: www.gov.uk/government/publications/smi-b-6-investigation-of-specimens-for-bordetella-pertussis-and-bordetella-parapertussis

Altunaiji S, Kukuruzovic R, Curtis N, Massie J. Antibiotics for whooping cough (pertussis). *Cochrane Database Syst Rev.* 2007;(3):CD004404.

A1.24 Answer A: *Klebsiella pneumoniae*

K. pneumoniae is a Gram-negative member of the Enterobacteriales family. It is a lactose-fermenting coliform and is a common commensal of the gastrointestinal tract. It has the ability to acquire resistance mechanisms including plasmid mediated ESBLs. The spread of metallo-beta-lactamases such as KPC (Klebsiella producing carbapenemases) and NDM (New Delhi Metallo-beta-lactamase) within *K. pneumoniae* is of worldwide concern. *Enterobacter* spp., *C freundii* and *M. morganii* can acquire such plasmid-mediated mechanisms, but more commonly clinically relevant antimicrobial resistance is due to Ambler class C AmpC type beta-lactamases.

Further Reading

Jacoby GA, Munoz-Price LS. The new beta-lactamases. *N Engl J Med.* 2005;352(4):380–391.

Thomson KS. Extended-spectrum-beta-lactamase, AmpC, and Carbapenemase issues. *J Clin Microbiol.* 2010;48(4):1019–1025.

A1.25 **Answer C: *Pediculus humanus humanus***

Epidemic typhus (louse-borne typhus) causes epidemics following wars and natural disasters. The causative organism is *Rickettsia prowazekii*, transmitted by the human body louse (*Pediculus humanus humanus also known as Pediculosis humanus corporis*) in its faeces. The body louse is 2–4 mm in length, lives in clothes and lays eggs along the seams. The incubation period of epidemic typhus is 1–2 weeks. Symptoms include severe headache, a sustained high fever, cough, rash, severe myalgia, hypotension and delirium. The rash begins on the chest about five days after the fever appears, and spreads to the trunk and extremities. Louse infestation is often sufficiently treated by bathing the patient and heat treating the clothes and bed linen. Permethrin topically and oral ivermectin can be used in persistent cases. A randomised trial using permethrin impregnated underwear in homeless individuals failed to show sustained benefit.

Glossina spp. are known as Tsetse flies and transmit trypanosomiasis. *Aedes aegypti* is the vector for viruses such as dengue, chikungunya, Zika and yellow fever. *A. gambiae* is the vector for malaria. *Culex* spp. are the vectors for West Nile virus, Japanese encephalitis and Western and Eastern Equine encephalitis.

Further Reading

Benkouiten S, Drali R, Badiaga S, Veracx A, Giorgi R, Raoult D, Brouqui P. Effect of permethrin-impregnated underwear on body lice in sheltered homeless persons: a randomized controlled trial. *JAMA Dermatol.* 2014;150(3):273–279.

A1.26 **Answer B: Schistosomiasis**

The *Diphyllobothrium latum* intermediate host is a copepod (freshwater crustacean) then a fish. *Paragonamus* spp. intermediate host is a crab or crayfish. *Echinococcus* spp. (hydatid disease) has an intermediate host of sheep, goats and swine with the definitive host of canines. *Strongyloides stercoralis* a free-living organism. Each human infecting schistosome has a specific snail species for an intermediate host: *Schistosoma mansoni* with *Biomphalaria* spp.; *Schistosoma haematobium* and *Schistosoma intercalatum* with *Bulinus* spp.; *Schistosoma japonicum* with *Oncomelania* spp.; *Schistosoma mekongi* with *Tricula* spp.

Further Reading

Gryseels B, Polman K, Clerinx J, Kestens L. Human schistosomiasis. *Lancet* 2006;368:1106–1118.

Moore LSP, Chiodini PL. Tropical helminths. *Medicine.* 2010;38(1):47–51.

A1.27 **Answer A: *E. dispar***

E. histolytica is the causative agent of intestinal amoebiasis leading to clinical manifestations of amoebic dysentery or amoebic liver abscesses. *E. histolytica* has microscopic morphological similarity with two other species: *E. dispar* and *Entamoeba moshkovskii*. *Entamoeba dispar* is non-pathogenic but *Entamoeba moshkovskii* is reportedly associated with diarrhoea, but its pathogenic potential remains unclear. These can be diagnosed by stool samples but it is impossible to distinguish the three species by microscopy alone. Trophozoites may be seen in a fresh faecal smear and cysts in an ordinary stool sample. Antigen tests can distinguish between pathogenic and non-pathogenic species. Molecular techniques, such as PCR, can be used but are not widely available in clinical practice.

Further Reading

Parija SC, Mandal J, Ponnambath DK. Laboratory methods of identification of *Entamoeba histolytica* and its differentiation from look-alike *Entamoeba* spp. *Trop Parasitol.* 2014;4(2):90–95.

A1.28 Answer D: IgM

Immunoglobulins, composed of two heavy chains and two light chains in a Y shape, bind antigens in a variable domain and effect functions through a constant domain. There are five classes of constant domain, defining the five isotypes of immunoglobulins: IgA, IgD, IgE, IgG, IgM. IgM immunoglobulins are the first isotypes expressed during B-cell development; naïve B-cells express IgM as a monomer on their cell surface, then once stimulated by an antigen IgM is produced as a pentamer early in a primary viral infection. However, the heavy chains in IgM have not undergone much somatic mutation in response to antigens, and tend to be more poly-reactive than other immunoglobulin isotypes. IgG is the predominant isotype and are produced by activated B-cells (i.e. plasma cells) either part way through a primary viral infection (replacing IgM production) or upon activation of memory B-cells in response to later re-exposures or reactivation of viral infections. IgA occurs as a monomer in serum but as a dimer when secreted at mucosal surfaces and in breast milk where it acts to protect these mucosal surfaces from viruses, bacteria and toxins. IgE binds with high affinity to mast cells, basophils and eosinophils once activated by an antigen – typically a helminth, although it is also associated with hypersensitivity and allergic reactions. IgD functions as an antigen receptor on naïve B-cells and can also bind basophils and mast cells in respiratory immune defence.

Further Reading

Schroeder HW, Cavacini L. Structure and function of immunoglobulins. *J Allergy Clin Immunol.* 2010;125(202):S41–S52.

A1.29 Answer B: C7 deficiency

Adenosine deaminase deficiency is an autosomal recessive metabolic disorder. It leads to severe combined immunodeficiency (SCID) in 90% cases with T, B and natural killer cell dysfunction. It causes an accumulation of deoxyadenosine, which causes an increase in S-adenosylhomocysteine; both of which are toxic to immature lymphocytes leading to a complete lack of both T- and B-cells. Prognosis is poor and acute recurrent infections occur in particular *Pneumocystis jirovecii* (PCP) pneumonia, candidiasis, herpetic infections (CMV, EBV, VZV), parainfluenza and enterovirus. Job syndrome (autosomal dominant hyperimmunoglobulin E syndrome) is characterised by abnormally high levels of immunoglobulin E. It clinically appears with recurrent skin abscesses, cystic lung infections (primarily *Staphylococcus aureus* and *Candida*), eczematous dermatitis, eosinophilia and elevated IgE levels. Patients with C7 deficiency have markedly diminished total haemolytic complement activity and little if any C7 is in their serum. Serum bactericidal activity is markedly reduced and is responsible for the increased risk of *Neisseria* spp. (especially *Neisseria meningitidis*) infections. The cause of IgM deficiency is unknown but is characterised by an absence of IgM in the presence of normal levels of IgG and IgA. Serious recurrent bacterial infections can occur from *Staphylococcus aureus*, encapsulated organisms (*Streptococcus pneumoniae*, *Haemophilius influenzae*) and viral infections.

Further Reading

Corvini M, Randolph C, Aronin SI. Complement C7 deficiency presenting as recurrent aseptic meningitis. *Ann Allergy Asthma Immunol.* 2004;93(2):200–205.

A1.30   Answer B: Defect in phagocyte oxidase

Phagocytes use nicotinamide adenine dinucleotide phosphate (NADPH) oxidase to generate reactive species of oxygen. CGD is caused by mutations resulting in loss of function in this process. Neutrophils, monocytes and macrophages are unable to phagocytose bacteria such as *Staphylococcus aureus* leading to recurrent bacterial infections.

Further Reading

Chiriaco M, Salfa I, Matteo GD, Rossi P, Finocchi A. Chronic granulomatous disease: clinical, molecular and therapeutic aspects. *Pediatr Allergy Immunol.* 2015;27(3):242–253.

A1.31   Answer B: TLR4

TLRs are surface molecules on cells that detect and react to microbial antigens. The ligands for these receptors are parts of microbes and often called pathogen-associated molecular patterns (PAMPs). TLR4 is the principle receptor for LPS of the Gram-negative bacterium. TLR3 binds double-stranded RNA produced by many viruses. TLR5 recognises flagella of bacteria. TLR7 is similar to TLR8 and bind single-stranded RNA from viruses such as influenza and HIV. TLR10 function is not yet known.

Further Reading

Takeuchi O, Hoshino K, Kawai T, Sanjo H, Takada H, Ogawa T, Takeda K, Akira S. Differential roles of TLR2 and TLR4 in recognition of gram-negative and gram-positive bacterial cell wall components. *Immunity.* 1999;11(4):443–451.

A1.32   Answer C: IL2 and IFN-γ

A TH1-type response is generally associated with killing of intracellular organisms, either viruses or bacteria. Cytokines associated with a TH1 response are, therefore, typically pro-inflammatory and activate macrophages and induce opsonising/complement-fixing immunoglobulin production by B-lymphocytes. Interferon gamma is one of the main TH1 cytokines.

A TH2-type response occurs typically to combat extracellular bacteria and parasite. This leads to activation of eosinophils, basophils and dendritic cells through cytokines including interleukins 4, 5 and 13, and a degree of anti-inflammatory response through interleukin-10.

In hepatitis C, both IL-2 and IFN-γ are key cytokines associated with clearance of acute and chronic HCV. The impact of IL-2 is likely due to its role in differentiation of CD8+ T-lymphocytes into effector and long lived memory cells. The activity of IFN-γ in hepatitis C is likely attributable to its direct role in inhibiting viral replication. Untreated patients with hepatitis C who have primary clearance of the virus display high magnitude IL-2 and IFN-γ responses. Treated hepatitis C patients who display sustained virological response have a higher magnitude and maintenance levels of IL-2 and IFN-γ. Null-responder patients may have high magnitude IFN-γ responses early in infection but lack high maintenance levels.

Table 2 Cytokine profilesin TH1 and TH2 responses.

	TH1	TH2
Main partner cell	Macrophage	B cell
Cytokines	IL-2, IFN-γ, TNF-β	IL-2, -4, -5, -6, -10, -13
Immune system stimulated	Maximises cellular immune system (macrophages and CD8+ T cells)	Maximises humoral immune system (B cell antibody production and class switching)
Other functions	IFN-γ up regulates IL-12 (potentiating TH1 further) and down regulates IL-4 (inhibiting TH2 responses)	IL-10 inhibits IL-2, IL-12 and IFN-γ production

Further Reading

Flynn JK, Dore GJ, Hellard M, Yeung B, Rawlinson WD, White PA, Kaldor JM, Lloyd AR, Ffrench RA. Maintenance of TH1 HCV-specific responses in individuals with acute HCV who achieve sustained virological clearance after treatment. *J Gastroenterol Hepatol.* 2013;28(11):1770–1781.

Chapter 2

Microbiology and Virology Laboratory Practice

To provide an effective infection specialist service, practitioners must be conversant in pre-analytical, analytical and post-analytical elements of laboratory practice, irrespective of the specific areas of infectious diseases undertaken on a day-to-day basis. Pre-analytical skills and knowledge will include areas such as understanding the microbial differential diagnoses sufficiently to advise on and obtain the correct tests on the optimal sample types, be this for culture or for serological or genetic diagnostic tests. Pre-analytical skills also help practitioners identify where tests will not aid diagnosis, including for conditions which are currently diagnosed clinically and for which laboratory diagnostics do not currently exist. Analytical skills and understanding will vary depending on the area of practice, but will include safe laboratory work, the strengths and limitations of different tests, the impact of quality assurance and quality control and the cost implications of different modalities. Post-analytical skills and understanding will include contextualisation of results in each patients' care, awareness of positive and negative predictive values of different tests and implications for further diagnostics including reflex testing.

Questions

Q2.1 A 26-year-old male presents 3 days after a dog bite. What diagnostic test aids with ascertaining exposure to rabies?

A. Serum IgM
B. Skin biopsy
C. Mucosal IgA
D. Whole blood PCR
E. None

Q2.2 A 12-year-old male presents with trismus, vomiting and hypoxia. He reports a minor trauma while playing outside several days ago. Which of the following best achieves a diagnosis of tetanus?

A. Gram-stain of wound swab
B. Isolation of *Clostridium tetani* in blood culture
C. Isolation of *C. tetani* in wound swabs
D. Clinical diagnosis
E. Serology

Q2.3 A nursing home and a hospital in the same geographic area have an outbreak of diarrhoea and vomiting but all routine bacteriology and viral stool tests from affected patients return negative. What test should be requested?
A. Stool 16s rRNA PCR
B. Stool 16S rRNA PCR
C. Western blot of filtered stool
D. Stool electron microscopy
E. Norovirus PCR on vomitus

Q2.4 A 51-year-old female presents to the clinic for investigation of deranged liver function tests.

ALT 89

ALP 56

ALB 36

Which hepatitis B laboratory result is diagnostic of chronic active hepatitis?
A. HBe Ag
B. HBc IgG
C. HBc IgM
D. HBe Ab
E. HBs Ag

Q2.5 A 38-year-old male presents with acute-onset fever, headache and confusion. On examination, he has no neck stiffness and no focal neurological deficit is detectable. His Mini-Mental State Examination (MMSE) is 21/30. Magnetic resonance imaging of his brain is depicted in Figure 2.1.

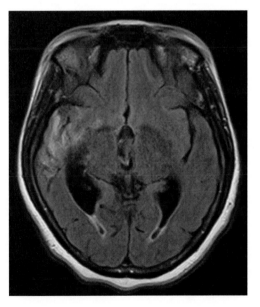

Figure 2.1 Magnetic resonance image of the brain with gadolinium contrast (Fluid Attenuated Inversion Recovery (FLAIR)).

A lumbar puncture is performed and his cerebrospinal fluid results are:

White cell count: 16
Red cell count: 450
Protein: 0.28
Glucose: 4.8
Plasma glucose: 5.1
Microscopy: no organisms seen

What is the most appropriate next investigation?
A. Serum sample for herpes serology
B. Throat swab for adenovirus
C. CSF PCR for herpesviridae
D. Stool PCR for enteroviridae
E. CSF viral antibody testing in 10 days

Q2.6 A 31-year-old woman delivers a female child on the second centile which at 8 months of age is found to have a patent ductus arteriosus and early bilateral cataracts. The paediatric team suspect congenitally-acquired rubella. Which laboratory test may help make the diagnosis?
A. Maternal rubella IgM
B. Maternal rubella IgG
C. Infant rubella IgM
D. Infant rubella IgG
E. Infant mucosal swab rubella IgA

Q2.7 A 27-year-old homosexual male presents after his partner was recently diagnosed with *Chlamydia trachomatis*. A rectal swab is sent from the patient for *C. trachomatis* testing. Which is the best laboratory method to diagnose this pathogen?
A. PCR
B. Reverse-transcriptase PCR
C. ELISA
D. Culture on McCoy cells
E. Immunofluorescence

Q2.8 A 17-year-old male presents with fever and oral pain. A swab is sent for microscopy, culture and sensitivity. A diagnosis can be made based solely on the Gram-stain morphology for which infection?
A. Diphtheria
B. *Arcanobacterium haemolyticum*
C. Vincent's angina
D. Group A Streptococcal disease
E. Actinomcycosis

Q2.9 A 23-year-old male presents with a fever of unknown origin.
A blood culture becomes culture-positive (Figure 2.2). The culture
is oxidase-positive, does not grow without blood and can ferment glucose
but not maltose.

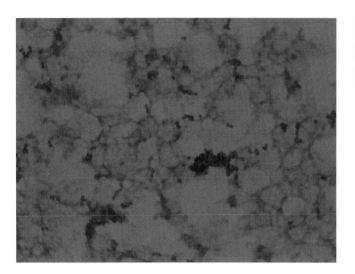

Figure 2.2 Gram stain from a positive blood culture. (A black and white version of this figure will appear in some formats. For the colour version, please refer to the plate section.)

What is the likely diagnosis?
A. *Neisseria sicca*
B. *Neisseria meningitidis*
C. *Neisseria gonorrhoeae*
D. *Moraxella catarrhalis*
E. *Acinetobacter* spp.

Q2.10 A 20-year-old male presents to a genitourinary clinic with an all over maculo-papular rash and a healing painless ulcer on his penis. His syphilis serology is negative. What is the prozone effect caused by?
A. Incorrect serum dilution
B. Low antigen titre
C. High antibody titre
D. Inhibitory factors
E. Incorrect diluent concentration

Q2.11 A 64-year-old male presents with altered sputum production. A computerised tomograph of his chest is undertaken (Figure 2.3). Sputum is submitted for mycobacterial examination. A *Mycobacterium* spp. grows on Löwenstein–Jensen medium at 37°C after 4 weeks and has bright yellow colonies.

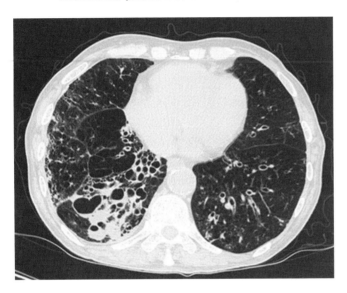

Figure 2.3 Mid thoracic high-resolution computerised tomograph, axial plane.

Which of the following is it likely to be?
A. *Mycobacterium fortuitum*
B. *Mycobacterium chelonae*
C. *Mycobacterium kansasii*
D. *Mycobacterium malmoense*
E. *Mycobacterium paratuberculosis*

Q2.12 A 56-year-old female who owns several caged birds is diagnosed with pneumonia. What is the best way to diagnose *Chlamydia psittaci* infection?
A. Sputum culture
B. Complement fixation
C. Antigen ELISA detection
D. Urinary antigen detection
E. Microimmunofluorescence

Q2.13 An 18-year-old male presents to the genitourinary clinic with penile discharge. Chlamydia cryptic plasmid PCR results show the specimen as negative and the internal positive control as negative. What is the significance of this result?
A. No patient DNA in the specimen
B. The PCR reaction has been inhibited
C. There is likely exogenous nucleic acid contamination of the PCR reaction
D. The reaction was not initiated
E. There was degradation of the target DNA in the specimen

Q2.14 A 36-year-old male presents with a ruptured dental abscess. A swab is sent of the pus. Which of the following antimicrobials is commonly used to make media selective for anaerobes?
A. Colistin
B. Neomycin
C. Chloramphenicol
D. Vancomycin
E. Metronidazole

Q2.15 Latex agglutination tests are commonly used in the lab for presumptive microbiological diagnoses. For which of the following bacteria is a latex agglutination test not commonly used?
A. *Staphylococcus aureus*
B. *Streptococcus pyogenes*
C. *Shigella sonnei*
D. *Pseudomonas aeruginosa*
E. *Salmonella* Typhi

Q2.16 A 16-year-old female presents with a sore throat and a beta-haemolytic *Streptococcus* is grown. Which of the following species is a Group C *Streptococcus*?
A. *Streptococcus dysgalactiae*
B. *Streptococcus pyogenes*
C. *Streptococcus canis*
D. *Streptococcus agalactiae*
E. *Streptococcus suis*

Q2.17 The healthcare-associated infection screening policy is undergoing revision. In screening for extended-spectrum beta-lactamase producing Enterobacteriales, which antimicrobial disk can be used?
A. Cefpodoxime
B. Cefotaxime
C. Ceftazidime
D. Cefalexin
E. Cefoxitin

Q2.18 A blood culture from a 7-year-old male with a haematological malignancy grows Gram-positive cocci. Initial laboratory investigations show the organism is catalase test positive, coagulase test negative and resistant to the antibiotic teicoplanin. Which of the following is the most likely identity?
A. *Staphylococcus aureus*
B. *Staphylococcus haemolyticus*
C. *Staphylococcus intermedius*
D. *Staphylococcus lugdunensis*
E. *Staphylococcus epidermidis*

Q2.19 A 5-year-old male is seen for review of his cystic fibrosis. He has a productive cough and a specimen is forwarded to the laboratory.
Which culture medium would be the most appropriate to isolate *Haemophilus influenzae*?
A. Blood agar
B. Chocolate bacitracin agar
C. MacConkey agar
D. Mannitol salt agar
E. XLD agar

Q2.20 An 18-year-old woman has symptoms of a lower urinary tract infection. Which of the following statements about the nitrate test is true?
A. Detects the presence of bacterial nitrate reductase
B. Specificity is below 80% for indicating a urinary tract infection
C. Sensitivity is above 90% for detecting a urinary tract infection
D. False positives arise with *Enterococcus* spp.
E. False positives arise when urine has been in the bladder for less than 4 hours

Q2.21 An 18-year-old woman has symptoms of a lower urinary tract infection. Which of the following statements about the leukocyte esterase test is true?
A. False negatives arise as a result of contamination with vaginal secretions
B. False positives arise in patients with neutropaenia
C. False positives arise in patients with proteinuria
D. A positive result can occur with damaged or lysed leukocytes
E. A positive result indicates a successful antimicrobial treatment course

Q2.22 An 18-year-old woman has symptoms of a lower urinary tract infection. Which of the following statements about specimen collection is true?
A. Unpreserved urine should be processed in less than 4 hours from collection time
B. Preservatives such as iodine stabilise bacterial counts for 24–72 hours from collection
C. A suprapubic aspirate should be obtained
D. The first void urine of the day should be collected
E. A pure growth of an organism in a mid-stream urine is indicative of a pathogen

Q2.23 An 18-year-old woman has a mid-stream urine sent to the lab. Which of the following statements about asymptomatic bacteriuria are true?
A. It describes a positive urinary dipstick test without clinical symptoms
B. It describes significant bacteriuria without urinary leukocytes
C. It is only present in pregnant women
D. It should be treated if $>10^5$ CFU/mL in two consecutive mid-stream urines
E. It should be treated if 10^5 CFU/mL in one mid-stream urine

Q2.24 Four patients in a general surgical ward are diagnosed with healthcare-associated meticillin-resistant *Staphylococcus aureus* wound infections in a week. What is the most useful method to determine the similarity of these isolates?
A. Phage-typing with international consensus phages
B. Multilocus sequence typing (MLST)
C. Bacterial antibiotic susceptibility profiles
D. Capsular antigen typing
E. Ribosomal 16S sequencing

Q2.25 Four neonates in the neonatal intensive care have colonisation with *Pseudomonas aeruginosa* identified over a 4-month period, but without clear evidence of co-location. Which is the optimal method for typing *P. aeruginosa* to investigate a possible outbreak?
A. Antimicrobial susceptibility patterns
B. Pyocin typing
C. Pulsed-field gel electrophoresis
D. Whole genome sequencing
E. Variable nucleotide tandem repeat

Q2.26 A 34-year-old male presents with haematuria several months after return from Lake Malawi. What is the optimal sample type for microscopy?
A. Mid-stream urine
B. Terminal void urine
C. Early morning urine
D. 24-hour urinary collection
E. Cystoscopy and biopsy

Q2.27 A 34-year-old male presents with haematuria several months after return from Lake Malawi. What would be your confirmatory diagnostic finding for Schistosomiasis?
A. Cysts
B. Larvae
C. Ova
D. Adults
E. Microfilariae

Q2.28 A 45-year-old man who keeps reptiles presents with enteritis. Which phenotypic aspects of *Salmonella* Arizonae must be considered during stool culture?
A. It does not grow on routine media
B. It is oxidase positive
C. It is a lactose fermenter
D. It is urease positive
E. It does not grow on xylose lysine desoxycholate (XLD) agar

Q2.29 A 45-year-old man presents with enteritis. On examination of stool for ova, cysts and parasites, 8–10 mm spheres with refractile internal globules are seen. What is the likely diagnosis?
A. *Giardia intestinalis*
B. *Cryptosporidium parvum*
C. *Necator americanus*
D. *Cyclospora cayetanensis*
E. *Schistosoma mansoni*

Q2.30 A 27-year-old male presents with fever 10 days after return from India. Which would be the highest yielding sample to isolate *Salmonella* Typhi?
A. Nasopharyngeal aspirate
B. Blood
C. Stool
D. Bone marrow
E. Urine

Q2.31 A 27-year-old male presents with fever 10 days after return from India. A blood culture grows a Gram-negative bacilli, and a matrix-assisted laser desorption ionisation time-of-flight (MALDI-TOF) suggests the isolate to be *Salmonella* Typhi. How would you rapidly confirm the identity of the isolate?
A. Use a biochemical kit (e.g. API® 20E)
B. Send it to reference laboratory
C. No additional tests are necessary, the MALDI-TOF spectra is enough
D. Perform serology (±Vi 0:9,12 H:d)
E. Perform serology (Group W)

Q2.32 A 27-year-old male reports enteritis after eating at a local restaurant to the local health protection team. Which of the following is not involved in the laboratory detection of food-borne intoxication?
A. Qualitative culture of the enteric pathogen from faeces
B. Quantitative culture of the enteric pathogen from faeces
C. Detection of enterotoxin in faeces
D. Detection of enterotoxin in vomit
E. Qualitative culture of the enteric pathogen from food

Q2.33 A 27-year-old male at a refugee camp reports enteritis. Which is the best transport media for faecal specimens?
A. Cary-Blair
B. Amies
C. Stuart
D. Alkaline peptone water
E. Buffered glycerol saline

Q2.34 A 27-year-old male presents with enteritis and a *Salmonella* Paratyphi A is grown. Why is *S.* Paratyphi A notable among the *Salmonella* spp.?
A. Lysine decarboxylase negative
B. Hydrogen sulphide negative

    C. Gas negative

    D. Urea positive

    E. Phenylalanine deaminase positive

Q2.35 A 27-year-old male presents with enteritis. From a stool sample a yellow colony is growing on thiosulfate-citrate-bile-sucrose (TCBS) agar. What is the likely diagnosis?

    A. *Vibrio cholerae*

    B. *Vibrio parahaemolyticus*

    C. *Vibrio mimicus*

    D. *Escherichia coli*

    E. *Yersinia enterocolitica*

Q2.36 A 27-year-old male presents with enteritis and *Shigella dysenteriae* serotype 1 is grown. Why is *S. dysenteriae* serotype 1 notable among the Enterobacteriales?

    A. It is oxidase positive

    B. It is catalase positive

    C. It is catalase negative

    D. It does not grow on XLD

    E. It is not a member of the Enterobacteriales

Q2.37 A 27-year-old male with known HIV presents with enteritis. Which *Campylobacter* spp. particularly relevant in HIV positive individuals may not be identified at standard *Campylobacter* spp. incubation temperatures?

    A. *Campylobacter jejuni*

    B. *Campylobacter fetus*

    C. *Campylobacter coli*

    D. *Campylobacter lari*

    E. *Campylobacter ureolyticus*

Q2.38 A 72-year-old male presents with fever and tachycardia. A blood culture grows a Gram-positive coccus and it is demonstrated to be catalase negative, hydrolyse aesculin in the presence of bile, latex agglutinate with group D and be sensitive to penicillin. Which of the following is the most likely identity?

    A. *Enterococcus faecium*

    B. *Leuconostoc lactis*

    C. *Streptococcus gallolyticus*

    D. *Streptococcus agalactiae*

    E. *Streptococcus constellatus*

Q2.39 A 60-year-old female is diagnosed with *Listeria monocytogenes* bacteraemia. Which growth characteristic defines a psychrophilic organism?

    A. It grows at 4°C incubation

    B. It grows at 40°C incubation

    C. It grows in the absence of light

    D. It grows only in aerobic incubation

    E. It grows only in carbon dioxide incubation

Q2.40 A 22-year-old female presents with diarrhoea. A stool sample grows red colonies with black centres on XLD agar. What is the laboratory importance of deoxycholate?

    A. Enables faecal coliform count

    B. Discerns *Campylobacter* spp.

    C. Discerns *Salmonella* spp. and *Shigella* spp.

    D. Discerns *Escherichia coli* O157

    E. Discerns *Yersinia* spp.

Q2.41 A 70-year-old female with chronic obstructive pulmonary disease presents with an exacerbation. A sputum sample grows Gram-negative cocci which are oxidase positive. What further test would you do to identify the organism?

    A. Catalase

    B. DNAse

    C. Coagulase

    D. Oxidase

    E. Indole

Q2.42 A concern is raised over the cleaning of endoscopes from the washer-disinfector unit. How would you quantify the number of live bacteria within a broth culture?

    A. Cell count

    B. Flow cytometry

    C. Miles–Misra method

    D. Optical density

    E. Quantification of DNA

Q2.43 A 65-year-old with suspected infective endocarditis has blood cultures taken. What has the least impact on whether a blood culture will grow an organism?

    A. Volume of blood taken

    B. Technique of culture

    C. Fastidiousness of organism

    D. Number of patient white cells

    E. Duration of culture

Q2.44 A 3-year-old male presents with a fine scaly rash with skin depigmentation. Microscopy of a skin biopsy with a potassium hydroxide (KOH) stain shows yeasts and small hyphae. What is the most likely diagnosis?

    A. *Trichophyton rubrum*

    B. *Microsporum canis*

    C. *Candida albicans*

    D. *Malassezia furfur*

    E. *Coccidiomycoides immitis*

Q2.45 A 61-year-old male with diabetes presents with severe sinusitis and a decreased Glasgow coma score. What is the best laboratory method for the rapid identification of fungi responsible for rhinocerebral mucormycosis?
   A. Calcofluor staining
   B. Haematoxylin-eosin staining
   C. Potassium hydroxide staining
   D. Periodic acid-Schiff staining
   E. Methenamine-silver staining

Q2.46 A 64-year-old male presents with altered sputum production. He undergoes a computerised tomography of his chest (Figure 2.4).

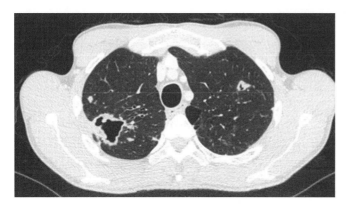

Figure 2.4 Upper thoracic high resolution computerised tomograph, axial plane.

Which is the best stain to visualise fungal elements from his bronchoalveolar lavage?
   A. Periodic acid-Schiff stain
   B. Albert's stain
   C. Haematoxylin-eosin stain
   D. Gram stain
   E. Giemsa stain

Q2.47 A 58-year-old female with a chronic cough has a bronchoalveolar lavage. Microscopy is non-contributory, but subsequently a filamentous fungi grows on a Sabouraud agar. What is the most useful method for speciation of the filamentous fungi?
   A. Calcofluor white stain
   B. Gram stain
   C. Lactophenol cotton blue stain
   D. Periodic acid-Schiff stain
   E. Potassium hydroxide wet preparation

Q2.48 A 31-year-old female presents with iron-deficiency anaemia. A stool specimen for ova, cysts and parasites examination is undertaken (Figure 2.5; diameter 60 μm).

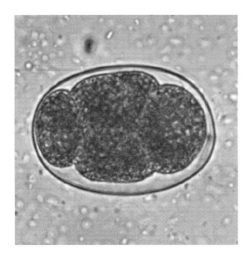

Figure 2.5 Light microscopy of stool sample prepared in 10% (v/v) formalin in water.

What is the most likely diagnosis?
A. *Ascaris lumbricoides*
B. *Trichuris trichuria*
C. *Strongyloides stercoralis*
D. *Enterobius vermicularis*
E. *Ancylostoma duodenale*

Q2.49 A 31-year-old female presents with pruritis ani. What is the best method of diagnosing *Enterobius vermicularis* infection?
A. Light microscopy
B. Latex agglutination
C. Serology
D. Immunofluoresence
E. Polymerase chain reaction

Q2.50 A 31-year-old male presents with high fever after return from rural India. What is the most useful method for rapid identification of *Plasmodium falciparum*?
A. Thick blood film with Field's stain
B. Thin blood film with Geimsa stain
C. Thin blood film with Field's stain
D. Polymerase chain reaction
E. Rapid serum agglutination test

Answers

A2.1 Answer E: None

Worldwide, canine (and to a lesser extent rodent and monkey) transmission of Rabies virus poses the most significant risk, with dog bites the leading cause of rabies. In the United Kingdom, while terrestrial animals are free from Rabies virus, bats have been found to be carriers of Lyssavirus, and exposure to their secretions may constitute a significant exposure. Ascertaining potential exposure to rabies is dependent upon an accurate history of the geographic location, animal type and nature of the exposure. Ascertaining the risk enables a decision on the type of post-exposure prophylaxis that needs to be given – vaccination or human rabies immunoglobulin (HRIG). A live vaccine is available for animals, but a killed formulation is available for human use. Post-exposure prophylaxis is highly successful in preventing the disease if administered within 10 days of infection.

There is no diagnostic test to determine exposure to rabies. However, once encephalomyelitis is established, the reference method for diagnosing rabies is by performing PCR/viral culture on post-mortem brain samples. Ante-mortem, the diagnosis can also be made from skin samples (classically taken from the nape of the neck), or from saliva, urine and cerebrospinal fluid samples, but these are not as sensitive. Inclusion bodies called Negri bodies are 100% diagnostic for rabies infection, but found only in 20% of cases.

Further Reading

Udow SJ, Marrie RA, Jackson AC. Clinical features of dog- and bat-acquired rabies in humans. *Clin Infect Dis.* 2013;57(5):689–696.

A2.2 Answer D: Clinical diagnosis

Tetanus is caused by a neurotoxin produced by the bacterium *C. tetani.* Tetanus spores are widespread in the environment and survive hostile conditions for prolonged periods of time. Transmission occurs when spores enter the body from wounds, and the incubation time is 3–21 days. The diagnosis is based on the presentation of tetanus symptoms and does not depend upon isolation of the bacteria, which is recovered from the wound in only 30% of cases and can be isolated from patients who do not have tetanus. Clinical diagnosis is defined as trismus with one or more of the following: dysphagia, respiratory involvement, spasms, autonomic dysfunction or spasticity. It can be graded as mild, moderate, severe or very severe. Provided serum is collected prior to therapeutic administration of antitoxin, determination of tetanus immunity status can be useful in confirming a clinical diagnosis of tetanus. Absence of detectable antibody or levels below or close to the minimum protective level lends support to the clinical diagnosis while higher levels do not. A bio-assay on serum can be performed for detection of toxin only when antibody levels are below the protective threshold. Direct PCR or culture techniques can detect *C. tetani*, but a negative result does not exclude tetanus. Clinical management involves wound debridement, anti-anaerobic antibiotic (metronidazole), intravenous tetanus immunoglobulin or human normal immunoglobulin.

Further Reading

Rodrigo C, Fernando D, Rajapakse S. Pharmacological management of tetanus: an evidence-based review. *Crit Care.* 2014;18(2):217.

Salisbury D, Ramsay M, Noakes K. The Green Book Chapter 30. Immunisation against infectious disease. 2006. Available at: www.gov.uk/government/collections/immunisation-against-infectious-disease-the-green-book

A2.3 Answer D: Stool electron microscopy

Stool culture typically only identifies *Salmonella* spp., *Shigella* spp., *Campylobacter* spp. and cytotoxic *Escherichia coli*. Other bacterial pathogens are not usually looked for. Rotavirus and norovirus testing (either by ELISA or PCR) is sometimes conducted on stool specimens where there is concern over an outbreak, or cross-transmission; however, the sensitivity of these viral tests is not high and the test is not valid on vomitus. Added to this, rarer or previously unknown viruses may also cause outbreaks of enteritis that would not be conducted through conventional diagnostic tests. PCR-based tests for bacterial causes of diarrhoea may be useful on occasion, but in this case where there are epidemiologically linked outbreaks in two institutes, a circulating community viral cause is more likely.

Further Reading

Goldsmith CS, Miller SE. Modern uses of electron microscopy for detection of viruses. *Clin Microbiol Rev*. 2009;22(4):552–563.

A2.4 Answer E: HBsAg

The Hepatitis B surface antigen (HBsAg) is a protein on the surface of the virus which can be detected in high levels during acute or chronic Hepatitis B infection, and indicates that the person is infectious. It is the first detectable marker of infection and is present as early as the incubation period. Hepatitis B surface antibody (HBsAb) indicates the patient is immune to hepatitis B, either through vaccination (when the hepatitis B core antibody is absent) or through natural infection which has been cleared (when hepatitis B core antibody is present). Hepatitis B core antibody (HBcAb) can also help distinguish between acute and chronic infection, through discerning whether HBc IgM or IgG is present (the former indicates a recent acute infection; the latter is present for life). Hepatitis B envelope antigen (HBeAg) is detectable during acute and chronic hepatitis B infection where there is active viral replication and indicates the infected person has high levels of the hepatitis B virus. Hepatitis B envelope antibody (HBeAb) is detectable during acute HBV infection or in chronic hepatitis during or after a burst in viral replication. Serological conversion from HBeAg to HBeAb is more likely to achieve long-term clearance of the virus.

Immune escape variants of hepatitis B virus do occur; an example are the precore mutants. These HBV variants occur during HBeAg seroconversion, where despite continuing production of infectious virions, mutations arise in the precore region preventing HBeAg synthesis. This mutation is more prevalent where hepatitis B genotypes B, C and D are predominant, representing up to 50% of individuals with chronic hepatitis B in Asia and the Mediterranean area. Pre core mutants do not occur in hepatitis B genotype A, and so are significantly less prevalent in North America and Europe. A diagnosis of a precore mutant should be considered where HBeAg is negative, HBsAg is positive, HBeAb is positive but HBV DNA is high (over 2,000) and there is evidence of ongoing transaminitis.

Table 3 Clinical interpretation of hepatitis B virus serological markers.

HBsAg	HBc IgG	HBc IgM	HBsAb	Interpretation
−	−	−	−	Susceptible
−	+	−	+	Immune (following natural infection)
−	−	−	+	Immune (following vaccination)
+	+	+	−	Acute infection
+	+	−	−	Chronic infection
−	+	−	−	Several possibilities, including: • recovering from acute HBV • immune but with very low levels of HBsAb • susceptible with false-positive HBcAb • chronic infection but with very low levels of HBsAg

Further Reading

Trépo C, Chan HLY, Lok A. Hepatitis B virus infection. *Lancet.* 2014;384(9959):2053–2063.

A2.5 Answer C: CSF PCR for herpesviridae

This patient presents with encephalitis; in the United Kingdom, the most common cause of this is herpes virus 1 and 2, although other causes including other herpesviridae, *Listeria monocytogenes*, enterovirus (particularly enterovirus 71) and travel-associated viruses should also be considered (including, for example, West Nile virus or Japanese encephalitis virus). Herpes simplex encephalitis is caused by retrograde transmission from a peripheral site on the face following HSV-1 reactivation, along a nerve axon, to the brain. An electroencephalogram might first show abnormalities in one temporal lobe, spreading to the other contralateral lobe 7–10 days later. The MRI scan, as in this case, may similarly show temporal lobe changes. CSF PCR is useful until about 10–20 days after the onset of neurological disease before it typically becomes negative. After this time detection of HSV antibody in the CSF can be used. Without treatment, HSE results in rapid death in up to half of the cases, with treatment reducing this to around 20%. In those who survive, serious long-term neurological damage in over half ensues. Only a small population of survivors (2.5%) regain completely normal brain function.

Further Reading

Solomon T, Michael BD, Smith PE, Sanderson F, Davies NWS, Hart IJ, Holland M, Easton A, Buckley C, Kneen R, Beeching NJ. Management of suspected viral encephalitis in adults – Association of British Neurologists and British Infection Association National Guidelines. *J Infect.* 2012;64:347–373.

A2.6 Answer D: Infant rubella IgG

The primary symptom of rubella virus infection is the appearance of exanthem on the face which spreads to the trunk and limbs and usually fades after 3 days. Other symptoms include fever (rarely >38°C), cervical lymphadenopathy, joint pains, headache and conjunctivitis. Forchheimer's sign (small, red papules on the area of the soft palate) occurs in

20% of cases. Rubella is rare in infants or those over the age of 40. Up to one-third of older girls or women experience joint pain or arthritic-type symptoms with rubella. Rubella can cause congenital rubella syndrome in the new born (particularly when acquired at under 20 weeks gestation) – comprising cardiac (frequently PDA), cerebral, ophthalmic (frequently cataracts) and auditory defects (sensorineural deafness). It may also cause prematurity, low birth weight and neonatal thrombocytopenia, anaemia and hepatitis. The diagnosis of congenitally acquired rubella is made by detecting (through Haemagglutination assay or EIA) the presence of rubella IgM in cord blood or serum samples taken in infancy, detection of rubella antibodies at a time when maternal antibodies should have disappeared (approx. 6 months of age) or isolation of rubella virus from infected infants in the first few months of life. Duration of virus excretion in infected infants is variable and can lead to transmission to susceptible adults.

Further Reading
Best JM, Enders G. Laboratory diagnosis of rubella and congenital rubella. *Perspect Med Virol.* 2006;15:39–77.

A2.7 Answer A: PCR
Rectal infection is usually asymptomatic but anal discharge and anorectal discomfort can occur. Rates of rectal infection in men who have sex with men (MSM) is up to 10%. Lymphogranuloma venereum (LGV) is caused by the L1, L2 and L3 serotypes of *C. trachomatis* and often presents with proctitis. Nucleic acid amplification tests (NAAT) are the current standard of care for all cases including extra-genital infections. These are known to be more sensitive and specific than EIAs. Screening via ELISA is no longer acceptable. NAATs include PCR, LCR and real-time PCR. Specific testing for LGV should be performed in individuals with proctitis and on HIV-positive MSM with or without symptoms. Self-taken extra-genital sampling of the pharynx and rectum have been favourably evaluated.

Further Reading
Nwokolo NC, Dragovic B, Patel S, Tong CY, Barker G, Radcliffe K. 2015 UK national guideline for the management of infection with *Chlamydia trachomatis. Int J STD AIDS.* 2016;27(4):251–267.

A2.8 Answer C: Vincent's angina
Acute necrotising ulcerative gingivitis (Vincent's angina) was known as trench mouth in the First World War. Gram staining is usually not performed on routine throat swabs. Numerous studies on the validity of direct Gram stain for Group A Streptococcal infections has shown poor sensitivity and specificity. For a patient with suspected anaerobic tonsillitis (Vincent's angina), a Gram stain may be performed looking for numerous fusiform Gram-negative bacilli and spirochaetes. The causative organisms of Vincent's angina include anaerobes such as *Bacteroides* spp. and *Fusobacterium* spp., as well as spirochaetes (*Borrelia* and *Treponema* spp.). The condition is caused by an overpopulation of established oral bacteria due to a number of interacting factors such as poor hygiene, poor diet, smoking and stress.

Further Reading
Hodgdon A. Dental and related infections. *Emerg Med Clin North Am.* 2013;31(2):465–480.

A2.9 Answer C: *Neisseria gonorrhoeae*

Laboratory tests for *N. gonorrhoea* for identification include catalase (3% hydrogen peroxide) positive, speroxol (30% hydrogen peroxide) positive, colistin resistant and nitrate reduction negative. Disseminated *N. gonorrhoeae* infections can occur resulting in endocarditis, meningitis or gonococcal dermatitis-arthritis syndrome. Dermatitis-arthritis syndrome presents with arthralgia, tenosynovitis and painless non-pruritic dermatitis. Infection of the genitals in females with *N. gonorrhoeae* can result in pelvic inflammatory disease, if left untreated, which can result in infertility. Fever is common but rarely exceeds 38°C. Disseminated gonococcal infection is more likely blood culture negative. Maltose-negative meningococci do appear and in some studies are thought to make up 3–4% of meningococci (predominantly serotype B).

Table 4 Carbohydrate utilisation profile from *Neisseria* spp. and *Moraxella* spp.

Species	Glucose	Maltose	Sucrose	Lactose
N. gonorrhoea	+	−	−	−
N. meningitidis	+	+	−	−
N. sicca	+	+	+	−
M. catarrhalis	−	−	−	−

Further Reading

Bignell C, Fitzgerald M; Guideline Development Group; British Association for Sexual Health and HIV UK. UK national guideline for the management of gonorrhoea in adults, 2011. *Int J STD AIDS*. 2011;22(10):541–547.

Centers for Disease Control and Prevention (CDC). Characteristics of N. gonorrhoeae and related species of human origin. Available at: www.cdc.gov/std/gonorrhea/lab/ngon.htm

A2.10 Answer C: High antibody titre

The prozone effect is the phenomenon in which mixtures of specific antigen and antibody do not agglutinate or precipitate visibly because of an excess of either antibody or antigen. This can lead to reporting of a false negative result, unless sufficient dilutions of the serum are undertaken to enable the agglutination reaction/precipitation to occur.

Further Reading

Liu LL, Lin LR, Tong ML, Zhang HL, Huang SJ, Chen YY, Guo XJ, Xi Y, Liu L, Chen FY, Zhang YF, Zhang Q, Yang TC. Incidence and risk factors for the prozone phenomenon in serologic testing for syphilis in a large cohort. *Clin Infect Dis*. 2014;59(3):384–389.

A2.11 Answer C: *Mycobacterium kansasii*

Mycobacteria are aerobic, capsulated organisms which are acid-fast. There are nearly 200 species recognised, varying from environmental organisms, to opportunistic pathogens. They display differing phenotypic characteristics on culture which allow differentiation of species to a certain degree, although increasingly speciation is now obtained through molecular methods. Two of the key characteristics of mycobacteria revolve around their speed of grown (rapid vs slow growers) and their reaction to light. For this later characteristic, some *Mycobacterium* spp. produce carotenoid pigments without light (scotochromogens), while some require initial photo-activation for the pigment to be produced (photochromogens). *M. kansasii* may be either a photochromogen or a scotochromogen. Some strains of *M. avium-intracellulare* can be pigmented. *M. szulgai* is a scotochromogen at 37°C but a photochromogen at 25°C. These characteristics are represented in the Runyon classification:

Table 5 Runyon classification system for non-tuberculous *Mycobacterium* spp.

Photochromogens (Non-pigmented colonies grown in the dark; pigmented colonies after exposure to light and re-incubation)	Scotochromogens (Deep yellow to orange colonies when grown in either the light or the dark)	Non-pigmented (Non-pigmented in the light or the dark – tan colonies that do not intensify after light exposure)	Rapid growers
←———————————————— *M. kansasii* ————————————————→			*M. fortuitum*
M. marinum	*M. scrofulaceum*	*M. avium-intracellulare*	*M. chelonae*
M. simiae	*M. gordonae*	*M. bovis*	*M. abscessus*
	M. xenopi	*M. ulcerans*	
←———————————————— *M. szulgai* ————————————→		*M. malmoense*	

Modified from Jarzembowski et al. (2008).

Further Reading
Jarzembowski JA, Young MB. Nontuberculous mycobacterial infections. *Arch Pathol Lab Med.* 2008;132(8):1333–1341.

A2.12   Answer E: Microimmunofluorescence
Chlamydia psittaci and *Chlamydia pneumoniae* are in the family Chlamydiaceae and are obligate intracellular bacteria, both of which can cause a respiratory infective process. "Avian" chlamydiosis (also known as psittacosis) can be caused by both avian and mammalian serovars. There is no gold standard laboratory diagnostic for psittacosis, and all current methods have drawbacks. Culture of *C. Psittaci* is possible, but as it is a category 3 pathogen, it is only possible in certain facilities. The complement fixation test was historically the mainstay, detecting antibodies to the chlamydial lipopolysaccharides. Enzyme-linked immunoassays for chlamydial antigen are not currently available, either from blood or urine. Microimmunofluoresence is the current optimal modality for serological investigation, and is more sensitive and specific than the complement fixation test. However, cross-reactivity means it is difficult to distinguish *C. psittaci*, *C. trachomatis* and *Cp. pneumoniae*, and some lipopolysaccharides from other genera

have also been known to cross-react. Although not widely available yet, molecular testing, predominantly through polymerase chain reaction, is likely to displace serological methods.

Further Reading

Public Health England. UK Standards for Microbiology Investigations: Chlamydial zoonotic infections. 2016. Available at: https://assets.publishing.service.gov.uk/government/uploads/system/uploads/attachment_data/file/563418/V_57i2.1.pdf

A2.13 Answer B: The PCR reaction has been inhibited

Nucleic acid amplification tests have been demonstrated to be more sensitive and specific than either enzyme immunoassays, cell culture or direct fluorescence assays for *Chlamydia trachomatis* diagnosis. The sample site should reflect the type of sexual activity undertaken. In women, vulvo-vaginal swabs have superior sensitivity to self-collected endocervical swabs or urine samples. In men, first void urine samples are more sensitive than urethral sampling. Although nucleic acid amplification tests are advocated in UK testing algorithms, care must be taken to optimise the analytic process. This includes having confirmatory testing methods (using a different genomic target) and valid internal and external quality controls. Organic and inorganic compounds that inhibit the amplification of nucleic acids by PCR are common contaminants in DNA samples from various origins. They can interfere with the reaction at several levels, leading to different degrees of attenuation and even to complete inhibition. Internal controls are used to detect inhibitors.

Further Reading

Public Health England. UK Standards for Microbiology Investigations. *Chlamydia trachomatis* infection – testing by Nucleic Acid Amplification Tests (NAAT). 2017. Available at: https://assets.publishing.service.gov.uk/government/uploads/system/uploads/attachment_data/file/583847/V_37i4.pdf

A2.14 Answer B: Neomycin

One of the key aspects of clinical laboratory microbiology is to discern commensal organisms from pathogens. This can be achieved in many circumstances through use of selective culture agar, providing a media which will suppress unwanted (commensal) organisms, thereby letting the suspected pathogens be identified more easily. Many different selective agar exist. To provide a selective environment for anaerobes, the addition of neomycin provides inhibition to facultative anaerobes (such as many of the Enterobacteriales), without inhibiting the growth of pure anaerobes (such as *Bacteroides* spp.). Colistin is often combined with nalidixic acid (CNA) to suppress the growth of Gram-negative organisms (such as the Enterobacteriales and *Pseudomonas*), enabling Gram-positive organisms and yeasts to grow. Chloramphenicol (Rose Bengal) agar is used to suppress all bacterial growth, enabling identification of fungi – it is particularly used in foodstuff investigation. Vancomycin can be added to agar for screening for glycopeptide-resistant enterococci.

Further Reading

Lagier JC, Edouard S, Pagnier I, Mediannikov O, Drancourt M, Raoult D. Current and past strategies for bacterial culture in clinical microbiology. *Clin Microbiol Rev.* 2015;28:208–236.

A2.15   Answer D: *Pseudomonas aeruginosa*

Latex agglutination kits, consisting of latex particles coated with specific antiserum, enables rapid bench-top identification of several different organisms with a reasonable degree of specificity. Such kits exist for *S. aureus* (detecting coagulase and/or protein A), the beta-haemolytic streptococci (enabling Lancefield grouping), *Shigella* spp. and *Salmonella* Typhi (directed against the Vi antigen). Agglutination tests for *S.* Typhi have had a chequered history, and even in the latest Cochrane review (2017) only moderate diagnostic accuracy was found. No latex agglutination text is in common use for *P. aeruginosa*.

Further Reading

Wijedoru L, Mallett S, Parry CM. Rapid diagnostic tests for typhoid and paratyphoid (enteric) fever. *Cochrane Database Syst Rev.* 2017;5:CD008892.

A2.16   Answer A: *Streptococcus dysgalactiae*

While Group A Streptococcus (*S. pyogenes*) is perhaps the most common bacterial cause of acute pharyngitis, Group C and Group G streptococci can also cause a similar syndrome. However, they are also frequent colonisers of the upper airway (and gastrointestinal tract and vagina). Group C and Group G streptococci from humans are now considered to be the same subspecies; *S. dysgalactiae* subsp. *equisimilis*, and is closely genetically related to *S. pyogenes*. To this end, Group C and Group G streptococci share similar virulence factors to Group A streptococci, including streptolysins O and S, streptokinase, M protein (antiphagocytic) and pyrogenic exotoxins (streptococcal toxic shock syndrome).

    S. canis was first isolated from dogs and groups with Group G Streptococcus antisera. *S. equi* and *S. zooepidemicus* were also originally isolated from animals, and do also group with Group C antisera. The milleri streptococci (*Streptococcus constellatus*, *S. anginosus* and *S. intermedius*) are typically alpha-haemolytic (although on occasion beta-haemolytic) but may also group with Group C or G antisera but have a different colonial morphology. *S. pyogenes* is Group A Streptococcus. *S. agalactiae* is Group B Streptococcus. *S. gallolyticus* (previously *S. bovis*; isolated from humans) and *S. equinus* (isolated from animals) are Group D streptococci. *S. suis* is an alpha-haemolytic *Streptococcus* spp.

Further Reading

Jensen A, Kilian M. Delineation of *Streptococcus dysgalactiae*, its subspecies, and its clinical and phylogenetic relationship to *Streptococcus pyogenes*. *J Clin Microbiol.* 2012;50:113.

A2.17   Answer A: Cefpodoxime

There are various different molecular mechanisms for beta lactamases, and each can manifest phenotypically through hydrolysis of different cephalosporins. TEM and

SHV-derived ESBLs demonstrate resistance to ceftazidime and variable resistance to cefotaxime. CTX-M ESBLs demonstrate resistance to cefotaxime, but variable resistance to ceftazidime. However, all ESBLs demonstrate resistance to cefpodoxime, and as such, this antimicrobial represents a good screening tool for detection of possible ESBL production. It is not absolutely specific, however, and confirmatory testing should be subsequently conducted where there are clinical concerns. Cefuroxime, cefalexin and cephradine are unreliable indicators for ESBL production. Cefoxitin is a screening antimicrobial for AmpC production.

Further Reading

Jacoby GA, Munoz-Price LS. The new beta-lactamases. *N Engl J Med.* 2005;352(4):380–391.

A2.18   Answer B: *Staphylococcus haemolyticus*

S. haemolyticus is an opportunistic pathogen with a particularly antimicrobial-resistant phenotype. It has been described as a cause of meningitis, skin and skin structure infections, prosthetic join infections and bacteraemia. Common antimicrobials found to be resistant in *S. haemolyticus* include meticillin, gentamicin and erythromycin, and uniquely among staphylococci, glycopeptide antibiotics such as teicoplanin.

While *S. aureus* is the most common coagulase-positive staphylococcus isolated in the clinical laboratory, *S. intermedius, S. delphini, S. schleiferi* subsp. *coagulans, S. lutrae* and some strains of *S. hyicus* are also coagulase positive. *S. intermedius* isolates are positive for free coagulase but are negative for protein A, and 14% of the isolates have a clumping factor, which would account for the positive slide coagulase and weak positive Staph latex. *S. intermedius* is a common commensal of oral, nasal and skin flora in healthy dogs and has been recognised as an invasive zoonotic pathogen being isolated from 18% of canine-inflicted wounds. Coagulase positivity is commonly used to attribute clinical significance and pathogenicity to isolates of *Staphylococcus* spp.

S. lugdunensis may produce a bound coagulase, a property which it shares with *S. aureus*, but unlike *S. aureus* it does not produce a free coagulase. In the laboratory it can give a positive slide-coagulase test but a negative tube-coagulase test.

Further Reading

John JF, Harvin AM. History and evolution of antibiotic resistance in coagulase-negative staphylococci: susceptibility profiles of new anti-staphylococcal agents. *Therapeut Clin Risk Manag.* 2007;3(6):1143–1152.

A2.19   Answer B: Chocolate bacitracin agar

Blood agar plates provide a non-selective culture medium for a broad range of bacterial and fungal organisms and enable determination of the haemolytic abilities of isolates. However, some organisms are more fastidious, and this includes some of the respiratory bacteria such *H. influenzae*. This organism needs two specific growth factors – nicotinamide adenine dinucleotide (NAD; factor V) and hemin (factor X). The addition of bacitracin inhibits the growth of staphylococci, streptococci, *Micrococcus* spp. and *Neisseria* spp., which represent common commensals of the upper respiratory tract and which, without bacitracin, may

Table 6 Growth requirements for *Haemophilus* spp. and associated genera.

Haemophilus species	Growth around disc		
	X	V	XV
H. influenzae	−	−	+
H. haemolyticus	−	−	+
H. aegyptius	−	−	+
H. aphrophilus	v/−	−	+
H. ducreyi	+	−	+
H. parahaemolyticus	−	+	+
H. parainfluenzae	−	+	+
Aggregatibacter aphrophilus	−	+	+

overgrow any *H. influenzae* present. Discriminating *H. influenzae* from other *Haemophilus* spp. requires subculture onto a factor-free media (such as Mueller–Hinton) and then separate factor X, factor V and combined factor X/V discs. The growth around each disc then enables identification to species level.

MacConkey agar is a selective media for Gram-negative organisms, and allows differentiation based upon their ability to ferment lactose. Mannitol salt agar is a selective agar for Gram-positive organisms, specifically *Staphylococcus* spp. and *Micrococcus* spp., and allows differentiation based on mannitol fermentation (*S. aureus* turns yellow). Xylose lysine desoxycholate agar (XLD) is a selective media for *Salmonella* spp. and *Shigella* spp. (*Salmonella* spp. are red colonies, some of which have black centres; *Shigella* spp. are red colonies, and other coliforms are yellow to orange in colour).

Further Reading

Nørskov-Lauritsen N. Classification, identification, and clinical significance of *Haemophilus* and *Aggregatibacter* species with host specificity for humans. *Clin Microbiol Rev.* 2014;27(2):214–240.

A2.20 **Answer A: Detects the presence of bacterial nitrate reductase**
Nitrate reductase is produced by organisms belonging to the Enterobacteriales family, and production of this during urinary tract infections leads to the build-up of nitrites in the urine; these react with p-arsanilic acid on urine dipsticks. The reported sensitivity of a positive nitrate on a urine dipstick being indicative of a urinary tract infection is 30–80% but the specificity is higher at 92–100%. The reagent is highly sensitive to air exposure, which may cause a false-positive response. False-negative results may be seen where bladder incubation time is shortened (less than 4 hours), in the absence of dietary nitrate, in the presence of nitrate-reductase negative organisms (such as *Enterococcus* spp., *Staphylococcus* spp. and *Acinetobacter* spp.), when urine specific gravity is elevated, where pH is less than 6.0 and in the presence of urobilinogen and urinary vitamin C.

Further Reading

Sharp VJ, Lee DK, Askeland EJ. Urinalysis: case presentations for the primary care physician. *Am Fam Physician.* 2014;90(8):542–547.

A2.21 Answer D: A positive result can occur with damaged or lysed leukocytes
Leukocyte esterase is present in neutrophils and macrophages and is released when those cells are damaged or lysed. The leukocyte esterase test is more sensitive than the nitrate test with a sensitivity of 75–96% and a specificity of 94–98%. The test is, however, prone to false positives particularly from vaginal secretions and trichomonal infections. False-negative results can occur in the context of high levels of urinary protein or urinary vitamin C or in neutropaenic patients. Combining the leukocyte esterase and nitrate tests results in higher specificity than using either test alone.

Further Reading
Sharp VJ, Lee DK, Askeland EJ. Urinalysis: case presentations for the primary care physician. *Am Fam Physician*. 2014;90(8):542–547.

A2.22 Answer A: Unpreserved urine should be processed in less than 4 hours from collection time
For adults suspected of having a lower urinary tract infection, a mid-stream urine, consisting of urine after the first 10–20 mL have been voided, is recommended. Early morning urine (first void of the day) is only recommended for the investigation of renal tract tuberculosis. For young children, discerning between commensal organisms from the external genitalia and organisms from higher up the urological tract can be difficult in a "mid"-stream urine and suprapubic aspirates may be warranted.

Microscopy and subculture of urine should occur within 4 hours of collection. However, chemical preservation (tartaric and boric acids being the most common) of urine specimens, or refrigeration, are available and allow urine to be stored for 48–96 hours, reducing bacterial overgrowth, which may lead to a false-positive result. Boric acid may be harmful to certain organisms and may inhibit the leukocyte esterase test.

Further Reading
Public Health England. UK Standards for Microbiology Investigations B 41: Investigation of urine. 2017. Available at: https://assets.publishing.service.gov.uk/government/uploads/system/uploads/attachment_data/file/638270/B_41i8.4.pdf

A2.23 Answer D: It should be treated if >10^5 CFU/mL in two consecutive mid-stream urines
The diagnosis of asymptomatic bacteriuria in women is appropriate only if the same species is present in quantities of at least 100,000 CFU/mL of urine in at least two consecutive voided specimens. Women who are pregnant should be screened for asymptomatic bacteriuria in the first trimester and treated, if positive. Treating asymptomatic bacteriuria in patients with diabetes, older persons, patients with indwelling catheters or patients with spinal cord injuries has not been found to improve outcomes.

Further Reading
Cormican M, Murphy AW, Vellinga A. Interpreting asymptomatic bacteriuria. *BMJ*. 2011;343:d4780.

A2.24 Answer B: Multilocus sequence typing (MLST)

Numerous techniques are available to differentiate *S. aureus* isolates. Historically, phenotypic methods such as antibiotic susceptibility testing and bacteriophage typing were used but these have marked limitations. Strain typing now focuses on DNA-based methods. Initial techniques compared restriction endonuclease patterns of chromosomal or plasmid DNA. The second generation of genotyping methods included Southern blot hybridisation using gene-specific probes, ribotyping, PCR-based approaches and pulsed-field gel electrophoresis but these remain difficult to standardise between laboratories. DNA sequence analysis is an objective genotyping method; it is highly portable and easily stored and analysed in a relational database, and rapid, affordable, high-throughput systems may make it possible for sequencing to be considered as a viable typing method.

Further Reading

Melles DC, van Leeuwen WB, Snijders SV, Horst-Kreft D, Peeters JK, Verbrugh HA, van Belkum A. Comparison of multilocus sequence typing (MLST), pulsed-field gel electrophoresis (PFGE), and amplified fragment length polymorphism (AFLP) for genetic typing of *Staphylococcus aureus*. *J Microbiol Methods*. 2007;69(2):371–375.

A2.25   Answer D: Whole genome sequencing

P. aeruginosa is a common healthcare-associated pathogen and can be the cause of outbreaks in inpatient settings, either from patient-to-patient transmission or from a point source as a water outlet. Investigating these outbreaks through appropriate clinical and molecular epidemiology enables appropriate infection control interventions to be made.

Early methods used to investigate *Pseudomonas* spp. epidemiology included pyocin production, comparison of antimicrobial susceptibility patterns and phage typing. However, these phenotypic methods lacked reproducibility, particularly because phenotypic expression of elements of interest may change during an outbreak or under differing laboratory incubation conditions. Molecular methods have now become the mainstay and include ribotyping, pulsed-field gel electrophoresis (PGFE) and variable nucleotide tandem repeats (VNTR). VNTR and PFGE provide a comparable level of isolate discriminatory power, but VNTR enables a faster turn-around-time and greater reproducibility for *Pseudomonas* spp. Where there is clear clinical epidemiology to support possible cross transmission, either of these modalities may be sufficient to suggest strain similarity. Whole genome sequencing, although slower and currently costlier than VNTR or PFGE, may be of particular use where there are no clear clinical epidemiological links or the cases are separated over prolonged periods of time, as in this case.

Further Reading

Parcell BJ, Oravcova K, Pinheiro M, Holden MTG, Phillips G, Turton JF, Gillespie SH. *Pseudomonas aeruginosa* intensive care unit outbreak: winnowing of transmissions with molecular and genomic typing. *J Hosp Infect*. 2018;98(3):282–288.

A2.26   Answer B: Terminal void urine

Schistosoma haematobium infection results in adult worms residing in the venous plexus of bladder (in other *Schistosoma* spp. infections the adult worms reside in mesenteric venules in various locations). Detection depends upon microscopy or urine in *S. haematobium* stool in the other *Schistosoma* spp.). Terminal urine is the optimal sample type for microscopy for *S. haematobium* infection, but urine can only be investigated more than 5 weeks after exposure (no eggs are passed prior to this). Terminal urine samples should be collected between 10.00 am and 2.00 pm as this is the period of maximum activity. A 24-hour collection of terminal samples of urine can be obtained, but is often more technically difficult for patients to concord with.

Further Reading
Barsoum RS. Urinary schistosomiasis: review. *J Adv Res*. 2013;4(5):453–459.

A2.27 Answer C: Ova
Schistosoma haematobium infection causes egg (ova) release into the urinary tract causing granuloma, which over a prolonged period can lead to fibrosis, strictures and eventual urodynamic abnormalities. The eggs of *S. haematobium* are ellipsoidal with a terminal spine, *S. mansoni* eggs are also ellipsoidal but with a lateral spine, *S. japonicum* eggs are spheroidal with a small knob. Other helminthic infections are detected by looking for larvae or adults in stool or other samples types or microfilariae in skin scrapings. In protozoal infections, cysts can be seen in some sample types, including stool.

Further Reading
Barsoum RS. Urinary schistosomiasis: review. *J Adv Res*. 2013;4(5):453–459.

A2.28 Answer C: It is a lactose fermenter
Salmonella enterica subsp. Arizonae is a non-Typhi *Salmonella* spp., which has a particular association with reptiles, including tortoises and snakes. It can cause enteritis in humans, and has also been documented to cause meningitis and septic arthritis. *S.* Arizonae has several biochemical features which enable differentiation from other *Salmonella* spp. Specifically, *S.* Arizonae can ferment lactose, liquefy gelatine, are ONPG positive and are malonate positive. However, it is the lactose fermentation which complicates routine clinical microbiology as most selective media rely upon *Salmonella* spp. being lactose non-fermenters.

Further Reading
Lee YC, Hung -C, Hung SC, Wang SC, Wang HP, Cho HL, Lai MC, Wang JT. *Salmonella enterica* subspecies Arizonae infection of adult patients in Southern Taiwan: a case series in a non-endemic area and literature review. *BMC Infect Dis*. 2016;16:746.

A2.29 Answer D: *Cyclospora cayetanensis*
Cyclosporiasis usually presents as prolonged watery diarrhoea, starting several weeks after ingestion of contaminated food or water. Direct person-to-person transmission is unusual as the oocysts require several weeks in a favourable environment to sporulate. The oocysts are shed in variable amounts, and so sequential stool samples for microscopy for ova, cysts and parasites over several days may be required for diagnosis. Acid-fast staining (such as

Kinyoun's) is used for microscopy and has a sensitivity of 96%. However, both *Cryptosporidium* spp. and *Cyclospora* spp. appear highly refractile and differentiation is through size; *Cyclospora* spp. is larger at 8–10 μm whereas *Cryptosporidium* spp. is smaller at 4–5 μm. Alternatively, the oocysts of *Cyclospora* spp. are auto-fluorescent, such that when examined under an ultraviolet microscope the parasite appears blue or green. Molecular diagnostic methods, such as polymerase chain reaction, are also now becoming available for *Cyclospora* spp.

Further Reading
Came VA, Matheson BA. Infections by intestinal Coccidia and *Giardia duodenalis*. *Clin Lab Med*. 2015;35(2):423–444.

A2.30   Answer D: Bone marrow
Enteric fever is caused by *Salmonella* Typhi and *Salmonella* Paratyphi and presents with high fever, with or without disturbance to stool frequency (patients can have diarrhoea, constipation or indeed normal bowels). The occurrence of relative bradycardia and rose spots, although highly suggestive of enteric fever, is infrequent. Indirect methods for diagnosing enteric fever have suboptimal sensitivity and specificity, and culture of *S.* Typhi or *S.* Paratyphi remains the gold standard. This also enables susceptibility testing, and with high rates of antimicrobial resistance in this genus, this can be essential to aid treatment success.

Dependent upon local laboratory equipment, sample processing and technical skill, stool cultures yield *S.* Typhi in 45–65% of cases, while blood cultures (when multiple sets are taken) can provide an isolate in ~70% of cases. The highest yield is obtained from bone marrow aspirates, from which a pathogen can be obtained in 90–95% of cases.

Further Reading
Parry CM, Wijedoru L, Arjyal A, Baker S. The utility of diagnostic tests for enteric fever in endemic locations. *Expert Rev Anti Infect Ther*. 2011;9(6):711–725.

A2.31   Answer D: Perform serology (±Vi 0:9,12 H:d)
Salmonella spp. laboratory diagnosis predominantly follows several stages, with initial isolation using selective media (e.g. XLD), followed by biochemical (e.g. API®) or mass spectroscopy (e.g. MALDI-TOF) for presumptive identification to species level. However, both biochemical and mass spectroscopy struggle to definitively discern serovar assignment. Therefore, alternative methods to confirm presumptive diagnoses (in particular to discern *S.* Typhi/*S.* Paratyphi from the non-Typhi *Salmonella* spp.) are needed. Latex agglutination of somatic ("O"), flagellar ("H") and Vi antigens can aid further microbial identification with a rapid turn-around-time. In many settings, including the United Kingdom, definitive serovar assignment occurs at reference laboratories. Some commercial agglutination kits group *Salmonella serovars* together and denote these groups as letters such as "group W" (but specifically "group W" relates to "O-45," which does not include *S.* Typhi or *S.* Paratyphi).

Further Reading

Kang L, Li N, Li P, Zhou Y, Gao S, Gao H, Xin W, Wang J. MALDI-TOF mass spectrometry provides high accuracy in identification of Salmonella at species level but is limited to type or subtype *Salmonella serovars*. *Eur J Mass Spectro*. 2017;23(2):70–82.

A2.32 Answer D: Detection of enterotoxin in vomit

Qualitative culture of stool for faecal pathogens is useful for organisms that are not commensal to the gastrointestinal tract, including *Shigella* spp., *Salmonella* spp., verocytotoxic *Escherichia coli* and *Campylobacter* spp., as well as rarer causes of food-borne intoxication including *Plesiomonas shigelloides* and *Vibrio* spp. Although some organisms are found in small numbers in healthy individuals, they may also be the cause of food-borne enteritis. These include *Bacillus cereus* (predominantly from re-heated rice), *Clostridium perfringens* and *Staphylococcus aureus*.

Some causes of enteritis are determined through enterotoxin detection, including *C difficile* and *C botulinum* (the latter usually only undertaken at reference laboratories). Food samples can be both qualitatively and quantitatively cultured for enteric pathogens. Vomit is not an appropriate sample for enterotoxin detection.

Further Reading

Lindström M, Korkeala H. Laboratory diagnostics of botulism. *Clin Microbiol Rev*. 2006;19 (2):298–314.

Public Health England. UK Standards for Microbiology Investigations. B 30: Investigation of faecal specimens for enteric pathogens. 2014. Available at: https://assets.publishing.service.gov.uk/government/uploads/system/uploads/attachment_data/file/343955/B_30i8.1.pdf

A2.33 Answer A: Cary-Blair

Cary-Blair (CB) transport medium contains sodium thioglycollate, di-sodium hydrogen phosphate, sodium chloride and calcium chloride and agar. It has been shown to maintain better viability of bacteria than Stuart's or Amies medium. Alkaline peptone water can maintain the viability of *Vibrio* spp. but is inferior to CB media. Buffered glycerol saline can maintain the viability of *Shigella* spp., but not *Vibrio* spp.

CB media is recommended for the collection and transport of faecal and rectal samples to maintain viability of *Salmonella* spp., *Shigella* spp., *Vibrio* spp. and verocytotoxic *Escherichia coli*. CB medium has a low nutrient content, a phosphate buffer and sodium thioglycollate to inhibit growth of *E. coli* and *Klebsiella aerogenes*. CB medium has been described as especially good for epidemiological studies of *Vibrio parahaemolyticus*, allowing long-term survival (up to 35 days at temperatures from 22°C to 31°C) of rectal swabs. Long recovery times have been reported for *Pasteurella pestis* (75 days) as well as for *Salmonella* spp. and *Shigella* spp. (49 days).

Further Reading

Barber S, Lawson PJ, Grove DI. Evaluation of bacteriological transport swabs. *Pathology*. 1998;30:179–182.

A2.34 Answer A: Lysine decarboxylase negative

Benchtop biochemical tests are still frequently used to distinguish *Salmonella* spp. from other Enterobacterales. The lysine decarboxylase test is used to distinguish *Salmonella* spp. (and *Escherichia coli*, *Klebsiella* spp., *Serratia* spp., *Vibrio* spp., all usually positive) from *Shigella* spp. (usually negative). However, among the *Salmonella* spp., *S.* Paratyphi A is unusually lysine decarboxylase negative and can be mis-identified in clinical laboratory practice. Phenylalanine deaminase is used to differentiate *Proteus* spp., *Morganella morganii* and *Providencia* spp. (all positive) from the other Enterobacterales. The only *Salmonella* spp. found to be urea positive is *Salmonella Cubana*, all other *Salmonella* spp., *Shigella* spp. and *E. coli* should be negative (positive include *Proteus* spp. and *Yersinia* spp.).

Further Reading
Crump JA, Sjölund-Karlsson M, Gordon MA, Parry CM. Epidemiology, clinical presentation, laboratory diagnosis, antimicrobial resistance, and antimicrobial management of invasive *Salmonella* infections. *Clin Microbiol Rev*. 2015;28(4):901–937.

A2.35   **Answer A: *Vibrio cholerae***
Vibrio spp. are non-motile Gram-negative rods which often morphologically have a single, rigid curve. Most are oxidase and catalase positive and ferment glucose without producing gas. They are often associated with seafood or water contamination when causing enteritis (or seawater exposure when causing skin and skin structure infections with *Vibrio vulnificus*).

Thiosulfate-citrate-bile-sucrose (TCBS) agar is highly selective for the isolation of *Vibrio* spp., including *V. cholerae* and *V. parahaemolyticus*. TCBS has an alkaline growth medium (pH 8.5–9.5), which otherwise inhibits the growth of Enterobacterales and other intestinal flora. *V. cholerae* and the biotype Eltor ferment sucrose, which lowers the pH and produces yellow-brown colonies (most other *Vibrio* spp. produce yellow colonies), but *V. parahaemolyticus* will produce light bluish colonies and *V. mimicus* and *V. damsela* produce green-coloured colonies. Certain strains of *Proteus* and enterococci may grow and produce yellow colonies, but these are small and are easily distinguishable from *Vibrio* spp.

Further Reading
Baker-Austin C, Oliver JD. *Vibrio vulnificus*: new insights into a deadly opportunistic pathogen. *Environ Microbiol*. 2018;20(2):423–430.

Elbashir S, Parveen S, Schwarz J, Rippen T, Jahncke M, DePaola A. Seafood pathogens and information on antimicrobial resistance: a review. *Food Microbiol*. 2018;70:85–93.

A2.36   **Answer C: It is catalase negative**
Shigella spp. are Gram-negative, non-motile facultative anaerobes. They cause enteritis and colitis, also known as shigellosis, and are not gut commensals. The diarrhoea can be watery but can also present with fulminant dysentery. Most shigellosis is acquired through faeco-oral transmission (humans are the only natural host); *S. flexneri* in low- and middle-income countries (and among men who have sex with men globally) and *S. sonnei* in high-income countries (but not in low- and middle-income countries due to host immunogenicity from frequent population exposure to *Plesiomonas shigelloides* O17 which

has an almost identical O antigen to *S. sonnei*). *S. dysenteriae* type 1 usually emerges in emergency situations such as natural disasters and social disruption.

Diagnosis is through PCR, often as part of a multiplex enteric pathogen panel, or through stool culture and susceptibility. The latter is particularly useful for *S. flexneri* isolated from men who have sex with men because of frequent antimicrobial resistance seen in these circulating strains. Where cultured, laboratory identification is through either mass spectroscopy or biochemical tests (such as with API®). Predominantly, *Shigella* spp. are oxidase negative, urease negative, do not decarboxylate lysine and are catalase positive with the exception of *S. dysenteriae* type 1.

Further Reading

Kotloff KL, Riddle MS, Platts-Mills JA, Pavlinac P, Zaidi AKM. Shigellosis. *Lancet*. 2018;391 (10122):801–812.

A2.37   Answer B: *Campylobacter fetus*

Campylobacter spp. are motile rods, which most often appear spiral (*C. coli*) or S-shaped (*C. jejuni*), can be broadly divided into those that reside in the human oral cavity as commensals and infrequent causes of periodontitis (*C. ureolyticus*, *C. curvus*, *C. concisus*, *C. showae*, *C. gracilis*, *C. rectus*), and those that are zoonotic (predominantly *C. jejuni* and *C. coli*).

Culture is typically with charcoal cefoperazone deoxycholate agar (CCDA) incubated microaerobically at 42°C for 40–48 hours. At this standard *Campylobacter* spp. incubation temperature selectivity is increased and growth of *Campylobacter* spp. is faster. However, non-thermophilic strains will not grow, such as *C. fetus* subspecies *fetus*. *C. fetus* can lead to fatal septicaemia in new-borns and immunocompromised individuals such as those with HIV. *Campylobacter* spp. are oxidase positive, and analysis with matrix-assisted laser desorption/ionisation time-of-flight (MALDI-TOF) mass spectrometry provides identification with a good degree of confidence.

Further Reading

Lee S, Lee J, Ha J, Choi Y, Kim S, Lee H, Yoon Y, Choi KH. Clinical relevance of infections with zoonotic and human oral species of *Campylobacter*. *J Microbiol*. 2016;54(7):459–467.

Wagenaar JA, van Bergen MA, Blaser MJ, Tauxe RV, Newell DG, van Putten JP. *Campylobacter fetus* infections in humans: exposure and disease. *Clin Infect Dis*. 2014;58(11):1579–1586.

A2.38   Answer C: *Streptococcus gallolyticus*

S. gallolyticus (previously known as *S. bovis*) is a Gram-positive coccus which can demonstrate alpha, beta or non-haemolytic properties. It is catalase negative (as with all streptococci), hydrolyses aesculin (in common with enterococci and *Leuconostoc* spp.) and agglutinates with Group D antisera. Several biotypes of *S. gallolyticus* are recognised, and while all can cause endocarditis, urinary tract infections, neonatal meningitis and bacteraemia, only biotype-1 has a reasonably unambiguous association with colon cancer. Patients in whom an invasive *S. gallolyticus* infection is identified should undergo subsequent investigations for bowel cancer.

Leuconostoc spp. are Gram-positive cocci which are more oval than spherical. They are commensals and very infrequently cause disease. They are catalase negative (enabling them to be distinguished from *Staphylococcus* spp.), but are all intrinsically resistant to enterococci (and care must be taken to distinguish *Leuconostoc* spp. from glycopeptide-resistant enterococci). *S. agalactiae* is a Group B beta haemolytic *Streptococcus*. *S. constellatus* is one of the milleri streptococci, and therefore will be catalase negative, will not hydrolyse aesculin and is variably alpha or beta haemolytic. *S. constellatus*, as with the other milleri streptococci (*S. intermedius* and *S. anginosus*) can agglutinate with Group C and Group G antisera.

Further Reading

Dekker JP, Lau AF. An update on the *Streptococcus bovis* group: classification, identification, and disease associations. *J Clin Microbiol.* 2016;54(7):1694–1699.

A2.39 **Answer A:** It grows at 4°C incubation

L. monocytogenes is a Gram-positive rod which is facultatively anaerobic and catalase positive. It is associated with food-borne outbreaks, in part because it is found in soil and animals, and is a psychrophile (or cryophiles). This means that it is capable of growth and reproduction in cold temperatures (i.e. <15°C), and so can continue to reproduce, while food products, including packaged goods and cheeses, are refrigerated. Psychrophiles can be contrasted with thermophiles, which thrive at unusually hot temperatures (*Campylobacter* spp. are relative thermophiles, being able to reproduce at 42°C). In the laboratory, *L. monocytogenes* demonstrates tumbling motility under light microscopy at room temperature (20–25°C).

Clinically, *L. monocytogenes* causes listeriosis, which can include bacteraemia and meningitis. It particularly affects immunocompromised individuals, including those who are elderly or who have diabetes and alcohol dependency. It also particularly affects pregnant women, where it can cause intrauterine infections leading to spontaneous abortion.

Further Reading

Radoshevich L, Cossart P. *Listeria monocytogenes*: towards a complete picture of its physiology and pathogenesis. *Nat Rev Microbiol.* 2018;16(1):32–46.

A2.40 **Answer C: Discerns *Salmonella* spp. and *Shigella* spp.**

Xylose lysine deoxycholate agar (XLD) is a selective media for *Salmonella* spp. and *Shigella* spp. *Salmonella* spp. appear as red colonies with (for the majority of species) black centres; *Shigella* spp. appear as just red colonies. Deoxycholic acid is a secondary bile acid, a metabolic by-product of intestinal bacteria. In XLD and deoxycholate citrate (DCA) agar, it is selective for the isolation of *Shigella* sp. and *Salmonella* sp. The only fermentable carbohydrate is lactose.

Further Reading

Public Health England. UK Standards for Microbiology Investigations. ID 24: Identification of *Salmonella* species. 2015. Available at: www.gov.uk/government/publications/smi-id-24-identification-of-salmonella-species

A2.41   **Answer B: DNAse**
Infective exacerbations of chronic obstructive pulmonary disease (COPD) are associated with significant changes in the respiratory tract flora. However, even in stable COPD, the upper respiratory tract microbiome is significantly different to that of a healthy individual. In both stable COPD and during exacerbations, *Haemophilus influenzae*, *Moraxella catarrhalis*, *Staphylococcus aureus* and *Streptococcus pneumoniae* predominate over the non-pathogenic upper respiratory tract organisms. In addition, in infective exacerbations, *Pseudomonas aeruginosa* is also seen. Infective exacerbations may, therefore, be due to new acquisition of one of these organisms, increased bacterial load from already present commensals or a new strain or change in virulence factors among commensal species.

Given this, isolation of *H. influenzae*, *M. catarrhalis*, *S. aureus* and *S. pneumoniae* from sputum during an infective exacerbation of COPD should be viewed with caution. While *S. aureus* and *S. pneumoniae* both grow on blood agar, chocolate agar are needed for the more fastidious organisms. On chocolate plates, *H. influenzae* and *M. catarrhalis* will grow, but so will some commensal oropharyngeal organisms, including oral *Neisseria* spp. Both *Neisseria* spp. and *Moraxella* spp. are Gram-negative cocci which are catalase positive, but only *M. catarrhalis* has a DNAse. Alternatively, a tributyrin test can be used, with *M. catarrhalis* hydrolysing tributyrin and turning it yellow, and *Neisseria* spp. having no impact and hence no colour change.

Further Reading
Beasley V, Joshi PV, Singanayagam A, Molyneaux PL, Johnston SL, Mallia P. Lung microbiology and exacerbations in COPD. *Int J Chron Obstruct Pulmon Dis.* 2012;7:555–569.

A2.42   **Answer C: Miles–Misra plates**
The methods described by Miles and Misra is a technique for counting the number of colony forming units in a bacterial suspension. The procedure involves serial dilutions of the bacterial suspension, then inoculation on divided agar plates using a set method and incubation for 18–24 hours. Agar segments where more than 20 colonies are present without any confluence are utilised to make viable counts and can be calculated per mL, equating back to the initial inoculation drop volume.

Cell counts in broth solution are not consistent enough to enable total viable counts. Flow cytometry, optical density and quantification of DNA do not discern viable colony forming units.

Further Reading
Marek A, Smith A, Peat M, Connell A, Gillespie I, Morrison P, Hamilton A, Shaw D, Stewart A, Hamilton K, Smith I, Mead A, Howard P, Ingle D. Endoscopy supply water and final rinse testing: five years of experience. *J Hosp Infect.* 2014;88(4):207–212.

A2.43   **Answer D: Number of patient white cells**
Bacteraemia is associated with significant mortality, and appropriately identifying and managing patients can be optimised by appropriate blood culture sampling. Blood cultures are usually taken in the context of fever, raised inflammatory markers or suspicion of deep seating infections, such as infective endocarditis.

Multiple factors influence the sensitivity and specificity of this investigation. Sensitivity is impacted by the volume of blood, duration of culture (however prolonging cultures beyond

5 days also increases the likelihood of a contaminant organism growing), and the fastidiousness of the organisms causing the disease. Specificity (i.e., the likelihood that the organism grown in the blood culture is relevant to the patient's presentation) is predominantly influenced by the venepuncture technique.

Further Reading

Lamy B, Dargère S, Arendrup MC, Parienti J-J, Tattevin P. How to optimize the use of blood cultures for the diagnosis of bloodstream infections? A State-of-the Art. *Front Microbiol.* 2016;7:697.

A2.44 Answer D: *Malassezia furfur*

M. furfur and *M. globosa* are both associated with dermatological infections. *M. globosa* is a cause of dandruff, while *M. furfur* is the cause of tinea versicolor. Tinea versicolour, as in this case, typically presents as a fine scaling of the skin producing a very superficial ash-like scale with sharply demarcated pale or pink patches which can darken if the patient becomes flushed. There may be associated pruritis in affected area, sometimes described as a feeling of "pin-pricks," often when there is elevated body temperature from the environment or from exercise, which is relieved once sweating begins.

The dermatophyte filamentous fungi include the three genera *Trichophyton* spp., *Microsporum* spp. and *Epidermophyton* spp. *Candida* spp. (both *C. albicans* and non-albicans *Candida* spp.) is the cause of thrush which typically manifests as a pruritic exudate on mucous membranes (including oropharynx and genitalia) or the skin (typically in moist folds where it causes intertrigo). *C. immitis* is a dimorphic fungus (i.e. can exist as either a yeast or a mould), which is prevalent in the southern areas of North American, down through to the northern areas of South America. Coccidiomycosis can manifest as a pulmonary infection, but can also disseminate, including causing cutaneous lesions with distinct lesions containing the organism or through reactive manifestations including erythema nodosum and erythema multiforme.

Further Reading

Georgios Gaitanis, Prokopios Magiatis, Markus Hantschke, Ioannis D. Bassukas, Aristea Velegraki. The Malassezia genus in skin and systemic diseases. *Clin Microbiol Rev.* 2012;25(1):106–141.

A2.45 Answer A: Calcofluor staining

Rhinocerebral mucormycosis is caused by the saprophytic fungi *Rhizopus* spp., *Mucor* spp. and *Absidia* spp. These fungi cause a rapid and extensive destructive process, infecting the nasal mucosa and spreading into the turbinate bone. It particularly affects those who are immunocompromised, including patients with diabetes. Pulmonary and disseminated infections can also occur, and mortality without prompt surgical (including extensive debridement) and medical interventions is high.

Laboratory identification of the causative genera of fungi from a tissue biopsy is most rapidly achieved by light microscopy of a wet mount (the hyphae do not stain well with a Gram stain). The hyphae may be difficult to characterise on a simple potassium hydroxide wet preparation, and calcofluor or blancofluor with a fluorescent microscope enable identification of hyphae seen on initial potassium hydroxide wet mounts. To differentiate the hyphae of these genera from other fungi, they are broad (6–16 μm diameter), irregularly shaped and often described as "ribbon-like," and non- or sparsely septate with branches arising at right angles and non-dichotomously. The genera of these fungi are seen much more clearly with methenamine-silver, do not stain with periodic acid-Schiff and are difficult to observe on haematoxylin-eosin staining. However, these stains may all take some time to result, and the need for expediency makes calcofluor staining optimal in this case.

Further Reading

Walsh TJ, Gamaletsou MN, McGinnis MR, Hayden RT, Kontoyiannis DP. Early clinical and laboratory diagnosis of invasive pulmonary, extrapulmonary, and disseminated mucormycosis (zygomycosis), *Clin Infect Dis.* 2012;54(S1):S55–S60.

A2.46   Answer A: Periodic acid-Schiff stain

Respiratory specimens, such as bronchoalveolar lavage, should have appropriate microscopy and culture for fungal pathogens where clinical signs indicate possible mycotic disease (in this case the vignette suggests a possible aspergilloma or at least fungal invasion of an old upper lobe cavity). These specimens can be examined for fungal elements with wet mounts after partial clearance of the tissue with 10–20% potassium hydroxide. This allows visualisation of yeasts and the hyphae of filamentous fungi, but does not enable accurate discrimination to the level of genera or species. In addition, Calcofluor white stain can be added enabling fluorescence microscopy, which will enhance the detection of most fungi by binding to the fungal cell wall.

Among histopathological stains, Grocott methenamine silver (GMS), periodic acid-Schiff (PAS) and Gridley's fungus (GF) are particularly effective for visualising and discriminating between fungi. Among these three stains, GMS is more advantageous since it stains old and non-viable fungal elements more efficiently than either GF or PAS stains. Haematoxylin and eosin (H&E) stain enables visualisation of host response, but is not a particularly discriminatory fungal stain, not staining most of the fungi, with the exception of the *Aspergillus* spp. and the zygomycetes. Thus, a combination of GMS and H&E is usually employed to visualise both the tissue reaction and the infecting fungus.

Giemsa stain is used for the diagnosis of malaria and other parasites, but among the fungi, is only practically useful for *Histoplasma* spp. Gram stain is not useful for filamentous fungi, but can stain *Candida* spp. as Gram positive. Albert's stain can be used to identify the metachromatic granules in *Corynebacterium diphtheriae*.

Further Reading

Guarner J, Brandt ME. Histopathologic diagnosis of fungal infections in the 21st century. *Clin Microbiol Rev.* 2011;24:247–280.

Patterson TF, Thompson GR 3rd, Denning DW, Fishman JA, Hadley S, Herbrecht R, Kontoyiannis DP, Marr KA, Morrison VA, Nguyen MH, Segal BH, Steinbach WJ, Stevens DA, Walsh TJ, Wingard JR, Young JA, Bennett JE. Practice Guidelines for the Diagnosis and Management of Aspergillosis: 2016 Update by the Infectious Diseases Society of America. *Clin Infect Dis.* 2016;63(4):e1–e60.

A2.47   Answer C: Lactophenol cotton blue stain

While clearance with potassium hydroxide, with or without addition of calcofluor white stain, can be useful for identification of fungi from primary specimens, once a subculture of a fungi is available, alternative methods offer improved discriminatory power for speciation.

Lactophenol cotton blue, iodine glycerol and Congo red formaldehyde staining have all been used, but it is the former which is perhaps used most widely. The phenol inactivates the organisms and inactivates lytic cellular enzymes, meaning cells do not readily lyse. The cotton blue stain dyes the fungal wall chitin. Once stained, in conjunction with the colonial morphology, the appearance of mycelia and fruiting structures can be used to discriminate genera and in some instances species, although subsequent biochemical tests may be needed to confirm identification.

The Gram stain is not useful for discrimination of species from fungal cultures. Periodic acid-Schiff stain, while useful for identifying fungi from primary tissue samples, is not useful for fungal subcultures.

Further Reading

Patterson TF, Thompson GR 3rd, Denning DW, Fishman JA, Hadley S, Herbrecht R, Kontoyiannis DP, Marr KA, Morrison VA, Nguyen MH, Segal BH, Steinbach WJ, Stevens DA, Walsh TJ, Wingard JR, Young JA, Bennett JE. Practice Guidelines for the Diagnosis and Management of Aspergillosis: 2016 Update by the Infectious Diseases Society of America. *Clin Infect Dis.* 2016;63 (4):e1–e60.

A2.48   Answer E: *Ancylostoma duodenale*

Ancylostoma duodenale is very similar in morphology to *Necator americanus* (together both frequently called "hookworms"), with males usually 5–9 mm and females 10–13 mm long. These nematodes, along with the other soil transmitted nematodes, *Trichuris trichuria* (also known as "whipworm") and *A. lumbricoides* (also known as "roundworm") are considered soil-transmitted helminths, and together may infect in excess of 20% of the global population. Light hookworm infections are usually asymptomatic, but heavy hookworm burdens often cause abdominal bloating, altered bowel habit and on occasion malabsorption. Hookworm infestation can lead to anaemia, but usually only in conjunction with other factors, such as dietary insufficiency or menorrhagia. *S. stercoralis* (also known as "threadworm") and *E. vermicularis* (also known as "pinworm") are also nematodes, but do not usually contribute to anaemia.

The eggs of the two human hookworms – *A. duodenale* and *N. americanus* – are microscopically indistinguishable. In a wet preparation under light microscopy they are oval, measuring approximately 60–70 μm × 35–40 μm. *E. vermicularis* eggs are approximately 50–60 μm in length. *T. trichuria* eggs are approximately 50 × 20 μm. *A. lumbricoides* eggs are approximately 60 × 45 μm.

Further Reading

Moore LSP, Chiodini PL. Tropical helminths. *Medicine.* 2010;38(1):47–51.

A2.49   Answer A: Light microscopy

E. vermicularis ("pinworm") only infects humans, with most infestation being asymptomatic; however, where worm load is high, the predominating symptom is pruritis ani, particularly at night. In women, the presentation can on occasion be with vulvovaginitis. These symptoms are caused by the female nematode exiting the anus and laying eggs in the perianal folds, and on occasion the female genital tract. Onwards transmission is then through transmission of these eggs to the mouth, usually associated with the act of scratching.

Diagnosis can be made clinically by observing the female worm in the peri-anal region. However, more frequently the sellotape test is used, in which the sticky side of a strip of sellotape is pressed against the peri-anal skin first thing in the morning (prior to bathing), then examined under a microscope for pinworm eggs. Stool microscopy for ova, cysts and parasites can be used, but worm burden in a stool sample is much reduced. Vulval swabs can be smeared for microscopy where symptoms suggest infection there. *E. vermicularis* eggs are approximately 50–60 μm × 20–30 μm and are thick-walled. They are translucent and a developing embryo can often be seen within the egg.

Latex agglutination, serology, immunofluorescence and polymerase chain reaction are not currently useful in *E. vermicularis* clinical diagnosis.

Further Reading

L'Ollivier C, Piarroux R. Diagnosis of human nematode infections. *Expert Rev Anti Infect Ther.* 2013;11(12):1363–1376.

A2.50 Answer C: Thin blood film with Field's stain

In most laboratories in both the United Kingdom and in low- and middle-income countries, definitive diagnosis of malaria is still undertaken through microscopy of blood films; thick films to determine the presence or absence of malaria and thin films to allow speciation. Rapid diagnostic tests for malaria are available, with both polymerase chain reaction available in some settings, and lateral flow tests which detect specific antigens in blood, both enabling speciation of *Plasmodium* spp.

While either Giemsa or Field's stain may be used to examine thick malaria films for the presence or absence of *Plasmodium* spp., thin films (enabling speciation) should be stained with either Giemsa, Field's or Leishman stain. In the United Kingdom, the National Parasitology Reference Laboratory recommends Field's stain for examination of both thick and thin blood films. In particular, Field's stain of thin blood films enables rapid diagnosis of *P. falciparum*, however, Giemsa stain does enable precise identification of other non-falciparum *Plasmodium* spp. Field's stain is a version of a Romanowsky stain, incorporating two parts – Field's A: azure dye dissolved in phosphate buffer solution and Field's B: Eosin in a buffer solution.

Giemsa is a mixture of methylene blue and eosin and is specific for the phosphate groups of DNA, particularly where there are high amounts of adenine-thymine bonding. The UK National Parasitology Reference Laboratory recommends Giemsa use for staining blood for parasites other than malaria, including microfilariae (Giemsa stains *Wucheria bancrofti* and *Brugia* spp., but not *Loa loa* – for microfilariae of this latter organism Delafield's haematoxylin can be used), *Leishmania* spp. and *Trypanosoma* spp.

Further Reading

Bailey JW, Williams J, Bain BJ, Parker-Williams J, Chiodini PL; General Haematology Task Force of the British Committee for Standards in Haematology. Guideline: the laboratory diagnosis of malaria. General Haematology Task Force of the British Committee for Standards in Haematology. *Br J Haematol.* 2013;163(5):573–580.

Chapter 3

Health and Safety for Infectious Diseases, Microbiology and Virology

In a clinical setting, practising infectious diseases medicine must incorporate knowledge, skills and behaviour to prevent onward spread of communicable diseases to other patients and to members of staff. The mode of transmission of communicable diseases must be understood, and practitioners must be able to interrupt their onward transmission. This includes the use of personal protective equipment for clinical interactions; from the types of equipment available, to their indication and the legislation surrounding their use (including Health and Safety at work). This also includes the use of isolation facilities; the indications for side rooms, negative pressure ventilation rooms; and when and how to arrange transfer to high-consequence infectious diseases units.

In a laboratory setting, practising microbiology and virology must incorporate the knowledge, skills and behaviour to ensure the safety of all laboratory personnel. This includes scientific and medical laboratory staff involved with sample and isolate processing, but also mechanisms to decontaminate laboratory areas after isolate exposure, as well as methods for the safe disposal of clinical waste. Practitioners must be cognizant of the particular issues around category 3 and 4 pathogens, and be aware of the legislative requirements for handling of such pathogens in laboratory environments.

Questions

Q3.1 A biomedical scientist asks for advice on a clinical specimen. Which of the following must be handled in a safety cabinet at containment level 3 (CL3)?
A. Serum from an intravenous drug user
B. Toxoplasma serology
C. Sputum for mycobacterial culture
D. Blood from a hepatitis B positive patient
E. Blood cultures from a patient with fever with recent travel abroad

Q3.2 A 31-year-old male presents with a 3-month history of productive cough, night sweats and weight loss. A sputum sample is sent to the laboratory. Which of the following statements are true regarding processing this sample?
A. Ziehl–Neelsen stain components release toxic fumes
B. Auramine stain components release toxic fumes
C. The sputum should be prepared for staining in a Class III biosafety cabinet
D. The sputum should be prepared for staining in a Class I biosafety cabinet
E. The sputum should be prepared for staining in a Class II biosafety cabinet

Q3.3 A 33-year-old female is suspected of having brucellosis and a blood culture is sent to the laboratory. What are the mandatory requirements for a category 3 containment laboratory?
A. High-efficiency particulate air inlet
B. Laminated floor
C. Sealable for fumigation
D. Shower facilities
E. Air lock

Q3.4 A 34-year-old female presents unwell to occupational health and notes that she works in the microbiology and virology laboratory. What is the most commonly acquired workplace-associated infection among laboratory workers?
A. Human immunodeficiency virus
B. *Brucella* spp.
C. Methicillin-resistant *Staphylococcus aureus*
D. *Mycobacterium tuberculosis*
E. *Shigella* spp.

Q3.5 A 34-year-old female presents with acute pneumonitis after returning from Saudi Arabia. A nasopharyngeal aspirate is obtained for testing at the regional reference laboratory. To which standard must the packaging adhere to in order to safely courier this sample?
A. UN2814
B. UN2900
C. UN3291
D. UN3373
E. P650

Q3.6 Serum samples of a 38-year-old female with hepatitis B are sent for laboratory investigation. What are the minimum laboratory safety criteria for processing these samples?
A. Containment level 1
B. Containment level 2
C. Containment level 3
D. Class 3 safety cabinet
E. Class 2 safety cabinet

Q3.7 A blood sample from a 38-year-old female with known hepatitis B is spilled in the laboratory. What is the best method for disinfection of the blood spill?
A. Phenolic compounds
B. Alcohol
C. Glutaraldehyde
D. Hypochlorite
E. Peroxymonosulphate

Q3.8 The laboratory decontamination standard operating procedure is being revised. What is an acceptable use of formaldehyde in terms of health and safety regulations?
A. Bench top decontamination
B. Cleaning of the floor in the laboratory washing facilities
C. Fumigation following spillage of a positive tuberculosis culture in a containment level 3 laboratory
D. Cleaning of class 3 safety cabinets after fungal manipulation
E. Cleaning of class 2 safety cabinets after fungal manipulation

Answers

A3.1 Answer C: Sputum for mycobacterial culture
Biological agents are assigned to specific hazard groups according to their level of risk of infection to humans. *Mycobacterium tuberculosis* is classed within hazard group 3 indicating that it can cause severe human disease and may be a serious hazard to employees; it may also spread in the community but there is effective treatment. Hazard group 3 organisms should be processed within a CL3 laboratory. The Advisory Committee on Dangerous Pathogens produces an Approved List of biological agents at the request of the Health and Safety Executive.

Further Reading

Advisory Committee on Dangerous Pathogens. The Approved List of biological agents. Crown copyright; 2013. Available at: www.hse.gov.uk/pubns/misc208.pdf

A3.2 Answer E: The sputum should be prepared for staining in a Class II biosafety cabinet
Mycobacterium spp. are acid-fast organisms, whose lipid-rich cell walls resist staining by other methods, such as the Gram stain. Other stains are needed, therefore, to identify *Mycobacterium* spp. from clinical samples, and the most common for these are auramine, Ziehl–Neelsen and the modified Kinyoun cold (MKC) stain. The Ziehl–Neelsen has a poorer sensitivity than the auramine stain but is more specific. It uses carbol fuchsin (which stains acid-fast bacilli red), then acid-alcohol and finally methylene blue counterstain. While *Mycobacterium tuberculosis* is acid fast, and so will stain red, a red bacilli can be any *Mycobacterium* spp. and is not specific for *M. tuberculosis*. Some non-mycobacterial organisms also stain with Ziehl–Neelsen, including *Cryptosporidium* spp., *Isopoda* spp. and *Nocardia* spp.

Sputum and other potentially infective specimens should be prepared in an appropriately safe environment. A Class I biological safety cabinet offers protection for the user but no protection for the specimen (i.e. from contamination). A Class II cabinet protects the user, the environment and the specimen. It controls airborne contamination and reduces the risks of user exposure to dispersed airborne infective particles. A Class III cabinet provides total enclosure of the working area, and manipulation of the specimen is via gloves mechanically attached to the cabinet (these cabinets are for use for category 4 pathogens).

Further Reading

Caulfield AJ, Wengenack NL. Diagnosis of active tuberculosis disease: from microscopy to molecular techniques. *J Clin Tuberc Other Mycobact Dis.* 2016;4:33–43.

A3.3 Answer C: Sealable for fumigation

In the United Kingdom, the Advisory Committee on Dangerous Pathogens (ACDP) classifies and advises on organisms likely to be encountered in healthcare or scientific research. The ACDP categorises pathogens into hazard groups according to the likelihood of causing disease, the likelihood of the disease spreading to the community and the availability of any prophylaxis or treatment. The ACDP categorisation has implications for the Control of Substances Hazardous to Health (COSHH, 2002) legislation in the United Kingdom, but for the rest of Europe this is regulated by the European Directive 2000/54/EC. Hazard group 1 organisms are not considered to pose a risk to human health, group 2 may be hazardous, but are unlikely to spread and there is effective prophylaxis/treatment, group 3 may cause severe harm and may spread to the community, but there is effective treatment, while group 4 may cause severe harm, may spread and there is usually no effective therapy.

For a category 3 containment laboratory (i.e. one able to process infective pathogens such as *Brucella* spp. in this case), a continuous internal air flow must be maintained by extracting the laboratory air and the exhaust air from microbiological safety cabinets through independent ducting to the outside air through a high-efficiency particulate air (HEPA) filter. The ventilation system must incorporate a means of preventing reverse air flows, but inlet air does not have to be HEPA filtered. A category 3 containment laboratory must be maintained at a negative pressure to connecting areas. The laboratory must be sealable so as to permit fumigation, but must have some means (usually internal wall windows) of viewing the occupants. The laboratory must be equipped with a Class I, II or III safety cabinet, and all sample manipulations with live pathogens must be carried out within the cabinet. Specified pathogens should be stored within the category 3 containment laboratory, if needing to be stored at all, and this must be undertaken in suitable containers in a cabinet reserved for the specified pathogens. Entry and egress from the category 3 containment laboratory must be restricted. The laboratory must not allow entry or exit of insects or animals.

Further Reading

Advisory Committee on Dangerous Pathogens. The Approved List of biological agents. Crown copyright; 2013. Available at: www.hse.gov.uk/pubns/misc208.pdf

Health and Safety Executive. The management, design and operation of microbiological containment laboratories. Crown copyright; 2001. Available at: www.hse.gov.uk/pUbns/priced/microbiologyiac.pdf

A3.4 Answer B: *Brucella* spp.

Bacterial infections account for the largest proportion of workplace-associated infection among laboratory workers. While enteric disease is the most common presentation among laboratory workers, the additional risk/contribution from the workplace from this is unclear.

However, the incidence of brucellosis among laboratory workers has been suggested to convey an 8,000 relative risk over the risk in the general population in an American study. *Neisseria meningitidis* has also been found to have a higher incidence among laboratory workers than the general population, as has *M. tuberculosis*, but to a lesser degree than brucellosis.

For viral infections, near-universal hepatitis B vaccination has almost obviated laboratory acquisition of this disease. For areas where this vaccination is not mandated, however, hepatitis B is the most commonly acquired healthcare-associated viral infection. After hepatitis B, human immunodeficiency virus and hepatitis C cause the next most common workplace-associated viral infections.

Among the fungal infections, diamorphic fungi are responsible for the majority of workplace-associated infections, but outside endemic regions, this is particularly rare. Similarly rare are workplace-associated laboratory infections with parasites. Among the parasitic diseases, most workplace-associated infections have been documented from research rather than healthcare institutes. The most frequently reported have been *Toxoplasma gondii* and *Plasmodium* spp.

Further Reading

Weinstein RA, Singh K. Laboratory-acquired infections. *Clin Infect Dis.* 2009;49(1):142–147.

A3.5 **Answer D: UN3373**
Ensuring the safety of those who transport clinical specimens or infectious isolates, and the safety of any members of the public who may accidentally encounter the specimen en route, is essential. The Health and Safety Executive in the United Kingdom recognises the international Dangerous Goods Regulations classifications for shipment of potentially dangerous infectious agents. Specifically, there are four UN numbers which relate to the criteria for transporting various types of infectious substances.

UN2814: refers to infectious substances that can affect humans and is particularly used where there is a pure isolate of many of the most dangerous bacteria and viruses. Examples include *Brucella* spp., *Mycobacterium tuberculosis* and viral haemorrhagic fever. This category of transport is also used where there is not yet a confirmed pathogen, but where there is a strong likelihood of there being one of these pathogens.

UN2900: refers to infectious substances that can affect animals (otherwise similar to UN2814).

UN3291: is used to transport clinical waste such as Regulated Medical Waste and Bio Medical Waste.

UN3373: refers to diagnostic specimens where exposure to the specimen in its current form (i.e. whole blood, serum, or in this case nasopharyngeal aspirate) will not cause permanent disability or life-threatening disease in otherwise healthy animals and humans. P650 is the packing instructions for samples, which meet the criteria for transport in a UN3373-approved manner. This is the most common carriage regulations used by clinical microbiology and virology laboratories (Figure 3.1).

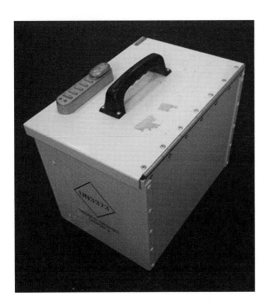

Figure 3.1 UN3373-approved container for transport of diagnostic specimens.

Further Reading

Health and Safety Executive. Infectious substances, clinical waste and diagnostic specimens. Available at: www.hse.gov.uk/biosafety/blood-borne-viruses/transportation-of-infectious-substances.htm

A3.6 Answer B: Containment level 2

Laboratory-acquired cases of blood-borne infections (human immunodeficiency virus, hepatitis B and hepatitis C) still occur intermittently. Clinical laboratories in most healthcare settings are, therefore, strictly regulated, and in the United Kingdom these regulations are directed by the Health and Safety Executive. Clinical laboratory diagnostic procedures with specimens that are known or suspected to contain blood-borne viruses may be carried out in an environment which meets the criteria for being containment level 2. Standard operating procedures should be in place to control the risk of sharps injuries and splashes to skin and mucous membranes. Laboratory works which seek to directly manipulate or increase the concentration of viable blood-borne viruses must be carried out in a laboratory which meets the criteria for containment level.

Further Reading

Health and Safety Executive. The management, design and operation of microbiological containment laboratories. Crown copyright; 2001. Available at: www.hse.gov.uk/pubns/priced/microbiologyiac.pdf

A3.7 Answer E: Peroxymonosulphate

A significant number of cases of nosocomial hepatitis B transmission have been reported worldwide. Although in many settings vaccination against hepatitis B is mandatory for healthcare workers, mechanisms to safely disinfect body fluid spills, preventing onward transmission of virus particles, is needed. Hepatitis B virus is readily inactivated by a variety of germicides, including quaternary ammonium compounds and formaldehyde. Two percent glutaraldehyde solution is also viricidal for hepatitis B, but a contact time of 15 minutes is needed, and its toxicity to humans makes its use undesirable. However, for chlorine bleach products, although there is laboratory evidence suggesting adequate viricidal effect against blood-borne pathogens, many are not registered by regulatory bodies for use as laboratory surface disinfectants. Peroxymonosulphate (e.g. Virkon®) has potent microbicidal activity, including having viricidal activity on hepatitis B virus.

Table 7 Common laboratory disinfectants and their antimicrobial activity.

Disinfectant	Bacteria	Bacterial spores	Myco-bacteria	Enveloped viruses	Non-enveloped viruses	Fungi	Prions
Hypochlorite	Activity	Limited activity	Limited activity	Activity	Activity	Activity	Activity
Alcohols (e.g. 70% ethanol)	Activity	No activity	Activity	Activity	Limited activity	Limited activity	No activity
Formaldehyde/ glutaraldehyde	Activity	Activity	Activity	Activity	Activity	Activity	No activity
Phenolics	Activity	No activity	Activity	Activity	Limited activity	Activity	No activity
Peroxygen-based (e.g. Virkon®)	Activity	Activity	Activity	Activity	Activity	Activity	No activity

Further Reading

Health and Safety Executive. Biological agents: managing the risks in laboratories and healthcare premises; 2005. Available at: www.hse.gov.uk/biosafety/biologagents.pdf

Sauerbrei A. Is hepatitis B-viricidal validation of biocides possible with the use of surrogates? *World J Gastroenterol.* 2014;20(2):436–444.

A3.8   Answer C: Fumigation following spillage of a positive tuberculosis culture in a containment level 3 laboratory

Formaldehyde has historically been the preferred fumigation method for laboratory decontamination. However, considering the toxicity to human health, need for prolonged periods where the laboratory is sealed (preferably 12 hours overnight) and the resultant surface residues, it is far from an ideal solution. While one of the defining criteria for a containment level 3 laboratory is that it must be sealable to enable gaseous fumigation, formaldehyde is classified as a schedule 1 chemical according to the Control of Substances Hazardous to Health (COSHH) regulations. This means that it is deemed a carcinogen and exposure to this chemical by employees should be avoided as far as is reasonably practicable. It has been suggested that hydrogen peroxide vapour demonstrates efficacy against *Mycobacterium* spp. and may be a useful alternative to formaldehyde fumigation.

There are other options for bench top and safety cabinet decontamination (such as peroxymonosulphate, alcohols, hypochlorite or phenolic compounds) and for cleaning wash-room floors (such as detergent).

Further Reading

Health and Safety Executive. Control of substances hazardous to health. Crown copyright; 2002. Available at: www.hse.gov.uk/pUbns/priced/l5.pdf

Kaspari O, Lemmer K, Becker S, Lochau P, Howaldt S, Nattermann H, Grunow R. Decontamination of a BSL3 laboratory by hydrogen peroxide fumigation using three different surrogates for *Bacillus anthracis* spores. *J Appl Microbiol.* 2014 Oct;117(4):1095–1103.

Principles of Public Health in Relation to Infectious Diseases, Microbiology and Virology

Chapter 4

Beyond safety considerations for other patients and staff in the immediate vicinity, those practising in the field of infectious diseases, microbiology and virology must have proficient knowledge, skills and behaviour relating to the public health considerations of communicable disease control. Practitioners must be able to describe the public health issues relating to communicable diseases and to specific infections (incubation periods, transmission routes, vaccinations available, need for mandatory notification), as well as understand basic epidemiological methods and the functions of health protection and environmental health teams.

Questions

Q4.1 A family who moved from Somalia and have lived in London for the past 10 years are seen in the tuberculosis clinic. The mother has recently been diagnosed with pulmonary tuberculosis and is on quadruple anti-tuberculous therapy. The father has had a renal transplant 5 years previously. The 4-year-old son has no symptoms, but the 7-year-old daughter has complained of a cough for the past week. They also live with an aunt who had a gastrectomy for stomach cancer last year and is convalescing in the house. Which family member does not have an increased risk of developing active TB?

A. The father
B. The 4-year-old son
C. The 7-year-old daughter
D. The aunt
E. None of the above

Q4.2 The manager of a nursing home calls. There is an outbreak of an itchy, scaly rash among the residents. What is the most likely cause?

A. *Sarcoptes scabiei*
B. *Pediculus humanus*
C. *Staphylococcus aureus*
D. Group A *Streptococcus*
E. *Molluscum contagiosum*

Q4.3 Infection control guidelines are being developed for the healthcare provider for which you work. Which organism is most likely to be spread from person to person?

A. *Salmonella* spp.
B. *Coxiella burnetii*

    C. *Bordetella pertussis*
    D. *Giardia lamblia*
    E. *Cryptosporidium parvum*

Q4.4 Following a wedding party, there are reports of most guests vomiting 24 hours later, but all report no further vomiting or diarrhoea after a further 48 hours. What is the most likely cause?
    A. *Campylobacter* spp.
    B. Adenovirus
    C. Norovirus
    D. *Bacillus cereus*
    E. *Staphylococcus aureus*

Q4.5 A 32-year-old male who works in an abattoir presents with fever. Which organism is least likely to be the cause?
    A. *Brucella abortus*
    B. *Salmonella* Typhi
    C. *Streptococcus suis*
    D. *Coxiella burnetii*
    E. *Mycobacterium bovis*

Q4.6 An 18-year-old female presents with headache, neck stiffness and a peripheral rash (Figure 4.1).

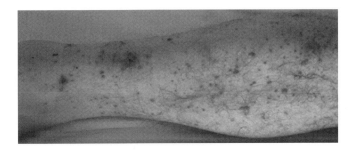

Figure 4.1 Clinical appearance of anterior lower left leg. (A black and white version of this figure will appear in some formats. For the colour version, please refer to the plate section.)

    Which member of the staff is most likely to be offered prophylaxis for this condition?
    A. Emergency department receptionist who registered the patient for 5 minutes
    B. Triage nurse who took history for 10 minutes
    C. Staff nurse who took observations five times, each for 5 minutes
    D. Medical doctor who took history and examined for 20 minutes
    E. Anaesthetist who intubated for 5 minutes

Q4.7 An 18-year-old female is diagnosed with meningococcal meningitis. Which community contacts are likely to need prophylaxis?
    A. Those who attended the same classes as the index case that day
    B. Those who ate lunch with the index case that day

C. Those who attended a party with the index case the evening before
D. Those who travelled on the bus next to the index case that day
E. Those who slept in the dormitory with the index case on a field trip last week

Q4.8 An 18-year-old female is diagnosed with meningococcal meningitis. What prophylaxis should be offered to close contacts?
A. Vaccination
B. Rifampicin
C. Ciprofloxacin
D. Erythromycin
E. Benzylpenicillin

Q4.9 A 30-year-old male presents with bloody diarrhoea, and a *Shigella* spp. is isolated and sent to the reference laboratory for sub-speciation. When should this be notified to public health practitioners?
A. On presentation
B. On discharge
C. On isolating the *Shigella* spp.
D. On receipt of the reference laboratory sub-speciation
E. This is not notifiable to public health

Q4.10 An outbreak of large volume watery diarrhoea, without discernible fever, occurs during winter in a daycare centre. The number of patients is growing every 24 hours. Which pathogen is most likely to be the cause?
A. Rotavirus
B. *Shigella* spp.
C. *Trichuris trichuria*
D. *Salmonella* Typhimurium
E. *Vibrio mimicus*

Q4.11 A 30-year-old male presents with suspected food-poisoning related bloody diarrhoea. What is the least appropriate action?
A. Submit stool specimens to the laboratory
B. Inform public health practitioners
C. Initiate oral rehydration therapy
D. Initiate empirical antimicrobial therapy
E. Encourage hand hygiene

Q4.12 A 30-year-old male presents with suspected food-poisoning related diarrhoea. Which cause of diarrhoea has the longest incubation period?
A. Enterotoxigenic *Escherichia coli* diarrhoea
B. *Salmonella* spp. enteritis
C. Giardiasis
D. *Shigella* spp. enteritis
E. *Bacillus cereus* emetic syndrome

Q4.13 A 30-year-old male presents with suspected food-poisoning related diarrhoea. Which enteric pathogens have a strictly human reservoir?
A. *Aeromonas hydrophila*
B. *Salmonella enteritidis*
C. *Salmonella* Typhi
D. *Shigella dysenteriae* serotype 1
E. *Vibrio cholerae*

Q4.14 A 9-year-old female is diagnosed with haemolytic-uraemic syndrome. Why may use of antibiotics in children with *Escherichia coli* 0157:H7 infection be contraindicated?
A. *E. coli* 0157:H7 is multi-resistant to conventional antimicrobials
B. Effective antimicrobials against *E. coli* 0157:H7 are nephrotoxic
C. Antimicrobials are not contraindicated and actually decrease illness severity
D. Antimicrobials may increase the risk of haemolytic-uraemic syndrome
E. *E. coli* 0157:H7 causes a prolonged diarrhoeal illness, especially in children

Q4.15 A 30-year-old male presents with suspected food-poisoning related bloody diarrhoea. In giving public health advice, *Shigella* spp. infection cannot be transmitted by which mode?
A. Sexual contact
B. Fomites
C. Food
D. Water
E. Inhalation

Answers

A4.1 Answer C: The 7-year-old daughter

Although the whole family are at risk as they have been living with the mother who has active pulmonary tuberculosis, there are specific groups who have an increased risk. According to current UK national recommendations, the following people are at risk of developing active TB:

- People with HIV, diabetes, chronic kidney disease, silicosis or haemodialysis
- Children younger than 5 years old
- People with excessive alcohol intake or injecting-drug users
- People who have haematological malignancy or are receiving chemotherapy
- People who have had a gastrectomy or jejuno-ileal bypass
- People who are having anti-tumour necrosis factor alpha or other biologic agents

Further Reading

Hoppe LE, Kettle R, Eisenhut M, Abubakar I. Tuberculosis – diagnosis, management, prevention, and control: summary of updated NICE guidance. *BMJ*. 2016;352:h6747.

A4.2 Answer A: *Sarcoptes scabiei*

Scabies is a contagious ectoparasite skin infection characterised by superficial burrows and intense pruritus caused by *S. scabiei*. It can be spread by skin-to-skin contact (although a relatively long contact is required) or through fomites including clothes and bedclothes. Diagnosis is usually clinical, although in indeterminate cases, skin scraping can be obtained for microscopy. Topical permethrin 5% is the medication of choice or alternatively malathion 0.5% is effective in killing both adults and eggs. Oral ivermectin has also been demonstrated to be effective and is particularly useful in crusted scabies. Pruritus can continue for up to 2 weeks after successful treatment for the initial scabies infestation. The appearance of new burrows, however, would suggest treatment failure.

In this case, public health advice should also be provided. This includes advice on the laundering of bedding, clothing and towels from patients with suspected infestation. These items should be laundered at high temperature and dried in a hot dryer. Alternatively, clothes should be sealed in a plastic bag for at least 72 hours. Where crusted scabies is being considered, patients should be isolated immediately and barrier nursing commenced. All household contacts (in this case one might argue all residents in the relevant areas of the nursing home) should be treated at the same time as the index case.

Further Reading

White LC, Lanza S, Middleton J, Hewitt K, Freire-Moran L, Edge C, Nicholls M, Rajan-Iyer J, Cassell JA. The management of scabies outbreaks in residential care facilities for the elderly in England: a review of current health protection guidelines. *Epidemiol Infect*. 2016;144 (15):3121–3130.

A4.3 Answer C: *Bordetella pertussis*

The R_0 of a disease relates to its infectivity. Specifically, in an unvaccinated/non-immune population, the R_0 relates to the average number of people who will catch the disease from an index case. The R_0 is dependent upon the infectious period, the contact rate and the mode of transmission. While the infectious period and mode of transmission cannot be readily modified, public health interventions should focus on the contact rate. This can be achieved through isolation of the index case or through personal protective equipment for those in close contact.

While the R_0 of diseases is debated, the highest among existing diseases are often considered to be measles (R_0 = 15–18), *Corynebacterium diphtheriae* (R_0 = 5–7), polio (R_0 = 5–7), rubella (R_0 = 5–7), mumps (R_0 = 4–7), HIV (R_0 = 2–5), *B. pertussis* (R_0 = 5–6), severe acute respiratory syndrome (R_0 = 2–5) and influenza (R_0 = 2–3). Where immunisation programmes exist, as in the United Kingdom, the R_0 of the vaccine-preventable diseases on this list falls dramatically.

B. pertussis is spread by contact with airborne discharges from the mucous membranes of those infected. Infected individuals are most contagious to others during the catarrhal stage. *C. burnetii* infection results from inhalation of contaminated particles in the air, and from contact with the milk, urine, faeces or other bodily secretions of infected animals. *Salmonella* spp., *G. lamblia* and *C. parvum* are spread through faeco-oral transmission.

Further Reading

Kretzschmar M, Teunis PFM, Pebody RG. Incidence and reproduction numbers of pertussis: estimates from serological and social contact data in five European countries. *Plos Med*. 2010;7(6): e1000291.

A4.4   Answer C: Norovirus

The nature of the food, incubation periods and symptom duration enables presumptive diagnoses of causative agents in food-borne enteritis outbreaks in many instances. This then facilitates appropriate environmental and food-stuff investigations, and prompts public health interventions.

Norovirus is characterised by diarrhoea and vomiting (often projectile) with sudden onset following an incubation period of 24–48 hours. The enteritis symptoms are generally short-lived (usually less than 48 hours). Rotavirus has an incubation period of 24–48 hours and produces watery diarrhoea lasting for 5–8 days, preceded by vomiting. Adenovirus serotypes 40 and 41 are an important cause of childhood viral gastroenteritis and have an incubation period of 8–10 days. *Campylobacter* spp. incubation period is 1–10 days (usually 2–5), and diarrhoeal and abdominal bloating symptoms usually last 2 days to 1 week. *Salmonella* spp. incubation is usually 12–48 hours, occasionally up to 4 days, and lasts up to 3 weeks with carrier states persisting for up to 12 weeks or longer. *B. cereus* usually causes symptoms in 1–5 hours and usually lasts no longer than 24 hours. *Escherichia coli* incubation is 10–18 hours and the duration of symptoms is variable but can last days to weeks. *Clostridium botulinum* has an incubation period of 2 hours to 5 days with symptoms lasting months. *Clostridium perfringens* causes symptoms in 8–18 hours and symptoms usually only last 24 hours with diarrhoea and cramps predominating. *S. aureus* food poisoning usually occurs 1–2 hours after ingestion and symptoms can resolve within 24 hours with vomiting predominating.

Further Reading

DuPont HL. Acute infectious diarrhoea in immunocompetent adults. *N Engl J Med.* 2014;370:1532–1540.

A4.5   Answer B: *Salmonella* Typhi

Those who work with animals, either alive or as part of the food industry, are at increased risk of acquiring zoonotic infections. Among abattoir or slaughterhouse workers, *B. abortus* (from cattle), *Brucella melitensis* (from goats), *S. suis* (from pigs), *C. burnetii* (from cattle, sheep or goats), *M. bovis* (from cattle), influenza (from chickens, other fowl and pigs), Nipah virus (from pigs and horses), *Campylobacter* spp. (from chickens) and others are the causative organisms.

Many *Salmonella* spp. are associated with animals, and there is an increased incidence among slaughterhouse workers. However, *S.* Typhi has no known reservoir outside of humans. For *Salmonella* Paratyphi, the main reservoir is humans, although some association with cattle has been reported.

Further Reading

Vayr F, Martin-Blondel G, Savall F, Soulat JM, Deffontaines G, Herin F. Occupational exposure to human *Mycobacterium bovis* infection: a systematic review. *PLoS Negl Trop Dis.* 2018;12(1):e0006208.

Helmy YA, El-Adawy H, Abdelwhab EM. A comprehensive review of common bacterial, parasitic and viral zoonoses at the human-animal interface in Egypt. *Pathogens.* 2017;6(3):pii:E33.

A4.6   Answer E: Anaesthetist who intubated for 5 minutes

This patient presents with what is likely to be meningococcal meningitis. *Neisseria meningitidis* is a Gram-negative cocci which is a commensal of the oropharynx in a proportion of individuals. Carriage is highest among teenagers and lowest in young children. Transmission occurs during kissing/transfer of saliva or through large particle droplet spread from the nose or mouth. Among healthcare workers caring for patients with meningococcal meningitis, this type of exposure will only occur to those who are working close to the face of the index case without wearing a mask. Procedures that are likely to cause this type of exposure include inserting an airway or intubating, suctioning oral secretions or if the patient coughs directly into the healthcare worker's face. Exposure of the eyes to respiratory droplets is not an indication for prophylaxis.

Further Reading

Public Health England. Guidance for public health management of meningococcal disease in the UK. 2018. Available at: https://assets.publishing.service.gov.uk/government/uploads/system/uploads/attachment_data/file/688835/Public_health_management_of_meningococcal_disease_guidelines.pdf

A4.7 Answer E: Those who slept in the dormitory with the index case on a field trip last week

A community close contact of a patient with *Neisseria meningitides* is defined as someone who has had prolonged close contact with the index case during the last 7 days of illness. This contact is described as being 'household', and includes those who live and sleep in the same house, students who stay in the same dormitory or use the same kitchen and girlfriends/boyfriends.

In the United Kingdom, it is suggested that some very specific contacts do not represent close contacts (and therefore do not warrant prophylaxis). These include students in the same class, work colleagues, friends including those seen at social engagements, residents of nursing homes, those who have shared kisses on the cheek (but not those who have kissed on the lips), those who have shared meals and those who co-located during travel (either in a car or on public transport).

Further Reading

Public Health England. Guidance for public health management of meningococcal disease in the UK. 2018. Available at: https://assets.publishing.service.gov.uk/government/uploads/system/uploads/attachment_data/file/688835/Public_health_management_of_meningococcal_disease_guidelines.pdf

A4.8 Answer C: Ciprofloxacin

Close contacts in the community and among healthcare staff, who have been deemed to warrant prophylaxis, should receive a single dose of ciprofloxacin. This is irrespective of the close contacts preceding vaccination status. For those in whom ciprofloxacin is contraindicated, rifampicin is a suitable alternative (twice daily for 2 days). In the United Kingdom, it has been deemed suitable, as a single dose, to also give ciprofloxacin to children for chemoprophylaxis. Particular care should be taken in evaluating the need for chemoprophylaxis in pregnant women, but where indicated, in the United Kingdom a single dose of ciprofloxacin has also been suggested as first line.

Chemoprophylaxis given to close contacts has been demonstrated to reduce secondary cases of invasive meningococcal disease by up to 84%, with a number-needed-to-treat of around 200. Chemoprophylaxis should ideally be given within 24 hours of diagnosis of the index case. For the index case, treatment with a third-generation cephalosporin is suitable for clearing carriage, and no further antimicrobial is warranted for this purpose. In benzylpenicillin therapy, however, although the antimicrobial suppresses growth in the oropharynx, it does not reliably clear carriage, and in these patients, other antimicrobials (such as ciprofloxacin) to clear carriage are indicated.

Further Reading

Public Health England. Guidance for public health management of meningococcal disease in the UK. 2018. Available at: https://assets.publishing.service.gov.uk/government/uploads/system/uploads/attachment_data/file/688835/Public_health_management_of_meningococcal_disease_guidelines.pdf

A4.9 Answer A: On presentation

Acute bloody diarrhoea may be inflammatory, ischaemic, drug-related or infective. It is most likely to arise from pathology in the colon. Infective acute bloody diarrhoea may be caused by *Shigella* spp., *Campylobacter* spp., *Salmonella* spp., *Entamoeba histolytica*, entero-invasive *Escherichia coli* or *Aeromonas* spp.

Taking a dietary history is essential, and where there is epidemiological evidence of a likely infective cause, cases of bloody diarrhoea should be immediately notified to public health practitioners by the identifying clinician. In the United Kingdom, the 2010 Health Protection Regulations stipulate that cases of acute infective bloody diarrhoea, food poisoning and haemolytic-uraemic syndrome should be notified immediately. Where causative organisms are subsequently isolated, the health protection practitioners should be updated, but first notification should not wait for laboratory results.

Further Reading

McNulty CAM, Lasseter G, Verlander NQ, Yoxall H, Moore P, O'Brien SJ, Evans M. Management of suspected infectious diarrhoea by English GPs: are they right? *Br J Gen Pract*. 2014;64 (618):24–30.

Department of Health. Health Protection Legislation (England) Guidance. 2010. Available at: http://webarchive.nationalarchives.gov.uk/20130107105354/http://www.dh.gov.uk/prod_consum_dh/groups/dh_digitalassets/@dh/@en/@ps/documents/digitalasset/dh_114589.pdf

A4.10 Answer A: Rotavirus

In contrast to acute bloody diarrhoea, large volume watery diarrhoea is more likely to be of small bowel origin. This may be due to malabsorption or infection. Among the latter, many of the viruses (norovirus, rotavirus, astrovirus, calicivirus) can be the causative agent, or among the bacteria, enterotoxigenic *Escherichia coli*, *Cholera* spp., *Vibrio* spp. may present with large volume. A similar presentation can occur with the parasites *Giardia lamblia* and *Cryptosporidium* spp.

Among the viral causes, rotavirus has a short incubation (of up to 2 days), and therefore rapid increases in patient numbers can occur in enclosed populations, such as residential homes or cruise ships. *Shigella* spp. and *Salmonella* spp. typically cause a lower intestine picture, often with small volume bloody diarrhoea. *Vibrio mimicus* can cause a small bowel, large volume diarrhoea, mimicking that of *V. cholerae*. However, cases are rare, particularly so in the United Kingdom and in day care settings. *T. trichuria* (or 'whipworm') is a typical cause of large volume diarrhoea, although it can cause outbreaks in long-term care facilities.

Further Reading

Lee RM, Lessler J, Lee RA, Rudolph KE, Reich NG, Perl TM, Cummings DA. Incubation periods of viral gastroenteritis: a systematic review. *BMC Infect Dis.* 2013;13:446.

A4.11   Answer D: Initiate empirical antimicrobial therapy

Acute infectious diarrhoea presents a risk to close contacts, and for those involved in the care of others or in the food industry, a risk to a much wider cohort of people. Advice about strict hand hygiene, abstaining from preparing food for others and notifying public health practitioners minimises the risk of onward transmission. Identifying the causative organism (be it viral, bacterial or parasitic) aids epidemiological analysis of the outbreak. This can help identify where in the food chain the organism was introduced, clarify the risk to others, and in some (the minority) of cases aid appropriate management of the individual themselves.

For the index case, fluid and electrolyte management is the mainstay of therapy. Antimicrobial therapy is not required in the majority of gastroenteritis cases and symptoms are usually self-limiting. Antimicrobials are usually reserved when there is fever associated with the diarrhoea, when the index case is immunocompromised, or when symptoms persist for more than a week.

Further Reading

Zollner-Schwetz I, Krause R. Therapy of acute gastroenteritis: role of antibiotics. *Clin Microbiol Infect.* 2015;21(8):744–749.

A4.12   Answer C: Giardiasis

Understanding the differential incubation periods of causes of infective enteritis enables more accurate epidemiological analysis. This in turn enables appropriate public health interventions to be put in place in community cases to understand and prevent outbreaks, and in healthcare environments to enable appropriate infection control interventions to limit further spread of the infectious diarrhoea.

Giardia lamblia incubation is the longest of those noted, typically 1–2 weeks. Amoebiasis (*Entamoeba histolyitica*) incubation is longer at 2–4 weeks. Salmonellosis usually has an incubation period of 6–72 hours, although prolonged incubation periods of up to 14 days have been reported. Shigellosis has a typical incubation period of 12 hours to 7 days, but usually presents within 24–72 hours of ingestion. Emetic syndrome associated with *B. cereus* has one of the shortest incubation periods at 30 minutes to 6 hours, while the diarrhoeal aspects of *B. cereus* infection typically present in 6–15 hours. Among the viral causes of enteritis (which are typically large volume rather than small volume and bloody), norovirus has an incubation period of 12–48 hours, while rotavirus has the same window, but typically is at the 2-day end of this spectrum. Astrovirus incubation may be slightly longer, with a median incubation period of 4.5 days.

Further Reading

Lee RM, Lessler J, Lee RA, Rudolph KE, Reich NG, Perl TM, Cummings DA. Incubation periods of viral gastroenteritis: a systematic review. *BMC Infect Dis.* 2013;13:446.

A4.13 Answer B: *Salmonella* Typhi

Similar to incubation periods, understanding the reservoirs of the pathogens causing enteritis enables appropriate epidemiological analysis leading to preventative measures and outbreak termination. *Salmonella* Typhi is adapted to humans and is not noted to occur in animals. *A. hydrophila* causes diseases associated with fish (and amphibians), including through dietary exposure, causing enteritis through an aerolysin cytotoxic enterotoxin. While humans are the predominant reservoir for *Shigella* spp., *S. dysenteriae* can cause disease in other primates. Non-serotype-O1 *Vibrio cholerae* has been isolated from many domesticated and wild animals. Among the *Salmonella* spp., only *S.* Typhi is noted to have a strict human reservoir, with all other sub-species having been noted in at least one other animal type, and often many.

Further Reading

Stratev D, Odeyemi OA. Antimicrobial resistance of *Aeromonas hydrophila* isolated from different food sources: a mini-review. *J Infect Public Health.* 2016;9(5):535–544.

A4.14 Answer D: Antimicrobials may increase the risk of haemolytic uraemic syndrome

Haemalytic uraemic syndrome (HUS) is a potentially fatal condition associated predominantly with *E. coli* O157:H7, although other non-O157:H7 serotypes of *E. coli* have been implicated, as have some isolates of *Shigella* spp. and even a *Campylobacter* spp. infection. Around 5–10% of those who are diagnosed with vero-cytotoxic *E. coli* (VTEC) infection develop HUS. While the diarrhoea symptoms are usually self-limiting, the haemolytic uraemic component of the disease may be life threatening.

Antimicrobial therapy has been shown to increase toxin production among *E. coli* 0157:H7, with ciprofloxacin inducing the largest increase, along with increases reported with co-trimoxazole, cephalosporins and tetracycline. While outbreaks have been associated with food-stuffs, it is farm workers and those who visit farms and petting zoos (such as school groups), which pose particularly difficult public health issues. Both the clinical syndrome of HUS and the isolation of *E. coli* O157 should be notified to public health practitioners.

Further Reading

Pennington TH. *E. coli* O157 outbreaks in the United Kingdom: past, present, and future. *Infect Drug Resist.* 2014;7:211–222.

A4.15 Answer E: Inhalation

Shigellosis typically present with bloody diarrhoea as opposed to the large volume diarrhoea often seen in small bowel enteritis. Four species of *Shigella* spp. are commonly described: *S. dysenteriae*, *S. flexneri*, *S. boydii* and *S. sonnei*. *S. flexneri* is the most frequently isolated species worldwide and accounts for 60% of cases in the developing world; *S. sonnei* causes 77% of cases in the developed world compared to only 15% in the developing world; and *S. dysenteriae* is usually the cause of dysentery epidemics, particularly in confined populations such as refugee camps.

Transmission of *Shigella* spp. is limited by its predilection for humans and primates, but only a very low infectious dose is needed (as low as 10 colony forming units have been cited). Transmission is through the faeco-oral route, typically person-to-person through poor hand hygiene or through contamination during sexual encounters. Contaminated water, food and fomites are all recognised sources of acquisition.

Further Reading

Kotloff KL, Riddle MS, Platts-Mills JA, Pavlinac P, Zaidi AKM. Shigellosis. *Lancet.* 2018;391(10122):801–812.

Chapter 5

Infection Prevention and Control

Limiting the spread of communicable diseases within a healthcare setting is integral to patient safety and clinical practice. Practitioners in infectious diseases, microbiology and virology often lead infection prevention and control teams, and are often responsible for creating and implementing policies and ensuring their effectiveness. They are also often responsible for investigating outbreaks when there are lapses in practice, or other causes for onwards transmission of infectious agents.

To this end, practitioners in infectious diseases, microbiology and virology must understand the principles of infection prevention and control in order to reduce the risk of acquiring infections in healthcare settings and to control their spread. They must be aware of the organisation of infection prevention and control teams, their reporting structures and their responsibilities within organisations and to public health. This includes the management and reporting of healthcare-associated infections (HCAIs) including of organisms of concern, resistance patterns of concern and of surgical site and device-related infections. Practitioners should have appropriate skills in epidemiological analysis of outbreaks and in running surveillance schemes to aid with infection prevention and control activities.

Questions

Q5.1 Use of alcohol-hand gel is being advocated to aid hand hygiene compliance. Which virus is not killed by alcohol hand gels?

 A. Coxsackie virus

 B. Influenza A virus

 C. Hepatitis C virus

 D. Respiratory syncytial virus

 E. Hepatitis B virus

Q5.2 A 50-year-old male from China underwent vascular graft insertion for a large intra-abdominal aneurysm. During his prolonged inpatient admission, he developed a vascular graft infection requiring drainage of a peri-graft collection. He required prolonged antibiotic courses for multiple hospital-acquired infections including carbapenems. He was colonised with carbapenemase-producing *Klebsiella pneumoniae* which was confirmed colistin resistant. Two further patients on the ward tested positive for the same organism on rectal swabs during active surveillance and an outbreak was declared. What is the most likely mechanism of colistin resistance in this organism?

A. Expression of chromosomal carbapenemase gene
B. Expression of plasmid containing *mcr*-1 gene
C. Porin loss with hyper-expression of AmpC cephalosporinase
D. Alteration of target site in Gram-negative outer membrane
E. Expression of *bla*-kpc gene

Q5.3 A 65-year-old female in critical care is found to have a glycopeptide-resistant *Enterococcus* spp. on a rectal screening swab. What is the greatest predisposing risk factor for glycopeptide-resistant *Enterococcus* spp. acquisition?

A. Repeated enemas
B. Metronidazole use
C. Persistent diarrhoea
D. Urinary catheterisation
E. Inflammatory bowel disease

Q5.4 A 65-year-old female in critical care is found to have a meticillin-resistant *Staphylococcus aureus* on a rectal screening swab. What is the greatest predisposing risk factor for meticillin-resistant *S. aureus* acquisition?

A. Volunteer in day care centre
B. Resident in elderly care home
C. Two pet dogs at home
D. Lives with extended family including two school-age children
E. Uncomplicated elective hip operation 12 months ago

Q5.5 A 65-year-old female in critical care develops diarrhoea. *Clostridioides difficile* tests are negative. What is the greatest predisposing risk factor for healthcare-associated diarrhoea?

A. Preceding use of probiotics
B. Preceding use of proton pump inhibitor
C. Preceding use of metformin
D. Preceding use of H2 antagonist
E. Preceding use of octreotide

Q5.6   A 65-year-old female in the care of an elderly ward develops diarrhoea.
She has dementia but no known ischaemic heart disease and does
not have atrial fibrillation. She undergoes a flexible sigmoidoscopy
(Figure 5.1).

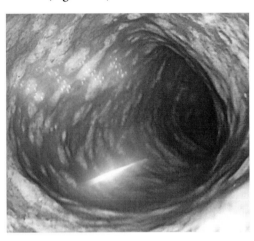

Figure 5.1 Endoscopic appearance of sigmoid
colon. (A black and white version of this figure will
appear in some formats. For the colour version,
please refer to the plate section.)

What is the greatest predisposing risk factor for this disease process?
A. Previous cephalosporin use
B. Previous co-amoxiclav use
C. Previous clindamycin use
D. Previous ciprofloxacin use
E. Previous proton pump use

Q5.7   A 65-year-old female in a care of the elderly ward develops diarrhoea and is
diagnosed with a second episode of *Clostridioides difficile* colitis. The first
episode, 2 months ago, was treated with oral metronidazole. What would be the
most suitable treatment?
A. 10 days of oral vancomycin
B. 10 days of oral vancomycin followed by a 6-week tapering dose
C. 10 days of fidaxomicin
D. 10 days of teicoplanin and rifamixin
E. Faecal microbiota transplant

Q5.8   A new sterile services protocol is being developed for operating theatre instru-
ments. How should sterilisation best be defined?
A. The process of destroying all microorganisms and their pathogenic
products
B. The reduction of the number of microorganisms to a level at which they are not
harmful
C. The removal of microbes that pose a threat to public health
D. The state of being free from biological contaminants
E. The disinfection of living tissues

Q5.9   The infection prevention and control team take a 1-day snap shot
       of all the infections in inpatient wards at any one time. What type
       of study is this?
       A. Case-finding study
       B. Case-control study
       C. Cohort study
       D. Prevalence study
       E. Controlled trial

Q5.10 There is an outbreak of diarrhoea and vomiting among some guests at a
       wedding. Clinical, epidemiological and dietary information is available about all
       guests. What is the most appropriate epidemiological investigation to investigate
       the cause?
       A. Case-control study
       B. Correlational study
       C. Cross-sectional study
       D. Randomised controlled trial
       E. Retrospective cohort study

Q5.11 Over a period of 3 weeks multiple wards identify patients with
       symptomatic *Clostridioides difficile* infection. A total of 24 patients are
       affected with clear epidemiological links suggesting nosocomial
       transmission. What is the best option to rapidly bring a *C. difficile* outbreak to
       a close?
       A. Change antimicrobial prescribing policy
       B. Encourage hand sanitation with alcohol gel
       C. Close the affected wards to admissions
       D. Screen all staff for carriage
       E. Move symptomatic patients to side rooms throughout the hospital

Q5.12 A 34-year-old female is being investigated as an inpatient for
       possible tuberculosis. What is the correct infection prevention and
       control advice?
       A. Patients with weeping scrofulous tuberculosis but who are not coughing and
          have a clear chest radiograph may be nursed in an open bay
       B. Patients with no risk factors for multi-drug-resistant tuberculosis and who are
          negative for HIV but are still sputum smear-positive after 2 weeks of treatment
          should continue to be isolated
       C. Patients with covered non-pulmonary tuberculosis can be nursed in open bays
       D. Patients with risk factors for multi-drug-resistant tuberculosis can be allowed
          out of negative pressure isolation and into a bay after 2 weeks of Directly
          Observed Therapy
       E. Patients with no risk factors for multi-drug-resistant tuberculosis who are only
          smear positive on a broncho-alveolar lavage need to be isolated in a negative
          pressure side room

Q5.13 A 34-year-old female is being investigated as an inpatient for possible tuberculosis. What is the correct advice on contact tracing?
  A. Contact tracing for a tuberculosis index case should stretch back 6 weeks from the first smear-positive sputum if the duration of symptoms is unknown
  B. Contact tracing for a tuberculosis index case should stretch back 3 months from the first smear-positive sputum if the duration of symptoms is unknown
  C. Contact tracing for a tuberculosis index case should be limited to an elispot and a chest radiograph
  D. Contact tracing for a tuberculosis index case should be limited to a tuberculin skin test and a chest radiograph
  E. Contact tracing for a tuberculosis index case should only result in significant contacts being given chemoprophylaxis if they are under 35 years of age

Q5.14 The clinical lead for anaesthetics asks for an infection control opinion on a potential new reusable anaesthetic airway device. Which disinfection might be most appropriate?
  A. 70% alcohol
  B. Gluteraldehyde
  C. Porous load autoclave
  D. 125 ppm hypochlorite
  E. Chlorhexidine

Q5.15 A 34-year-old male is diagnosed with food poisoning and a stool sample grows *Salmonella* Typhimurium. What advice should be given regarding return to work?
  A. After three negative stool cultures
  B. After six negative stool cultures
  C. Immediately as long as strict hand hygiene is observed
  D. Immediately after symptoms have resolved
  E. 48 hours after symptoms have resolved

Q5.16 A 34-year-old male is diagnosed with enteric fever and a stool sample grows *Salmonella* Typhi. He works as a nurse in a general medical ward. What advice should be given regarding return to work?
  A. After three negative stool cultures
  B. After six negative stool cultures
  C. Immediately as long as strict hand hygiene is observed
  D. Immediately after symptoms have resolved
  E. 48 hours after symptoms have resolved

Q5.17 The hospital staff food preparation policy is being revised. Which organism is allowed to grow up to 10^2 cfu/g in coleslaw?
  A. *Escherichia coli*
  B. *Campylobacter coli*
  C. *Listeria monocytogenes*

D. *Vibrio haemolyticum*

E. *Salmonella* Typhimurium

Q5.18 There is an outbreak of diarrhoea in a medical ward in your hospital. Sixteen out of thirty patients and five staff are affected. What action should be taken?

A. Close the hospital

B. Clean the ward and admit patients only into asymptomatic deep cleaned bays

C. Close the ward to admissions and restrict staff to that ward

D. Base decisions upon results of subsequent laboratory culture and PCR

E. Move symptomatic patients to side rooms where they are available on different wards

Q5.19 There is an outbreak of diarrhoea on a medical ward in your hospital. Sixteen out of thirty patients and five staff are affected. Norovirus is identified as the causative agent. What action should be taken?

A. Substitute general cleaning solutions with peroxygen compounds

B. Substitute general cleaning solutions with 100,000 ppm available chlorine

C. Use liquid soap and warm water as per WHO 5 moments

D. Use alcohol hand gel as per WHO 5 moments

E. Use gloves, aprons and masks for interactions with patients with diarrhoea

Q5.20 The operating theatres in your hospital are being reconditioned and a decision needs to be made about how many should have laminar flow air units fitted. Which patient group may benefit from having their procedures in theatres with laminar air flow?

A. Brain biopsy

B. Renal transplant

C. Total knee joint replacement

D. Coronary artery bypass graft surgery

E. Open reduction and internal fixation of hip fracture

Q5.21 The operating theatres in your hospital are being reconditioned and the air quality must be checked. How is this best achieved?

A. Air sampling

B. Environmental swabs

C. Air filter swabs

D. Quantification of air circulation per hour

E. Epidemiological survey of patient infection rates

Answers

A5.1 **Answer A: Coxsackie virus**

Viral envelopes are derived from the host cell membranes during the budding process. They predominantly include phospholipids and proteins but also some viral glycoproteins, which aid receptor site identification and binding. Functionally, the envelope is used to help viruses enter target cells by fusing with the host cell membrane. The viral envelope is

Table 8 Classification of viruses based upon nucleic acid composition and presence of envelope.

	Enveloped	Non-enveloped
DNA	Poxviridae Hepadnaviridae	Papovavirus Adenovirus Parvovirus
RNA	Coronaviridae Orthomyxoviridae Paramyxoviridae Flaviviridae Togaviridae Rhabdoviridae Bunyaviridae Filoviridae	Picornavirus Calicivirus Reovirus
Retroviruses	Retroviridae Hepadnaviridae	

relatively sensitive to detergents (including alcohol), heat and desiccation, meaning enveloped viruses typically have poor survivability outside of the host and are easier to control in healthcare environments than non-enveloped viruses.

Further Reading

Luangasanatip N, Hongsuwan M, Limmathurotsakul D, Lubell Y, Lee AS, Harbarth S, Day NP, Graves N, Cooper BS. Comparative efficacy of interventions to promote hand hygiene in hospital: systematic review and network meta-analysis. *BMJ*. 2015;351:h3728.

A5.2   Answer B: Expression of plasmid-containing *mcr*-1 gene

In 2016, a plasmid-carried gene conferring resistance to polymyxins including colistin was discovered in China. The gene called *mcr-1* has been found in both human and animal populations and is the first known plasmid-mediated resistance found in *Enterobacteriaceae*. This mechanism of resistance has now been found in five continents. Plasmids can spread rapidly between species, and therefore there are concerns about its ability to spread among populations and in healthcare settings. Some species, such as *Proteus* spp., are inherently resistant to colistin and do not pose the same infection control concern.

Further Reading

Liu YY, Wang Y, Walsh TR, Yi LX, Zhang R, Spencer J, Doi Y, Tian G, Dong B, Huang X, Yu LF, Gu D, Ren H, Chen X, Lv L, He D, Zhou H, Liang Z, Liu JH, Shen J. Emergence of plasmid-mediated colistin resistance mechanism MCR-1 in animals and human beings in China: a microbiological and molecular biological study. *Lancet Infect Dis*. 2016;16(2):161–168.

Marston HD, Dixon DM, Knisely JM. Antimicrobial resistance. *JAMA*. 2016;316(11):1193–1204.

A5.3   Answer B: Metronidazole use

Antimicrobial therapy with clindamycin, cephalosporins, aztreonam, quinolones, aminoglycosides or metronidazole are all at least equally associated with colonisation or infection with glycopeptide-resistant enterococci (GRE) than preceding glycopeptide prescription. Other risk factors for GRE acquisition have been identified, including prolonged hospitalisation, high severity of illness score, intra-abdominal surgery, renal insufficiency, enteral tube feedings and exposure to specific hospital units, healthcare professional groups or contaminated objects and surfaces within patient-care areas.

Inflammatory bowel disease, repeated use of enemas and persisting diarrhoea have not been associated with increased incidence of GRE. Similarly, neither has urethral catheterisation been associated with its acquisition when considered independent of the other noted risk factors (such as antimicrobial use).

Further Reading

Gouliouris T, Warne B, Cartwright EJP, Bedford L, Weerasuriya CK, Raven KE, Brown NM, Török ME, Limmathurotsakul D, Peacock SJ. Duration of exposure to multiple antibiotics is associated with increased risk of VRE bacteraemia: a nested case-control study. *J Antimicrob Chemother.* 2018;73(6):1692–1699.

A5.4 Answer B: Resident in elderly care home

S. aureus colonisation among the general public is considered to approximate 20–30%. However meticillin resistant *S. aureus* (MRSA) prevalence in the United Kingdom is much lower, at 1–2% of patients in the general population who live at home. Among those who reside in a long-term care facility, however, this climbs to up to 20%. Among healthcare professionals, levels of staff MRSA carriage are difficult to interpret from published studies and markedly varies between settings and between countries. There is also evidence of within-day variation in staff MRSA carriage among healthcare professionals, with staff becoming transiently colonised from patients during a shift, but without persisting carriage.

While there is an association between animals (both livestock and domesticated small animals) and MRSA (specifically mediated via the *mecC* gene), this is not as great a risk factor as that of being a resident in a long-term care facility. Similarly, day-case and short-stay operations are associated with a small increased risk of MRSA acquisition, as is any healthcare contact, but this is again likely to be much smaller than being in a residential home.

Further Reading

Hidron AI, Kourbatova EV, Halvosa JS, Terrell BJ, McDougal LK, Tenover FC, Blumberg HM, King MD. Risk factors for colonization with methicillin-resistant *Staphylococcus aureus* (MRSA) in patients admitted to an urban hospital: emergence of community-associated MRSA nasal carriage. *Clin Infect Dis.* 2005;41(2):159–166.

A5.5 Answer B: Preceding use of proton pump inhibitor

The causes of diarrhoea within healthcare facilities are significantly different from causes of community-associated diarrhoeal disease. Healthcare-associated (or nosocomial) diarrhoea is defined as new-onset increased frequency of passing stool of a looser consistency than normal, occurring in any inpatient that has been in hospital for more than 48 hours. The most likely cause is iatrogenic from medications, including antimicrobials, as well as chemotherapeutic agents, metformin, immunosuppressants, and in some circumstances, purposeful aperients. Non-infectious causes of healthcare-associated diarrhoea are thought to contribute to up to 70–90% of all cases, with infectious causes the remainder.

Among the infective causes, *C. difficile* may be one of the more frequent, but *Klebsiella oxytoca*, *C. perfringens* and *Staphylococcus aureus* have all been attributed as causes. Among non-infective causes, colchicine (80% of patients), chemotherapy (30–80%), immunosuppressants (30–60%), metformin (>20%), selective serotonin reuptake inhibitors (>20%) and octreotide (5–13%) are some of the more commonly associated. Proton pump inhibitors (and to a lesser degree H2 receptor antagonists) have been associated with an increased incidence of *C. difficile*, but as a primary cause of diarrhoea, it is more the magnesium-containing antacids for which this is a problem.

Further Reading

Elseviers MM, Van Camp Y, Nayaert S, Duré K, Annemans L, Tanghe A, Vermeersch S. Prevalence and management of antibiotic associated diarrhoea in general hospitals. *BMC Infect Dis.* 2015;15:129.

Polage CR, Solnick JV, Cohen SH. Nosocomial diarrhoea: evaluation and treatment of causes other than *Clostridium difficile*. *Clin Infect Dis.* 2012;55(7):982–989.

A5.6 Answer C: Previous clindamycin use

The flexible sigmoidoscope image is in keeping with a pan-colitis, and in the absence of ischaemic or other identifiable causes, *Clostridioides difficile* infection is likely. The risk of *C. difficile* infection is markedly increased by preceding antimicrobial use. Yet, not all antimicrobials contribute equally to this increased risk. A meta-analysis of the different effects of antimicrobials on the risk of *C. difficile* infection suggests clindamycin has the greatest impact (odds ratio 16.8 compared to no antimicrobials) compared to quinolones (OR 5.5), cephalosporins and carbapenems (OR 5.7), penicillins (OR 2.7) and sulphonamides and trimethoprim (OR 1.8). In comparison, a meta-analysis of proton pump inhibitors and the risk of developing *C. difficile* infection suggests the odds ratio was 1.29 in the community, rising to 1.43 in critical care settings.

Further Reading

Brown KA, Khanafer N, Daneman N, Fisman DN. Meta-analysis of antibiotics and the risk of community-associated *Clostridium difficile* infection. *Antimicrob Agents Chemother.* 2013;57 (5):2326–2332.

Cao F, Chen CX, Wang M, Liao HR, Wang MX, Hua SZ, Huang B, Xiong Y, Zhang JY, Xu YL. Updated meta-analysis of controlled observational studies: proton-pump inhibitors and risk of *Clostridium difficile* infection. *J Hosp Infect.* 2018;98(1):4–13.

A5.7 Answer A: 10 days of oral vancomycin

Treatment of a first episode of *C. difficile* infection is dependent upon making an assessment of severity. In the United Kingdom, this involves assessing for the presence of any of the following: severe colitis (either clinically or from radiological investigations), temperature above 38.5°C, white cell count above 15×10^9/L or an acutely rising creatinine (i.e. greater than 50% increase above baseline). The 2017 guidelines from the United States differ from those from the United Kingdom published in 2013, in that the new guidelines do not now include metronidazole as a first line regime, even for non-severe disease, instead suggesting vancomycin or fidaxomicin orally. These two agents are also advocated for severe disease.

The 2017 US guidelines suggest that for a first recurrence, where metronidazole was used for the first episode, a 10-day course of vancomycin should be used. Where vancomycin was used for the first episode, a tapering course of vancomycin should be administered after the initial vancomycin regime, or fidaxomicin should be used. For second or subsequent relapses, the greatest strength of recommendation in the 2017 guidelines is for faecal microbiota transplant. Where this is not feasible or practicable, vancomycin with a tapering dose, or vancomycin followed by rifamixin (for a further 20 days) or fidaxomicin are all possible.

Further Reading

Georghegan O, Eades C, Moore LSP, Gilchrist M. *Clostridium difficile*: diagnosis and treatment update. *Clin Pharm.* 2017;9(2):online.

McDonald LC, Gerding DN, Johnson S, Bakken JS, Carroll KC, Coffin SE, Dubberke ER, Garey KW, Gould CV, Kelly C, Loo V, Shaklee Sammons J, Sandora TJ, Wilcox MH. Clinical Practice Guidelines for *Clostridium difficile* Infection in Adults and Children: 2017 Update by the Infectious Diseases Society of America (IDSA) and Society for Healthcare Epidemiology of America (SHEA). *Clin Infect Dis.* 2018;66(7):987–994.

A5.8 Answer A: The process of destroying all microorganisms and their pathogenic products

Sterilisation refers to the process of destroying all biological agents and their pathogenic products including spores. Disinfection involves the reduction of the number of microorganisms to a level at which the infection hazard is removed so they are not harmful to humans. Sanitisation alludes to the removal of microbes that pose a threat to the public health. Asepsis relates to the disinfection of living tissues.

In healthcare, sterilisation is favourable wherever feasible, and can be achieved with autoclaves or steam. However, for many items in healthcare environments, sterilisation may be unnecessary, impractical or may damage the item in question. In these cases, disinfection may be suitable. While disinfection reduces microbial load to below infectious levels, it does not usually destroy bacterial spores.

Further Reading

Health and Safety Executive. Safe working and the prevention of infection in clinical laboratories and similar facilities; 2003. Available at: www.hse.gov.uk/pubns/clinical-laboratories.pdf

A5.9 Answer D: Prevalence study

Cross-sectional (prevalence) studies a "snapshot" of the frequency and characteristics of a disease in a population at a particular point in time. They do not allow investigation of association or causation, and in isolation do not allow inference of temporal changes. Serial (e.g. 6 monthly) cross-sectional studies may enable analysis of temporal trends, but controlling for confounding factors is difficult and frequently not done.

Case-finding is an active exploratory process to identify individuals with certain characteristics. In the context of infection prevention and control, this usually refers to patients at risk of, or with, a certain disease or constellation of symptoms. This type of investigation may be used, for example, in look back exercises after cases of *Mycobacterium tuberculosis* exposure, or when healthcare professionals are belatedly found to have blood-borne viruses.

Further Reading

Anglemyer A, Horvath HT, Bero L. Healthcare outcomes assessed with observational study designs compared with those assessed in randomized trials. *Cochrane Database Syst Rev.* 2014;(4): MR000034.

A5.10   **Answer A: Case-control study**
Unlike prevalence (or cross-sectional) studies, a case-control study is a study design that enables a degree of association to be inferred from the findings. Case-control studies are particularly useful where there is a rare outcome (e.g. guests with suspected food poisoning at this wedding as in this case). In contrast, cohort studies, while also enabling association to be inferred, are a useful study design for rare risk factors for a disease (e.g. in this case, if there was a strong suspicion of one food type being infectious, individuals who ate that food could be followed).

However, any association which may be derived from either a case-control or a cohort study does not necessarily indicate a causal link between a risk factor or intervention and any given outcome. Instead, for causation to be inferred, the most robust study design is often a controlled trial. In these study designs, confounding factors are often controlled by randomisation, and some biases are controlled by blinding participants and healthcare professionals.

Further Reading

Anglemyer A, Horvath HT, Bero L. Healthcare outcomes assessed with observational study designs compared with those assessed in randomized trials. *Cochrane Database Syst Rev.* 2014;(4): MR000034.

A5.11   **Answer C: Close the affected wards to admissions**
Ward closure is often then most effective method of rapidly bringing an infectious diseases outbreak under control. Other infection control measures such as policy change and change in behavioural practice take more time to have an impact, although these can bring sustained control and prevention of further outbreaks.

Antimicrobial usage often precedes *C. difficile* infection, with certain antimicrobials such as third-generation cephalosporins and fluoroquinolones particularly implicated, although any antimicrobial is a risk. As a control measure, there is evidence that national restriction of fluoroquinolones in English primary and secondary care settings coincided with reduction of *C. difficile* strains resistant to fluoroquinolones. Although this was at the same time as multiple infection prevention and control measures, this may suggest that restriction of particular high risk antimicrobials may be one of the most effective control measures for *C. difficile* infection.

Further Reading

Dingle KE, Didelot X, Quan TP et al. Modernising Medical Microbiology Informatics Group. Effects of control interventions on *Clostridium difficile* infection in England: an observational study. *Lancet Infect Dis.* 2017;17(4):411–421.

A5.12 Answer C: Patients with covered non-pulmonary tuberculosis can be nursed in open bays

Patients with non-pulmonary tuberculosis may be nursed in an open bay, but if the patient undergoes an aerosol-generating procedure (this includes airway manipulation such as induced sputum generation but also if tuberculous abscesses are going to be incised and irrigated, or if they are open and weeping), they should be placed in a single room. Patients with suspected pulmonary tuberculosis should be admitted to a single room until their sputum acid-fast bacilli stain result is available. In deciding on the nature of the single room (no pressure differential or negative pressure) and the duration of isolation, a risk assessment must be undertaken on the likelihood of multidrug-resistant (MDR) tuberculosis. The risk factors for MDR tuberculosis include close contact with a case of known MDR tuberculosis, co-infection with human immunodeficiency virus (HIV), previous failed course of therapy for tuberculosis, prolonged conversion to sputum smear-negative (considered to be 4 months in many settings) or culture-negative once therapy has started. Patients whose bronchial washings are smear-positive can be managed as non-infectious (i.e. isolation in a side room is not mandatory) unless their sputum is also smear-positive (or becomes so after the bronchoscopy), or the patients is suspected of having MDR tuberculosis or they are being nursed on a ward where there are immunocompromised patients. Unlike for bronchoscopy smear-positive patients, those who are smear-positive following induced sputum must be managed as infectious and nursed in a single room.

Patients with drug-susceptible tuberculosis usually become non-infectious after 2 weeks of drug therapy which includes rifampicin and isoniazid, even though smear positivity may persist for several weeks. Therefore, for these patients, de-isolation from a single room is generally considered acceptable after 2 weeks of therapy, as long as the ward area does not contain other immunocompromised patients.

Patients with suspected MDR tuberculosis should be admitted to a negative pressure ventilation single room, and if none are available, they must be transferred to a facility where such isolation can be enacted. Patients with suspected or proven MDR tuberculosis are often cared for in isolation until they become proven culture-negative, but may on occasion be de-isolated if several criteria are met, including having

- a minimum of 2 weeks of appropriate multiple drug therapy;
- three negative sputum microscopic smears on separate occasions over at least a 14-day period;
- tolerance and adherence to the drug-regime;
- complete resolution of cough or definite clinical improvement to treatment.

Further Reading

NICE Guideline NG33. Tuberculosis. 2016. Available at: www.nice.org.uk/guidance/ng33

A5.13 Answer B: Contact tracing for a tuberculosis index case should stretch back 3 months from the first smear-positive sputum if the duration of symptoms is unknown

Contact tracing should be undertaken for all cases of tuberculosis, but is likely to be particularly limited in the majority of non-pulmonary cases. For index patients with pulmonary tuberculosis, contact tracing should aim to identify or recommend review of close contacts for the period of time that the patient has had a cough or other respiratory symptoms. Close contacts should be considered as those who have had frequent, prolonged or intense contact with the index case. This might include those who share a house (including sharing a kitchen or bathroom), sexual partners and on occasion co-workers, although the geography of the workspace and the nature of the co-working should be examined.

Where the duration of the cough is unknown, contact tracing should extend for 3 months before the first positive sputum smear or culture. If the contact tracing during this 3-month period identifies higher than expected numbers of contacts with latent or active disease, contact tracing should be extended further by a month at a time.

Investigations of contacts identified through contact tracing should include inquiry into symptoms consistent with active tuberculosis, evidence of BCG vaccination, quantiferon testing and chest radiography. Close contacts under 65 years of age who do not have demonstrable latent tuberculosis should have consideration of BCG vaccine, while those who do have findings consistent with latent tuberculosis should have consideration for chemoprophylaxis. Those close contacts with symptoms consistent with active tuberculosis should be referred for rapid consideration of full tuberculosis treatment.

Further Reading

NICE Guideline NG33. Tuberculosis. 2016. Available at: www.nice.org.uk/guidance/ng33

A5.14   Answer C: Porous load autoclave

Anaesthetic airway devices, although usually not in contact with blood, still become grossly contaminated with secretions. They have been identified as contributing to cross-transmission of infecting pathogens when improperly sterilised between patients. The device used to secure the airway (laryngeal mask, endotracheal tube, etc.) should be for single patient use (i.e. disposable), or where this cannot be achieved they should be sterilised between patients (i.e. not just disinfected). Where this is done, manufacturers' recommendations should stipulate a maximum number of times the device can be sterilised.

Low-level disinfection (e.g. with hypochlorite, 70% alcohol or chlorhexidine) is microbicidal for most bacteria (with the exception of *Mycobacterial* spp. and bacterial spores), fungi and some viruses. High-level disinfection (e.g. with glutaraldehyde or peroxyacetic acid) offers additional activity against *Mycobacteria* spp. and a wider range of fungi and viruses (but still not bacterial spores). Only with processes that sterilise (such as an autoclave) can an item be deemed completely free from all microbes and be suitable for repeated patient airway manipulation.

Further Reading

Association of Anaesthetists of Great Britain and Ireland. Guidelines-infection control in anaesthesia. *Anaesthesia*. 2008;63:1027–1036.

Rutala WA, Weber DJ. Disinfection and sterilization: an overview. *Am J Infect Control*. 2013;41(S5): S2–S5.

A5.15   Answer E: 48 hours after symptoms have resolved

Public health measures around suspected and confirmed cases of infectious diarrhoea are necessarily strict. Food poisoning is statutorily notifiable, and should be notified on clinical suspicion. If this has not been done, isolation of a *Salmonella* spp. should prompt further discussion with public health practitioners. Where a patient is diagnosed with a non-typhoid *Salmonella* spp., they should self-exclude from work for 48 hours after their first normal stool. Laboratory confirmation of microbiological clearance is not required.

Further Reading

PHLS Advisory Committee on Gastrointestinal Infections. Preventing person-to-person spread following gastrointestinal infections: guidelines for public health physicians and environmental health officers. *Commun Dis Public Health*. 2004;7(4):362–384.

A5.16 Answer A: After three negative stool cultures

Where a diagnosis of enteric fever is made (*Salmonella* Typhi, *S.* Paratyphi A, B or C), patients must be excluded from work until microbiological clearance has been confirmed. Defining microbiological clearance required depends upon the individual patient and the nature of any employment they hold:

Group A: Individuals where there is doubt over personal hygiene or where there are suboptimal toileting or hand-washing facilities either at home or at school/work.

Group B: Children who attend nursery or pre-school.

Group C: Individuals employed in the preparation or serving of foods which won't subsequently be cooked.

Group D: Individuals employed in clinical or social care with direct contact with patients with an increased susceptibility or frailty.

Patients with enteric fever need to have demonstrated six (if in group C) or three (if in groups A, B or D) consecutive negative stool specimens. The stool samples should be taken 1 week apart, and cannot be collected until 3 weeks after completion of treatment. In the case of a contact of a case of enteric fever (whether symptomatic or an asymptomatic excreter) only two negative stool specimens are required and these can be taken 48 hours apart.

Further Reading

PHLS Advisory Committee on Gastrointestinal Infections. Preventing person-to-person spread following gastrointestinal infections: guidelines for public health physicians and environmental health officers. *Commun Dis Public Health*. 2004;7(4):362–384.

Public Health England. Interim – public health operational guidelines for typhoid and paratyphoid (enteric fever). Crown Copyright; 2017. Available at: https://assets.publishing.service.gov.uk/government/uploads/system/uploads/attachment_data/file/614875/Public_Health_Operational_Guidelines_for_Typhoid_and_Paratyphoid.pdf

A5.17 Answer C: *Listeria monocytogenes*

L. monocytogenes is a commonly occurring Gram-positive rod which is frequently identifiable from environmental sources including many raw foods. Because of this, *L. monocytogenes* can on occasion be isolated from food preparation areas and enter the food chain in cooked or processed foods. Despite refrigeration of these food products, because *L. monocytogenes* can grow at temperatures between 0°C and 45°C, a significant inoculum can develop where the bacterium is not killed by later cooking.

Food-borne *L. monocytogenes* is a particular problem among vulnerable groups (including the immunosuppressed, the elderly, pregnant women and many inpatients). Food noted to be at particular risk of harbouring *L. monocytogenes* include soft ripened cheese, sliced cooked meats and pâté and these should be avoided by those considered at risk. In inpatient settings, food for inpatients must be demonstrated to contain no *L. monocytogenes* in 25 g portions of the foodstuff. For non-vulnerable groups, which includes well and non-pregnant staff, regulations stipulate quantitative culture should demonstrate *L. monocytogenes* does not exceed 10^2 cfu/g within the shelf-life of the foodstuff.

Further Reading

Health Protection Agency. Guidelines for assessing the microbiological safety of ready-to-eat foods placed on the market. 2009. Available at: https://assets.publishing.service.gov.uk/government/uploads/system/uploads/attachment_data/file/363146/Guidelines_for_assessing_the_microbiological_safety_of_ready-to-eat_foods_on_the_market.pdf

A5.18   **Answer C: Close the ward to admissions and restrict staff to that ward**
Patient safety must be placed paramount in all healthcare decision making, and this applies equally to decisions about ward closures. Stopping admissions to a clinical area may prevent new admissions from becoming exposed to any outbreak organism, but if excessive, may inhibit the ability to appropriately care for those new admissions elsewhere. Risk assessment of these levels of decisions must be made based upon the number of patients affected, the locations of these patients, the number with ongoing symptoms/deemed contagious, the ability to segregate/subdivide the clinical area physically and with appropriate staffing and access to separate toilets, etc. the nature of the pathogen (where known, although frequently these decisions must be made prior to definitive laboratory diagnosis), and the wider context of the healthcare provider.

If there is one patient symptomatic in one open ward area, then they may be able to be isolated and that one bed blocked while the other exposed patients wait out the incubation period. In an open plan ward, or one with multiple symptomatic patients across multiple different bays, it is likely to be necessary to close the entire ward. Other environmental infection prevention and control precautions should be adhered to, including keeping side room doors closed, placing appropriate signage at the entrance to the ward and judicious use of terminal cleaning. Food should not be consumed on the ward. In terms of staff, all healthcare professionals working in or possibly visiting the affected area should be made aware of the outbreak, and understand the work exclusion policy and the need to absent themselves from work at the onset of first symptoms. Staff whos primary work is in the affected area should not work additional hours in other healthcare settings until the outbreak is over.

Further Reading

Norovirus Working Party. Guidelines for the management of norovirus outbreaks in acute and community health and social care settings. 2012. Available at: https://assets.publishing.service.gov.uk/government/uploads/system/uploads/attachment_data/file/322943/Guidance_for_managing_norovirus_outbreaks_in_healthcare_settings.pdf

A5.19   **Answer C: Use liquid soap and warm water as per WHO 5 moments**
Norovirus is a frequent cause of outbreaks of diarrhoea and vomiting in inpatient settings and long-term care facilities. Norovirus is a non-enveloped virus, and as such alcohol gels

and alcohol-based cleaning solutions are not effective at interrupting transmission. Instead, soap and water should be used to decontaminate hands at each of the World Health Organisation five-moments of hand hygiene. Stringent hand hygiene should apply to patients and relatives (considering that visitors should be minimised as much as possible) as well as staff. In addition to hand hygiene, appropriate personal protective equipment should be worn. This includes gloves and aprons for interactions with patients with diarrhoea, but masks are superfluous unless there is a risk of droplets or aerosols.

The environment should be decontaminated with detergent and disinfectant containing 1,000 ppm of available chlorine. Cleaning protocols should be increased in frequency and in areas cleaned, paying particular attention to toilets. Single-use equipment should be used wherever feasible, and all re-usable equipment must be disinfected immediately after use in line with manufacturers' guidelines and using 1,000 ppm chlorine where possible.

Further Reading

Norovirus Working Party. Guidelines for the management of norovirus outbreaks in acute and community health and social care settings. 2012. Available at: https://assets.publishing.service.gov.uk/government/uploads/system/uploads/attachment_data/file/322943/Guidance_for_managing_norovirus_outbreaks_in_healthcare_settings.pdf

A5.20 **Answer C: Total knee joint replacement**
Ultra-clean ventilated (UCV) theatres with high efficiency particulate air (HEPA) laminar flow were demonstrated in 1969 to reduce surgical site infections in prosthetic joint replacement surgery. Use of UCVs for joint replacement surgery has subsequently become widespread in many high-resource healthcare settings. The evidence for use of UCV outside of joint replacement surgery is limited, however, and the expense of the air handling systems means careful consideration should be given to whether they should be installed, or where already present, how many should be reconditioned.

The actual added value from these air handling systems in reducing surgical site infections, over and above optimising surgical practice, antimicrobial prophylaxis, theatre discipline including restricting movement of personnel and dressing protocols remains contentious, however. In 2017, a systematic review and meta-analysis which looked at 12 observational studies and suggested that there was no reduction in surgical site infections from laminar flow ventilation in operating theatres compared with conventional turbulent ventilation in total hip and knee joint replacement. This systematic review is still being debated, however, and in the United Kingdom UCV theatres are still in place in many healthcare providers.

Further Reading

Bischoff P, Kubilay NZ, Allegranzi B, Egger M, Gastmeier P. Effect of laminar airflow ventilation on surgical site infections: a systematic review and meta-analysis. *Lancet Infect Dis.* 2017;17 (5):553–561.

A5.21 **Answer A: Air sampling**
To monitor the microbiological content of the air, either active or passive methods may be used. Passive monitoring can be undertaken using standard (non-selective) agar as "settle-plates", which when exposed to air for a specified amount of time, can then be incubated and colony counts undertaken. While simple, settle plates can only identify microbes

which sediment out of the air flow, and may under-estimate microbial contamination of air. In contrast, active air sampling, using an impinger (which uses an air pump to accelerate air towards a liquid- or gel-capture system, which can then be cultured and colonies enumerated) or an impacter (which similarly accelerates air via a pump, but this time producing a laminar air flow over a solid agar). Both the Casella Slit Sampler and the Surface Air System are examples of impacter methods, but the latter is more portable and convenient.

Further Reading

Napoli C, Marcotrigiano V, Montagna MT. Air sampling procedures to evaluate microbial contamination: a comparison between active and passive methods in operating theatres. *BMC Public Health*. 2012;12:594.

Important Clinical Syndromes Presenting from the Community and within Healthcare Organisations

The cornerstone of practice for practitioners in infectious diseases, microbiology and virology is the ability to diagnose and manage important clinical syndromes where infection is in the differential diagnosis. Practitioners must hold a detailed knowledge (covering the epidemiology, clinical presentation, relevant investigations and management and prognosis) of both community-acquired and healthcare-associated infections. This knowledge must cover infections in all body compartments and those causing systemic infections (such as blood-borne viruses). This must incorporate patients presenting from the community, and infections which develop among those already undergoing healthcare treatment for other conditions. In this latter group, infections among surgical patients and those colonised and infected with multi-drug-resistant organisms must be able to be managed with confidence. Similarly, common clinical infection syndromes presenting among patients returning from travel abroad must be able to be recognised, investigated appropriately and treated promptly. Practitioners must also be able to manage infections among special populations, including itinerant populations, those who may misuse drugs or alcohol, those at the extremes of age or who are pregnant and immunocompromised individuals. Specific to immunocompromised individuals, this should encompass both those with primary and with secondary immunocompromise.

Practitioners must have the skills to be able to elicit appropriate clinical histories, including aspects of travel, dietary and sexual activity. They must be able to perform clinical examinations of all body systems and to characterise their findings, particularly with reference to dermatological findings. Practitioners must be able to select and interpret appropriate investigations and utilise these in the context of available national guidelines relevant to the area and setting of practice. They must be able to interpret and explain the results of investigations and subsequent management plans to patients and to fellow clinicians. With reference to less frequently encountered infections, particularly those in returned travellers, many primary and secondary care practitioners may have little or no experience of these conditions, and practitioners in infections must be able to work effectively and lead in these instances. Given the communicable nature of many of the conditions encountered in the fields of infectious diseases, microbiology and virology, practitioners must maintain a non-judgemental attitude towards patients no matter the mode of acquisition.

Questions

Q6.1 A 27-year-old male presents with a progressive subacute confusional state with some myoclonus. An electroencephalogram (EEG) demonstrated periodic high voltage discharges and magnetic resonance imaging (MRI) of the brain was suggestive of an encephalomyelitis. Cerebrospinal fluid was obtained and demonstrated:

CSF white cell count 1×10^6/L
CSF red cell count 1×10^6/L
CSF glucose 4.5 mmol/L
CSF protein 0.50 g/L
CSF IgG 40 mg/L
Plasma glucose 5.8 mmol/L

Which of the following viruses is the most likely cause?
A. Measles virus
B. Mumps virus
C. Enterovirus
D. Herpes simplex 1 virus
E. Rubella

Q6.2 A 53-year-old male from Jamaica presents with lower limb weakness. Human T-lymphotropic virus 1 (HTLV-1) serology is positive. Which condition may account for this?
A. Burkitt's lymphoma
B. Acute lymphobastic leukaemia
C. Spastic paraparesis
D. Multiple sclerosis
E. Hodgkin's lymphoma

Q6.3 A 29-year-old male presents with weight loss, night sweats, adenopathy and fatigue. His Epstein-Barr virus (EBV) serology is positive. Which malignancy is EBV most associated with?
A. Acute myeloid leukaemia
B. Hodgkin's lymphoma
C. Acute lymphoblastic leukaemia
D. Chronic lymphoblastic leukaemia
E. Non-Hodgkin's lymphoma

Q6.4 A 51-year-old male from Egypt presents with a fever and a vesicular rash that covers multiple dermatomes on his face, chest and abdomen (Figure 6.1). His observations include temperature 38.9°C, pulse 89 beats per minute, blood pressure 115/68 mmHg, respiratory rate 16 per minute, oxygen saturations 97% on room air. His rapid HIV test is negative.

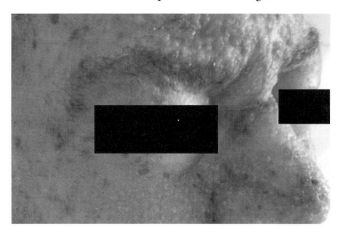

Figure 6.1 Clinical appearance of facial rash. (A black and white version of this figure will appear in some formats. For the colour version, please refer to the plate section.)

What is the next management priority for this patient?
A. Intravenous aciclovir
B. Oral aciclovir
C. High-flow oxygen
D. Positive pressure isolation
E. Varicella zoster immunoglobulin

Q6.5 During a ward round on the neonatal unit the team discuss a baby who had failed initial hearing test. During pregnancy the mother describes a flu-like illness with fever and fatigue but did not seek medical attention. She has a 3-year-old daughter who is not potty trained yet and wears nappies. On examination, the baby has evidence of hepatomegaly confirmed on ultrasonography. There are no other signs of central nervous system dysfunction and MRI brain is normal.
Investigations:
- Haemoglobin 165 g/L
- Platelet count – 110 × 10⁹/L
- Alanine transferase 70 U/L
- Bilirubin 20 mmol/L
- Saliva sample – cytomegalovirus PCR positive
- Maternal IgM and IgG positive for cytomegalovirus with low avidity

What would be your recommendation?
A. Referral to paediatric infectious diseases on discharge
B. Intravenous ganciclovir for 2 weeks
C. Oral valganciclovir for 6 weeks

D. Oral valganciclovir for 6 months
E. Cytomegalovirus immunoglobulin

Q6.6 An 80-year-old female was admitted through general medicine with a diagnosis of community-acquired pneumonia. She complained of 7 days of increased sputum production, 2 days of fever and pleuritic sounding chest pain. She has a background history of type 2 diabetes, chronic obstructive airways disease, gastric reflux, gout, hypertension and a previous stroke. She takes multiple different medications for her chronic illnesses which have been prescribed on her admission record. She has an unknown penicillin allergy and, therefore, commenced on a respiratory fluoroquinolone antibiotic. On a similar admission a year previously she developed symptomatic *Clostridioides difficile* infection which required prolonged treatment with vancomycin. The admitted physician was concerned about her risk of developing *C. difficile* infection and wants to know if there are any medications she is taking that might be stopped to reduce her risk. Which one of the following medications would you advice to withhold to reduce the risk of developing recurrent *C. difficile* infection?
A. Clopidogrel
B. Metformin
C. Lansoprazole
D. Allopurinol
E. Simvastatin

Q6.7 A 25-year-old male with cystic fibrosis (CF) presented with progressive worsening shortness of breath and reduced exercise tolerance. His spirometry had deteriorated and he was bringing up more phlegm than usual. Due to the severity of his respiratory condition he was admitted to the local CF unit and started on systemic intravenous antibiotic therapy. Severe respiratory failure in cystic fibrosis is commonly precipitated by infection with which organism?
A. *Pseudomonas aeruginosa*
B. *Staphylococcus aureus*
C. *Burkholderia cepacia*
D. *Haemophilus influenzae*
E. *Burkholderia pseudomallei*

Q6.8 A 30-year-old male presented to his GP with a lesion on his skin 15 days are walking in the New Forest with his family. He describes some flu-like symptoms and a rash that started off small, which he presumed was an insect bite. This had expanded to a larger single lesion on his calf. The GP thought the most likely diagnosis was Lyme's disease and prescribed oral doxycycline for 21 days. Which skin manifestations characterises Lyme's disease?
A. Erythema marginatum
B. Erythema chronicum migrans
C. Erythema nodosum
D. Erythema multiforme
E. Lesions on palms and soles

Q6.9 A 36-year-old male present with a non-painful erythema of his leg (Figure 6.2). Otherwise, he reported no other current focal symptoms. His observations are normal. The lesion was not hot and there was no proximal adenopathy. His blood results demonstrate:

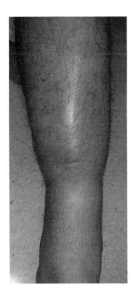

Figure 6.2 Clinical appearance of left lower leg.

CRP: 10.6 mg/L

ESR: 95 mm/1st hour

Which is the most likely organism associated with this?

A. *Staphylococcus aureus*

B. *Streptococcus pyogenes*

C. *Yersinia enterocolitica*

D. *Mycoplasma pneumoniae*

E. *Mycobacterium tuberculosis*

Q6.10 A 35-year-old female of Iranian origin presented with a 4-month history of fever, weight loss and night sweats. An annular blanching rash affected the upper torso and face. On examination, there was a single enlarged lymph node in the cervical region. Computed tomography showed a single necrotic lymph node which was excised showing features of a large infiltrate of histiocytes and necrosis. Her symptoms settled and she remains well. What is the most likely cause of the underlying illness?

A. Kikuchi's disease

B. Toxoplasmosis

C. Lymphoma

D. Tuberculosis

E. Sarcoidosis

Q6.11 A 30-year-old male presents with fever, weight loss and mild abdominal pain. He is a cameraman for a documentary channel and has an extensive travel history including Central America, North America, northern Africa and Central Asia. He has no past medical history. He denies illicit drug usage but consumes a moderate quantity of alcohol. He is not in a current relationship and is bisexual.

On examination, there is no remarkable features except pyrexia. His abdomen was soft, non-distended with normal bowel sounds. Chest X-ray showed no abnormalities. Computed tomography of the abdomen revealed bilateral adrenal masses, which were biopsied during the admission. Investigations included the following:

Interferon gamma release assay: negative

Adrenal node tissue:

Histopathology – granulomatous inflammation with histiocytes

Mycobacterial tuberculosis complex PCR: negative

Auramine and Ziehl–Neelsen staining: No acid-fast bacilli identified

What is the most likely underlying cause for this granulomatous disease?
A. Dirofilariasis
B. *Mycobacterium tuberculosis*
C. Histoplasmosis
D. Wegener's granulomatosis
E. Sarcoidosis

Q6.12 A 42-year-old female presented to her GP with a couple of subcutaneous lesions she noticed over the last few weeks and a lesion in her eye. She was concerned about skin cancer as her mother had a suspicious lump removed a few years ago. She was otherwise well with no significant past medical history. She takes no regular medication and has no known allergies. She described some childhood asthma, but this was not present in adulthood. She got married the previous year and went for honeymoon in Northern Italy. No other foreign travel in the past 5 years.

On examination, there were two subcutaneous nodules, one on the chest wall and the other on her right thigh. These were firm, non-tender with no overlying erythema. The lesion of the eye was periorbital with some erythema. Eye movements and visual acuity were normal. Full systems examination was unremarkable.

She was prescribed some oral antibiotics for a bacterial conjunctivitis with some chloramphenicol eye drops. She was referred to the local dermatologist who arranged for a biopsy of the subcutaneous lesion on the thigh.

Investigations revealed
- Haemoglobin: 119 g/L
- Platelet count: 427×10^9/L
- Total white cell count: 8.3×10^9/L
- Total neutrophil count: 6.8×10^9/L
- Total lymphocyte count: 0.4×10^9/L
- Total eosinophil count: 0.6×10^9/L

Thigh biopsy histopathology: granulomatous inflammation

What is the most likely diagnosis?
A. Sarcoidosis
B. Dirofilariasis
C. Loa Loa
D. Penicilliosis
E. Cutaneous tuberculosis

Q6.13 A 23-year-old male was bought into the emergency department with severe headache, nausea, vomiting and seizures. He had no previous medical history of significance. He was seen in the department with his regular female partner of 2 years. She denied that he took illicit substances and was a moderate drinker of alcohol. He was a good sportsman and played regular football and cricket. He had been on a stag party weekend 5 days previously where they had been white water rafting and canyoning. His partner denied any significant trauma. She described him complaining of a severe headache and then found him on the floor an hour later incontinent of urine and confused, believing he had had a seizure. On examination, he had a Glasgow Coma Scale of 13/15. There were some bruises on the arms with some healed small abrasions. There was no rash. Examination was difficult as he was confused and hallucinating. He was tachycardic in sinus rhythm.

Investigations revealed

- Haemoglobin: 139 g/L
- Platelet count: 120×10^9/L
- Total white cell count: 18.3×10^9/L
- Total neutrophil count: 16.8×10^9/L
- Creatinine: 230 U/L

CSF sample – macroscopically blood stained

- CSF white cell count: $2,330 \times 10^6$/L, red cell count $13,500 \times 10^6$/L
- CSF Gram stain: no organisms seen
- CSF culture: no growth following 2 days incubation

Computed tomography imaging showed an oedematous brain with mild hydrocephalus. The patient deteriorated over the next 2 days despite treatment with broad-spectrum antibiotics, antivirals and admission to the intensive care department. He was intubated and ventilated but despite maximal organ support he died 5 days following admission. On post-mortem examination, both macroscopically and microscopically, a purulent exudative inflammation was noted along the leptomeninges and extensive necrosis and haemorrhage of the temporal lobe parenchyma.

What is the most likely cause?
A. Primary amoebic meningoencephalitis
B. Granulomatous amoebic meningoencephalitis
C. Leptospirosis
D. Herpes simplex encephalitis
E. Autoimmune encephalitis

Q6.14 A 35-year-old female with a background of non-Hodgkin's lymphoma presents with fever, headache and photophobia which developed over the last few days. She is currently undergoing chemotherapy and is known to be neutropenic. On examination, she was febrile, tachycardic and photophobic. Kernigs' sign positive. She had a central venous catheter in situ which was non-tender with no signs of infection at the exit site.

Computed tomography of the head revealed no abnormality. An urgent lumbar puncture was performed showing:
- Opening pressure of 40 mmHg
- CSF white cell count 130×10^6/L
- CSF red cell count 16×10^6/L
- CSF protein 0.85 g/L
- CSF Gram-stain did not show any organisms
- CSF *Mycobacterium tuberculosis* complex PCR was negative

What is the most likely cause?
A. *Mycobacterium tuberculosis*
B. *Staphylococcus capitis*
C. *Cryptococcus neoformans*
D. *Candida auris*
E. *Nocardia species*

Q6.15 A 44-year-old male presents with painful, discharging lesions in his scrotal region. He has been suffering for months with pus discharging from multiple points of his perineum, associated with scrotal swelling, pain and difficulty walking. He has had multiple courses of oral antibiotics by his GP including flucloxacillin and clindamycin. He reports transient improvement with the antibiotics, but the condition keeps getting worse. Multiple swabs taken by the GP have either not grown any bacteria or grown *Staphylococcus aureus.*

On examination of the perineum there is scrotal swelling with erythema which is tender. There are discharging lesions in a tunnel-like formation with normal looking skin between the lesions. What is the most likely diagnosis?
A. Abscesses caused by Panton–Valentine leucocidin producing *S. aureus*
B. Cutaneous Crohn's disease
C. Hidradenitis suppurativa
D. Fournier's gangrene
E. Steatocystoma multiplex

Q6.16 A 60-year-old male presents with fever, lethargy and shortness of breath. He underwent mitral valve replacement 6 weeks previously due to severe mitral valve regurgitation. On examination, he was tachypnoeic, febrile with a pansystolic murmur and bibasal crepitations on auscultation.

He was commenced on intravenous antibiotic therapy with vancomycin, gentamicin and rifampicin. Echocardiography revealed moderate mitral regurgitation. Three sets of blood cultures grow Gram-positive bacilli 2 days into admission. What is the most likely organism?
A. *Corynebacterium jeikeium*
B. *Corynebacterium striatum*
C. *Staphylococcus epidermidis*

D. *Arcanobacterium haemolyticum*
E. *Corynebacterium pseudodiphtheriticum*

Q6.17 A 4-year-old female was admitted to hospital with a history of ear discharge, fever, seizures and subtle neurological symptoms. Her mother noticed that she thought a white cat was black in their backyard. Her nursery noted that the normally cheery girl was more withdrawn and playing with less enthusiasm. She has no pets and her parents work at Heathrow airport. Ophthalmological assessment noted features consistent with optic neuritis and papilloedema. She was treated with methylprednisolone, intravenous immunoglobulin, meropenem and clarithromycin.

Investigations revealed (prior to intravenous immunoglobulin administration):

Cerebrospinal fluid examination on day 2 of admission

– White cell count: 19×10^6/L
– Red cell count: 21×10^6/L
– Protein level: 1.4 g/L
– No organisms seen on Gram stain
– White cell differential predominance of mononuclear cells
– PCRs for herpes simplex virus, varicella zoster virus and enterovirus were negative

Borrelia burgdorferi IgG/IgM (C6 EIA) and IgM to Borrelia P41 antigen: positive
Bartonella henselae: positive with a titre 1,280 (<320 normal cut off)
Bartonella quintana: negative
Anti-streptolysin antibody titre (ASOT): positive 200–400 (<200 IU/mL normal cut off)

MRI head: brainstem changes consistent with encephalitis with enhancement around optic nerves suggesting pachymeningeal involvement.

What is the most likely diagnosis?
A. Neuroborreliosis (neuro-Lyme disease)
B. Bartonella neuroretinitis and encephalitis
C. Autoimmune encephalitis with cross-reacting antibodies
D. Paediatric autoimmune neuropsychiatric disorder associated with streptococcal infection (PANDAS)
E. Herpes simplex encephalitis

Q6.18 A 32-year-old man presented with a 24-hour history of necrosis and swelling over the left buttock and swollen genitalia. He had skin popped heroin to his left buttock 1 week prior; he also reported shivers, fever and malaise. He was given broad-spectrum antibiotics and was taken immediately to theatre for extensive debridement (image) with a suspected severe soft tissue infection. He required ventilatory and renal support. Blood cultures and tissue taken from debridement showed Gram-positive bacilli (Figure 6.3a and 6.3b).

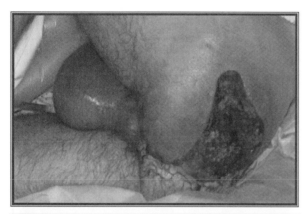

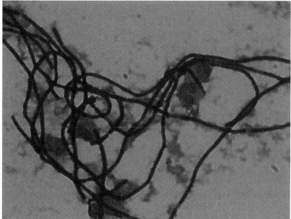

Figure 6.3 (a) Clinical appearance of perineum. (b) Gram stain of a positive blood culture.

What is the most likely diagnosis?
A. Anthrax
B. Fournier's gangrene
C. Gas gangrene
D. Type 1 (polymicrobial) necrotising fasciitis
E. *Clostridium sordellii*

Q6.19 A 29-year-old pregnant woman presents with fever and jaundice. Her viral serology is awaited. Her blood results demonstrate:

ALT 9856 U/L

ALP 246 U/L

Albumin 26 g/L

CRP 58 mg/L

Which viral cause of hepatitis has the worst prognosis for the mother?
A. Cytomegalovirus
B. Epstein-Barr virus
C. Hepatitis A virus
D. Hepatitis E virus
E. Rubella virus

Q6.20 A 3-year-old child presents with fever, stridor and a barking cough. Croup is diagnosed. What is the most common cause of laryngotracheobronchitis?
A. Respiratory syncytial virus
B. Influenza A virus
C. Parainfluenza virus 1
D. Coronavirus
E. Rhinovirus

Q6.21 A 32-year-old male presents with fever, myalgia, and severe left-sided pleuritic chest pain. ECG, echocardiogram, high-resolution CT scan of the chest and troponin T are all normal. A diagnosis of Bornholm's disease is made. What is the aetiology of this disease?
A. Adenovirus
B. Echovirus
C. Coxsackie virus A
D. Coxsackie virus B
E. Poliovirus

Q6.22 A 32-year-old female presents with a fever and cervical adenopathy. Examination confirms a temperature of 38.8°C and multiple small cervical lymph nodes are palpable. Her blood tests demonstrate:

Monospot positive

Cytomegalovirus IgM positive

Cytomegalovirus IgG negative

Epstein-Barr virus IgM negative

Epstein-Barr virus IgG positive

Urine βHCG positive

What advice should be given to her regarding her pregnancy?
A. CMV infection during pregnancy is not teratogenic
B. 40% of foetuses will demonstrate sensorineural deafness
C. 40% of foetuses will demonstrate congenital cataracts
D. 10% of foetuses are at risk of hydrops foetalis
E. 40% of foetuses become infected with cytomegalovirus

Q6.23 A 37 year of male goes surfing and suffers a laceration to his lower limb. Shortly afterwards he develops a wound infection and systemic sepsis (Figure 6.4). A Gram-negative bacillus is isolated from wound swab.

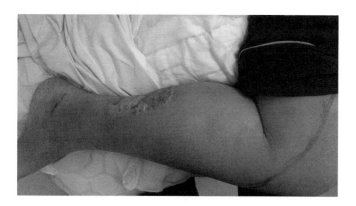

Figure 6.4 Clinical appearance of left lower leg. (A black and white version of this figure will appear in some formats. For the colour version, please refer to the plate section.)

Which of the following organisms is most likely the cause?
A. *Spirillum minus*
B. *Vibrio vulnificus*
C. *Mycobacteria marinum*
D. *Vibrio parahaemolyticum*
E. *Erysipelothrix rhusiopathiae*

Q6.24 A 7-year-old female presents with enlarged axillary lymph nodes having recently been given kittens as gift. Which of the following organisms is most likely the cause?
A. *Bartonella henselae*
B. *Bartonella quintana*
C. *Bartonella bacilliforrnis*
D. *Streptobacillus moniliformis*
E. *Bartonella rochalimae*

Q6.25 A 45-year-old male presents with a dog bite. He washed the wound on his hand and presented to the emergency department 5 days after the incident. On arrival, he was in septic shock complaining of abdominal pain and headache. He had a petechial rash on his extremities and mucous membranes. On examination, an old scar over the left flank was noted. Investigations showed:
WCC: 17.8×10^9/L
CRP: 265 mg/L
Lactate: 4.8 mmol/L
Hb: 112 g/L
Plts: 106×10^9/L

After 2 days a blood culture grew Gram-negative bacilli (Figure 6.5).
After 24 hours of aerobic incubation no growth had occurred on blood or chocolate agar.

Figure 6.5 Gram stain from a positive blood culture. (A black and white version of this figure will appear in some formats. For the colour version, please refer to the plate section.)

Which of the following organisms is most likely the cause?
A. *Capnocytophagia canimorsus*
B. *Pasteurella multocida*
C. *Fusobacterium necrophorum*
D. *Bacteroides fragilis*
E. *Streptococcus pyogenes*

Q6.26 A 20-year-old male presents with itching which is worse at night. He has recently returned from a beach holiday in Thailand. He swam in the sea and rivers.
He reports protected sexual intercourse with two female fellow travellers. He is HIV negative with no significant past medical history. On examination, he has erythematous papules on the hands, wrists, umbilicus and genital area. There were some short wavy greyish elevations of approximately 5 mm. What would be your initial treatment recommendation?
A. Ivermectin orally
B. Albendazole orally
C. Intramuscular benzathine penicillin
D. Permethrin 5% cream
E. Benzyl benzoate 25% emulsion

Q6.27 A 33-year-old mother presents with her 7-day-old baby who has bilateral conjunctivitis. A swab taken from the everted eyelid tested positive for *Chlamydia trachomatis* via nucleic acid amplification test (NAAT). The baby is otherwise well. What would be your recommended treatment?

A. Ofloxacin eye drops
B. Azithromycin orally
C. Erythromycin orally
D. Intramuscular ceftriaxone
E. Doxycycline orally

Q6.28 A 33-year-old female attends the local genito-urinary medicine (GUM) clinic complaining of vaginal discharge. She has been in a heterosexual relationship for 6 months and reports the partner has no symptoms she is aware of. On vaginal speculum examination, a swab was taken from the posterior fornix and in the GUM clinic microscopy was undertaken revealing motile flagellated organisms on high magnification. What is the most likely causative organism?

A. *Gardnerella vaginalis*
B. *Neisseria gonorrhoea*
C. *Chlamydia trachomatis*
D. *Trichomonas vaginalis*
E. *Treponema pallidum*

Q6.29 You are asked to review a 30-year-old woman in the obstetric ward who gave birth to a healthy baby boy 3 days previously. She was on holiday in the United Kingdom from the Caribbean. The obstetric team had performed syphilis screening due to lack of antenatal screening. The rapid plasma reagin (RPR) showed high titres with a positive specific treponemal test. The mother denies any genital ulceration or skin lesions and both the mother and baby have entirely normal physical examination with no clinical evidence of syphilis. The mother reports no known allergies. What is your recommendation to the obstetric team?

A. Reassure mother that the lack of clinical signs means no further action
B. Treat mother with benzathine penicillin intramuscularly and baby with intravenous benzylpenicillin
C. Treat mother and baby with intramuscular ceftriaxone
D. Treat mother with benzathine penicillin intramuscularly and baby with intravenous ceftriaxone
E. Treat mother with benzathine penicillin intramuscularly and baby with intravenous cefotaxime

Q6.30 A 22-year-old non-pregnant woman presents to the local GUM clinic with her fifth episode of genital herpes over the last year. These episodes are non-severe, have not needed previous hospitalisation and she is not distressed with the episodes. She is HIV negative and has no other known immunosuppressive conditions. She has previously had treatment with acyclovir to good effect. She is keen to reduce the frequency of her infections. What would your recommendation for further management?

A. Episodic course of oral acyclovir 400 mg thrice daily for 5 days
B. Episodic course of oral valaciclovir 500 mg twice daily for 3 days
C. Oral suppressive therapy with acyclovir 400 mg twice daily
D. Oral suppressive therapy with valaciclovir 500 mg once daily
E. Oral suppressive therapy with famciclovir 250 mg twice daily

Q6.31 A 25-year-old female has a 20-week antenatal scan which demonstrates microcephaly. She had received the full UK childhood immunisation schedule. There is no history of rash, ulcers, adenopathy or fever during the pregnancy. She has some blood tests sent:

CMV IgG positive
CMV IgM negative
CMV PCR <150 copies/ml
Rubella IgG positive
Toxoplasma IgG positive
Toxoplasma IgM positive
TPHA negative
RPR negative

What is the most likely cause?
A. *Rubella*
B. *Cytomegalovirus*
C. *Toxoplasma gondii*
D. *Herpes simplex*
E. *Treponemal disease*

Q6.32 A 22-year-old male presents with a painless rectal ulcer which has been present for 2 weeks. There is inguinal adenopathy but this has not ulcerated. There is no penile discharge. What is the most likely cause?
A. Herpes simplex virus
B. Lice
C. *Haemophilus ducreyi*
D. *Treponema pallidum*
E. *Neisseria gonorrhoeae*

Q6.33 A 23-year-old female presents complaining of fever, neck pain and a persistent sore throat for the past week. On arrival, she is hypotensive, tachycardic and febrile. On examination, a mild swelling over the left side of her neck and erythema of the posterior aspect of pharynx was noted. A chest radiograph demonstrates opacification at the left lower zone. An aspirate of the neck swelling has a Gram stain undertaken (Figure 6.6).

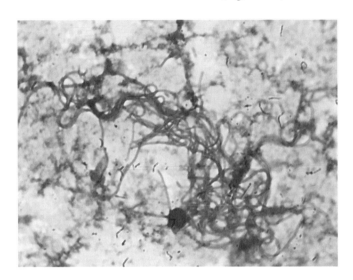

Figure 6.6 Gram stain from neck swelling aspirate. (A black and white version of this figure will appear in some formats. For the colour version, please refer to the plate section.)

Which is the most likely causative organism?
A. *Fusobacterium necrophorum*
B. Group A *Streptococcus*
C. *Corynebacterium diphtheriae*
D. *Staphylococcus aureus*
E. *Neisseria meningitidis*

Q6.34 A 29-week pregnant patient has spontaneous rupture of membranes and fever. The neonate is born with poor Apgar scores, floppy and admitted to the neonatal intensive care department. The neonatologists want to start empirical antibiotic therapy.

Which antimicrobial regimes would you recommend?
A. Cefotaxime
B. Cefotaxime and gentamicin
C. Piperacillin-tazobactam
D. Benzylpenicillin and gentamicin
E. Flucloxacillin and gentamicin

Q6.35 A 25-year-old female who is pregnant presents at 30 weeks gestation, having been with a new partner for 3 months. The venereal disease reference laboratory test is positive, but the treponemal fluorescent antibody test is negative. What is the optimal advice?
A. No need to screen partner
B. Treat with doxycycline
C. Treat with penicillin
D. Do nothing, this is latent syphilis
E. Increased frequency of antenatal ultrasound

Q6.36 A 30-year-old female who keeps tropical fish presents with violaceous hand nodules and swollen, painful lymph nodes at her elbow. What is the best way to culture a biopsy of the hand lesion to correctly diagnose this infection?
A. Culture on Lowenstein-Jensen at 30°C
B. Culture on Sabouraud's agar at 42°C
C. Culture on Sabouraud's agar at 37°C
D. Culture on Sabouraud's agar at 30°C
E. Culture on Lowenstein-Jensen at 37°C

Q6.37 A 6-month-old female who was previously fit and well and up to date with the UK immunisation schedule presents with sudden-onset respiratory failure.
The parents are not known to be immunocompromised. There is a marked lymphocytosis apparent in the full blood count (90% of WCC). What is the most likely cause?
A. *Bordetella pertussis*
B. *Listeria monocytogenes*
C. Cytomegalovirus
D. Respiratory syncytial virus
E. Human metapneumovirus

Q6.38 The peri-operative antimicrobial guidelines are undergoing review. What antimicrobial prophylaxis should be given to minimise the risk of infective endocarditis?
A. Amoxicillin should be given for dental prophylaxis in patients with metallic valves
B. Amoxicillin should be given for dental prophylaxis in patients with normal cardiac architecture
C. Antibiotics are not indicated for prevention of infective endocarditis in any circumstance
D. Transoesophageal echocardiography requires antibiotic prophylaxis
E. Where antibiotic prophylaxis for non-dental procedures is indicated, amoxicillin should be given pre- and post-procedure with a stat dose of gentamicin pre-procedure

Q6.39 A 71-year-old female develops a surgical site infection following a total hip replacement. She subsequently develops pain in the joint, but has no fevers and her inflammatory markers are normal. During a subsequent debridement and washout there is no visible pus, but five samples are taken for microbiological examination. Which is the most likely to confirm a prosthetic joint infection?

A. >3 leukocytes on microscopy on all five samples
B. *Cutibacterium acnes* in one sample
C. Meticillin-resistant *Staphylococcus aureus* in one sample
D. *S. aureus* isolates from two samples
E. *Staphylococcus epidermidis* in three different samples

Q6.40 A 45-year-old male patient presents with a 3-day history of fever, cough and breathlessness. He has raised inflammatory markers and has a chest radiograph (Figure 6.7).

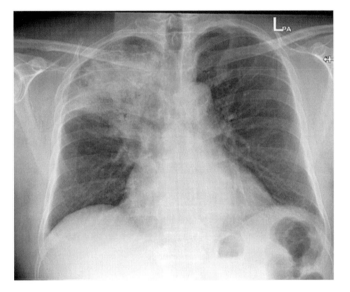

Figure 6.7 Posteroanterior chest radiograph.

Which of the following statements regarding this diagnosis is true?

A. Antimicrobials should not be given in primary care before admission
B. There is no requirement for *Legionella* spp. culture on invasive respiratory samples
C. *Legionella* urinary antigen should be undertaken on all severely ill patients
D. Chest radiography and clinical assessment are highly specific in identifying the pathogen
E. Co-amoxiclav as a single agent is advised

Q6.41 A 22-year-old female presents with dysuria, frequency and urgency. What is the main cause of community-acquired urinary tract infections?
A. *Klebsiella pneumoniae*
B. *Staphylococcus saprophyticus*
C. *Escherichia coli*
D. *Proteus mirabilis*
E. *Enterococcus faecalis*

Q6.42 A 55-year-old male presented to his general practitioner with fever. On examination, he was tachycardic and febrile. There were no localising signs or symptoms. A urine culture was sent and a pure growth of an organism was identified. Which bacteria are normally associated with haematogenous dissemination when found in a mid-stream urine?
A. *Staphylococcus aureus*
B. *Staphylococcus saprophyticus*
C. *Escherichia coli*
D. *Salmonella* Typhi
E. *Mycobacterium tuberculosis*

Q6.43 A 23-year-old female presents with a urinary tract infection. Why are urinary tract infections more common among women?
A. Density of bacterial receptors for uropathogens is higher in women
B. Urethral distance is shorter in women
C. Vulval conditions propagate bacterial growth
D. Rate of infection is the same in women and men
E. Men are more likely to urinate after sex

Q6.44 A 23-year-old female presents with a urinary tract infection. Which factor increases the frequency of urinary tract infection?
A. Use of a spermicidal gel
B. Avoiding anal sex
C. Use of a condom
D. Consumption of cranberry juice
E. Postcoital micturition

Q6.45 A 73-year-old male presents with a urinary tract infection. Why are urinary tract infections more common among elderly men?
A. Urethral catheterisation
B. Normal-sized prostate
C. Increase of prostatic secretions
D. Dilation of the ureter
E. Vesicoureteral reflux

Q6.46 A 73-year-old male presents with a urinary tract infection. He has a long-term catheter in situ. Which of the following statements are true regarding catheter-associated urinary tract infections?
   A. Catheter-associated urinary tract infections account for up to 40% nosocomial infections
   B. Bacteriuria is present in a minority of patients with indwelling catheters at 30 days
   C. Bacteriuria is frequently monomicrobial
   D. Asymptomatic bacteriuria should always be treated
   E. Patients with indwelling urinary catheters should receive antibiotic prophylaxis

Q6.47 A 73-year-old female presents with a urinary tract infection. Why are urinary tract infections more common among elderly women?
   A. Increased vaginal lactobacilli
   B. Vesicoureteric reflux
   C. Cognitive decline
   D. Increased albumin in urine
   E. Oestrogen replacement therapy

Q6.48 A 23-year-old pregnant woman has a mid-stream urine submitted. How should a mid-stream urine in a pregnant woman be interpreted?
   A. Asymptomatic bacteriuria develops in 20–40% of pregnant women
   B. Asymptomatic bacteriuria is diagnosed with a bacterial count higher than 10^5 CFU/mL
   C. Asymptomatic bacteriuria should always be treated in pregnancy
   D. Risk of pyelonephritis is comparable between pregnant and non-pregnant women
   E. Urinary tract infections in pregnancy have no effect on foetal development

Q6.49 A 23-year-old woman is symptomatic of a lower urinary tract infection but when a urine sample is sent is demonstrated to have sterile pyuria. What condition is sterile pyuria not characteristic of?
   A. Renal tract *Mycobacterium tuberculosis* infection
   B. *Chlamydia trachomatis* urethritis
   C. Antibiotic-treated *Escherichia coli* urinary tract infection
   D. *Neisseria gonorrhoeae* infection
   E. *Staphylococcus saprophyticus* urinary tract infection

Q6.50 A 54-year-old male with cirrhosis develops self-limited diarrhoea after consuming raw oysters. Two days later he presents with overwhelming sepsis, develops blistering skin lesions and dies. What is the most likely bacterial cause?
   A. *Bacillus cereus*
   B. *Salmonella* Heidelberg
   C. *Salmonella* Typhi
   D. *Vibrio vulnificus*
   E. *Cyclospora cayetanensis*

Q6.51   A 35-year-old male develops diarrhoea. He admits to purchasing two
        illegal turtles a week before the onset of symptoms. What is the most likely
        pathogen?
        A. *Plesiomonas shigelloides*
        B. *Strongyloides stercoralis*
        C. *Salmonella* Typhi
        D. *Salmonella* Arizonae
        E. *Vibrio cholerae*

Q6.52   A children's nursery manager calls to ask advice on diagnosing and managing an
        outbreak of diarrhoea at the nursey. Ten children aged between 4 and 7 years of
        age have become symptomatic in the last 2 weeks with diarrhoea characterised
        by low-volume stools but with blood and mucus. What is the most likely
        microbiological cause?
        A. *Shigella* spp.
        B. Enterotoxigenic *Escherichia coli*
        C. *Giardia intestinalis*
        D. Rotavirus
        E. Norovirus

Q6.53   A 49-year-old male takes his two children (11 years of age and 13 years of age) to
        a nearby farm and they eat pork chitterlings for lunch. Five days later the
        children develop diarrhoea (no blood or mucus) with abdominal pain and fever to
        38.5°C. What is the most likely microbiological cause?
        A. *Shigella* spp.
        B. Enterotoxigenic *Escherichia coli*
        C. *Campylobacter coli*
        D. *Yersinia enterocolitica*
        E. *Vibrio parahaemolyticus*

Q6.54   A 29-year-old female presents in the 33rd week of gestation with a temperature of
        38.8°C 1 day after having several episodes of diarrhoea. Which organism is a
        particularly dangerous potential cause of this presentation?
        A. *Salmonella* Typhimurium
        B. *Listeria monocytogenes*
        C. *Giardia intestinalis*
        D. *Taenia saginata*
        E. *Plesiomonas shigelloides*

Q6.55   A 29-year-old female presents in the 33rd week of gestation with a temperature of
        38.2°C and has a pre-term premature rupture of membranes. Which of the
        following organisms is most likely to be isolated?
        A. *Gardnerella vaginalis*
        B. *Ureaplasma urealyticum*
        C. *Bacteroides fragilis*
        D. *Escherichia coli*
        E. *Streptococcus agalactiae*

Q6.56 A 65-year-old male presents with fever after a catheter change. He is found to have a murmur and an *Enterococcus faecalis* is grown from blood cultures. Which of the following statements regarding enterococcal endocarditis is true?
A. It is more common in young females than old males
B. Treatment with vancomycin and gentamicin is optimal
C. Treatment with amoxicillin and gentamicin is optimal even where there is low-level gentamicin resistance
D. Where there is high level gentamicin resistance testing for tobramycin and amikacin is indicated
E. Where there is a *vanB* phenotype treatment with vancomycin rather than teicoplanin is advocated

Q6.57 A 77-year-old male is admitted with a stroke. His admission chest radiograph was clear. After 7 days in hospital he develops a pyrexia and breathlessness and has a repeat chest radiograph (Figure 6.8).

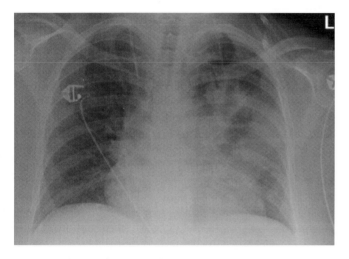

Figure 6.8 Anterioposterior chest radiograph.

What is the most likely cause?
A. *Clostridium perfringens*
B. *Staphylococcus aureus*
C. *Mycobacterium tuberculosis*
D. *Fusobacterium necrophorum*
E. *Klebsiella pneumoniae*

Q6.58 A 32-year-old female patient presents with fever associated with rigors and hypotension. A urine culture shows *Escherichia coli* resistant to amoxicillin, cefoxitin, cefuroxime and ciprofloxacin. What will you treat with pending further susceptibility?
A. Nitrofurantoin
B. Meropenem
C. Ceftazidime
D. Ceftriaxone
E. Amoxicillin-clavulanate

Q6.59 An 18-year-old male with cystic fibrosis complains of worsening shortness of breath. He has been colonised with *Pseudomonas aeruginosa* and *Staphylococcus aureus* in the past but not needed treatment for the past year. Sputum culture grows a pure isolate of *Stenotrophomonas maltophilia*. Which treatment is advised?

A. Amoxicillin

B. Gentamicin

C. Co-trimoxazole

D. Meropenem

E. Piperacillin-tazobactam

Q6.60 A 23-year-old male attended with upper respiratory tract symptoms and drooling. His vaccination status was unclear and a clinical diagnosis of diphtheria was suspected. What symptoms do you not see in diphtheria?

A. Cardiomyopathy

B. Peripheral neuropathy

C. Asphyxia

D. Septicaemia

E. Cervical lymphadenopathy

Q6.61 A 28-year-old male presents to the genitourinary medicine clinic with urethral discharge and dysuria. He is screened for sexually transmitted infections and is found to be VDRL negative but TPHA positive. What is the most likely explanation for this?

A. Primary syphilis

B. Secondary syphilis

C. Tertiary syphilis

D. Treated syphilis

E. *Treponema pallidum* ssp. pertenue infection

Q6.62 A 28-year-old male presents to the genitourinary medicine clinic with urethral discharge and dysuria. A Gram-negative diplococcus is seen on the urethral smear, however, the patient leaves without treatment. What is the likely outcome?

A. Septic arthritis

B. Urethral stricture

C. Epididymo-orchitis

D. Prostatitis

E. Septicaemia

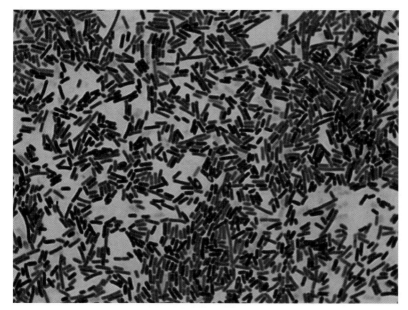

Figure 1.1 Gram stain from a positive blood culture.

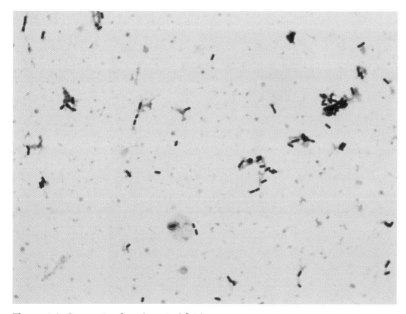

Figure 1.2 Gram stain of cerebrospinal fluid.

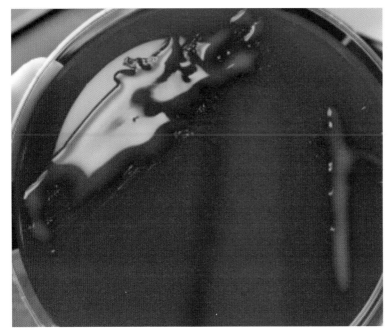

Figure 1.4 Growth on blood agar incubated in an aerobic environment at 37°C for 24 hours.

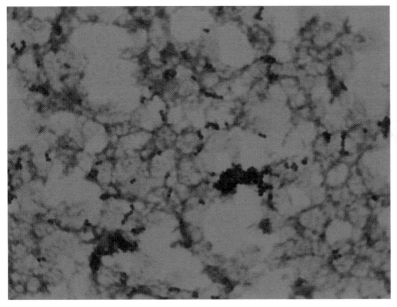

Figure 2.2 Gram stain from a positive blood culture.

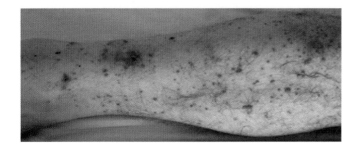

Figure 4.1 Clinical appearance of anterior lower left leg.

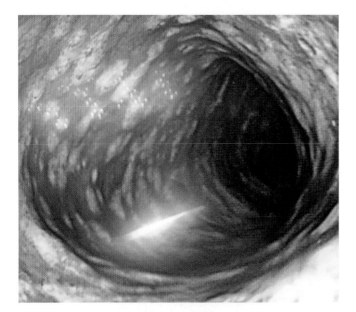

Figure 5.1 Endoscopic appearance of sigmoid colon.

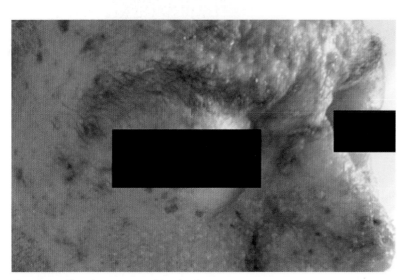

Figure 6.1 Clinical appearance of facial rash.

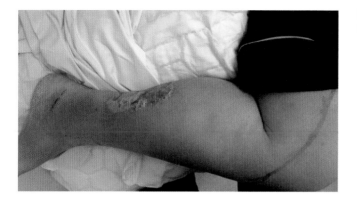

Figure 6.4 Clinical appearance of left lower leg.

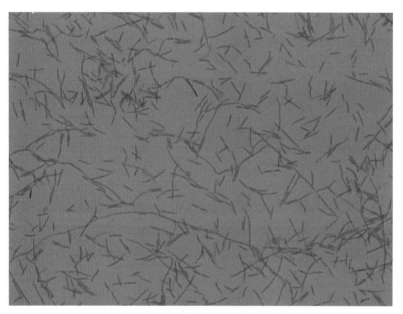

Figure 6.5 Gram stain from a positive blood culture.

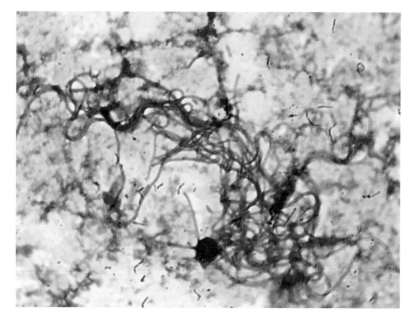

Figure 6.6 Gram stain from neck swelling aspirate.

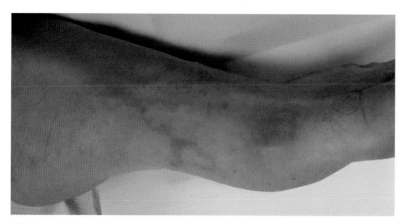

Figure 6.9 Clinical appearance of right foot.

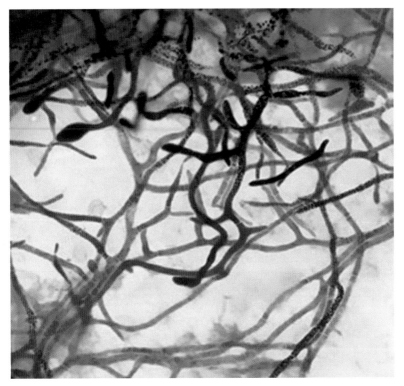

Figure 9.2 Gram stain from a positive blood culture.

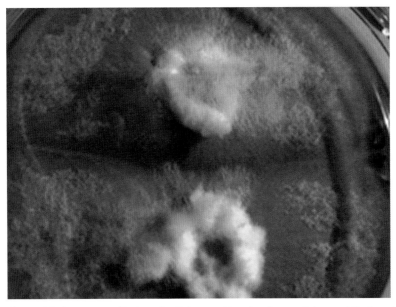

Figure 9.3 Appearance of isolate after 5 days aerobic sub-culture on Sabouraud Dextrose Agar at 25°C.

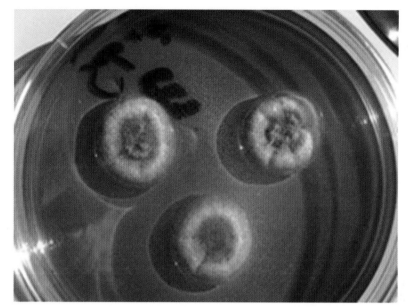

Figure 9.4 Appearance of isolate after 5 days aerobic sub-culture on Sabouraud Dextrose Agar at 30°C.

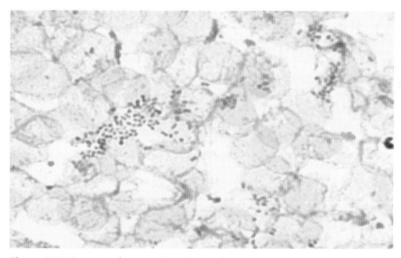

Figure 10.1 Gram stain from a positive blood culture.

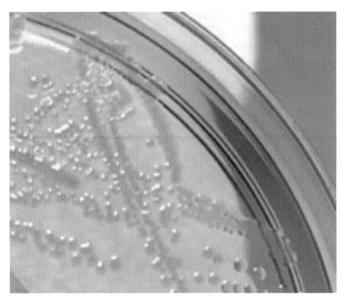

Figure 10.3b Growth on thiosulfate citrate bile salts sucrose incubated in an aerobic environment at 37°C for 24 hours.

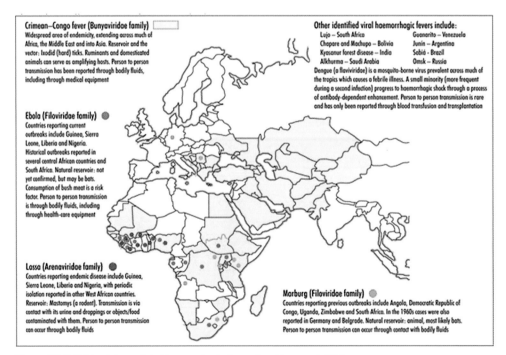

Crimean–Congo fever (Bunyaviridae family)
Widespread area of endemicity, extending across much of Africa, the Middle East and into Asia. Reservoir and the vector: Ixodid (hard) ticks. Ruminants and domesticated animals can serve as amplifying hosts. Person to person transmission has been reported through bodily fluids, including through medical equipment

Ebola (Filoviridae family)
Countries reporting current outbreaks include Guinea, Sierra Leone, Liberia and Nigeria. Historical outbreaks reported in several central African countries and South Africa. Natural reservoir: not yet confirmed, but may be bats. Consumption of bush meat is a risk factor. Person to person transmission is through bodily fluids, including through health-care equipment

Lassa (Arenaviridae family)
Countries reporting endemic disease include Guinea, Sierra Leone, Liberia and Nigeria, with periodic isolation reported in other West African countries. Reservoir: Mastomys (a rodent). Transmission is via contact with its urine and droppings or objects/food contaminated with them. Person to person transmission can occur through bodily fluids

Other identified viral haemorrhagic fevers include:

Lujo – South Africa	Guanarito – Venezuela
Chapare and Machupo – Bolivia	Junin – Argentina
Kyasanur forest disease – India	Sabiá - Brazil
Alkhurma – Saudi Arabia	Omsk – Russia

Dengue (a flaviviridae) is a mosquito-borne virus prevalent across much of the tropics which causes a febrile illness. A small minority (more frequent during a second infection) progress to haemorrhagic shock through a process of antibody-dependent enhancement. Person to person transmission is rare and has only been reported through blood transfusion and transplantation

Marburg (Filoviridae family)
Countries reporting previous outbreaks include Angola, Democratic Republic of Congo, Uganda, Zimbabwe and South Africa. In the 1960s cases were also reported in Germany and Belgrade. Natural reservoir: animal, most likely bats. Person to person transmission can occur through contact with bodily fluids

Figure 10.5 Epidemiology of viral haemorrhagic fevers (from Moore et al., 2014).

Q6.63 A 24-year-old male presents with a rash on his foot (Figure 6.9).
He denies any foreign travel, but admits to frequently going barefoot in
his local park.

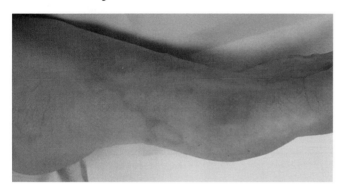

Figure 6.9 Clinical appearance of right foot. (A black and white version of this figure will appear in some formats. For the colour version, please refer to the plate section.)

Which is the most likely causative organism?
A. *Strongyloides stercoralis*
B. *Ancylostoma braziliense*
C. *Necator americanus*
D. *Borrelia burgdorferi*
E. *Clostridium perfringens*

Q6.64 A 37-year-old male who reports being an intravenous drug user presents with
an acutely swollen and painful right leg. He has a marked tachycardia and
hypotension, but on examination of the leg, there are no areas of necrosis.
Ultrasound imaging demonstrates patent veins. A subsequent computerised
tomographic scan of the thigh is depicted in Figure 6.10a, and a blood culture
subsequently becomes positive (Figure 6.10b).

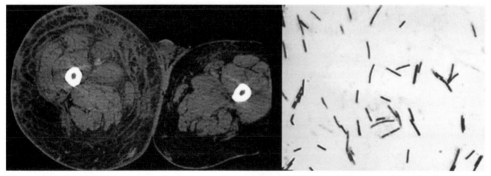

Figure 6.10 (a) Mid-thigh computerised tomograph, axial plane. (b) Gram stain from a positive blood culture.

What is the most likely microbiological diagnosis?
A. *Bacillus anthracis*
B. *Clostridium perfringens*
C. *Clostridium sordellii*
D. *Staphylococcus aureus*
E. *Streptococcus pyogenes*

Q6.65 A 31-year-old female presents with a history of several days of right sided headache and a new right cranial nerve VII palsy. She reports being an active swimmer. There is no neck stiffness. A computerised tomographic scan of her head is undertaken (Figure 6.11).

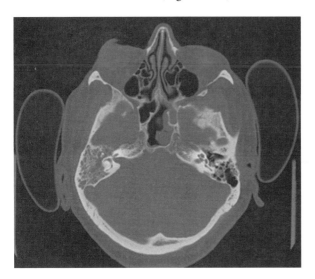

Figure 6.11 Skull base computerised tomograph, axial plane.

What is the clinical diagnosis?
A. Chronic sinusitis
B. Meningitis
C. Otitis externa
D. Mastoiditis
E. Cerebral abscess

Q6.66 A 31-year-old female with two small children gives a history of recurrent tonsillitis (Figure 6.12). She has had eight episodes in the last year, each necessitating antimicrobials.

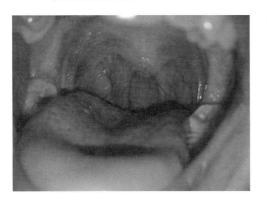

Figure 6.12 Clinical appearance of oropharynx.

What is the most appropriate curse of action in this case?
A. Prescribe lifelong penicillin V orally
B. Prescribe a further course of 1 week of amoxicillin
C. Refer to ear, nose and throat specialists for tonsillectomy
D. Prescribe a further course of 10 days of amoxicillin
E. Adopt a watch and wait approach

Q6.67 A 29-year-old female with no past medical history and no known cause of immunocompromise presents with a seizure. She has a negative point-of-care human immunodeficiency virus test. A computerised tomographic scan of her brain is undertaken (Figure 6.13).

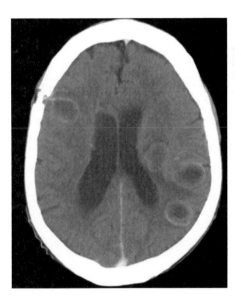

Figure 6.13 Brain computerised tomograph, with contrast, axial plane.

Which organism is the least likely to cause a cerebral abscess?
A. *Staphylococcus aureus*
B. *Peptostreptococcus* spp.
C. *Neisseria meningitidis*
D. *Nocardia brasiliensis*
E. *Actinomyces israelii*

Q6.68   A 38-year-old female is admitted with fever, right upper quadrant pain and lethargy. She is 18 weeks pregnant with her first child. She is originally from Greece and recently had a short admission to hospital in Greece for pyelonephritis 6 weeks ago while visiting family. On examination she looks unwell. She is tachycardic, hypotensive and febrile. A blood culture taken on admission grows a growth of *Klebsiella pneumoniae* >100,000 CFU/mL; resistant to amoxicillin, cephalexin, cefotaxime, ciprofloxacin, amikacin, meropenem, temocillin; sensitive to nitrofurantoin, colistin and tigecycline. Rapid PCR for the detection of carbapenemase enzymes detects the presence of KPC (*Klebsiella pneumonia* carbapenemase). Which of the following treatments would you recommend?
   A. Colistin
   B. Colistin and meropenem
   C. Colistin and tigecycline
   D. Nitrofurantoin
   E. Colistin and fosfomycin

Q6.69   A 66-year-old nun developed non-bloody diarrhoea which was self-limiting with bowel motions returning to normal. Two weeks following this episode she develops a swollen painful knee and presented to the local emergency department. The orthopaedic team performed a joint aspiration which was sterile. Inflammatory markers, including C-reactive protein, were raised and serum testing for HLA B27 was positive. Which of the following pathogens is the least likely to cause this condition?
   A. *Yersinia enterocolitica*
   B. *Shigella* spp.
   C. *Salmonella* spp.
   D. *Campylobacter* spp.
   E. *Giardia lamblia*

Q6.70   A 53-year-old male patient was bought into the emergency resus department via ambulance with a suspected infection. On arrival he looked unwell, confused and unkempt. Key signs and investigations showed:

   Blood pressure: 75/40 mmHg
   Heart rate: 140 bpm
   Respiratory rate: 30/min
   Glasgow Coma Scale: 12/15
   Temperature: 38.5°C
   Serum lactate: 5.5 mmol/L
   White cell count: 15×10^9/L

His qSOFA (Quick SOFA) score was 3 and he was initially diagnosed with severe sepsis and commenced on broad spectrum antibiotics, fluids and reviewed by the critical care team.

What are the three criteria that comprise the qSOFA?
   A. Respiratory rate, altered mentation, tachycardia
   B. Respiratory rate, tachycardia, hypotension
   C. Hypotension, raised inflammatory markers, tachycardia
   D. Respiratory rate, altered mentation, hypotension
   E. Hypotension, raised lactate, tachycardia

Answers

A6.1   Answer A: Measles virus

In contrast to the common enterovirus, and slightly less common herpes virus, encephalitidies which are caused by acute primary viral invasion, subacute sclerosing panencephalitis (SSPE) is a rare chronic, progressive encephalitis that primarily affects children and young adults. It is caused by a persistent infection of immune-resistant (mutated) measles virus affecting 1 in 100,000 people infected with primary measles. Patients with SSPE frequently have normal CSF results, other than a mildly raised protein, which is predominantly due to raised CSF IgG. This has been shown to be directed against measles virus. In the context of a compatible history and EEG findings (such as those described in this case), raised measles antibody titres of 1:4 or greater in CSF, or 1:256 or greater in serum is diagnostic of SSPE. Data examined by an expert World Health Organisation (WHO) committee in 2006 found no evidence to suggest that measles vaccine is a cause of SSPE.

Other myoclonic encephalopathies include juvenile Huntington's, Alzheimer's disease and Creutzfeldt–Jakob disease. If associated with ataxia, then Whipple's disease, Wilson's disease and spinocerebellar degeneration should also be considered. Other viruses, including those listed in this question stem, can all cause acute demyelinating encephalomyelitis (ADEM), which is characterised by fever and some degree of impairment of consciousness, with a history of recent infection or immunisation. CSF studies typically demonstrate a modest elevation in white cell count, unlike that seen here.

Further Reading

Fisher DL, Defres S, Solomon T. Measles-induced encephalitis. *Queensland J Med.* 2015;108 (3):177–182.

Rota PA, Moss WJ, Takeda M, de Swart RL, Thompson KM, Goodson JL. Measles. *Nat Rev Dis Primers.* 2016;2:16049.

A6.2   Answer C: Spastic paraparesis

HTLV-1 is predominantly found in CD4+ T cells, and other cell types in the peripheral blood can also be infected, including CD8+ T cells, dendritic cells and B cells. Cell entry is mediated via a virion envelope glycoprotein with the host cell receptor GLUT1. HTLV-1 has an immuno-stimulating effect, which, however, is also immunosuppressive. The virus causes TH1 cells to proliferate, leading to overproduction of TH1-related cytokines (mainly IFN-γ and TNF-α). These cytokines in turn suppress TH2 lymphocytes leading to reductions in TH2-related cytokines (mainly IL-4, IL-5, IL-10 and IL-13). The end result is a reduction in the ability to mount an adequate immune response to certain invading organisms (including for example *Strongyloides stercoralis*). HTLV-1 is also associated with adult T cell leukaemia/lymphoma, and is also associated with a progressive demyelinating upper motor neurone disease known as HAM/TSP (HTLV-1-associated myelopathy/ tropical spastic paraparesis).

Further Reading

Bangham CRM, Araujo A, Yamano Y, Taylor GP. HTLV-I-associated myelopathy/tropical spastic paraparesis. *Nat Rev Dis Primers.* 2015;1:15023.

A6.3   Answer B: Hodgkin's lymphoma

EBV has a seroprevalence of over 90% among UK adults, and results in latent B-lymphocytes infection, which is associated with potential induction of lymphoblastoid cell lines that are capable of indefinite growth. Through this mechanism EBV has been linked to nasopharyngeal carcinoma, Burkett's lymphoma, post-transplant lymphoma and Hodgkin's lymphoma. EBV has also been linked to oral hairy leukoplakia particularly in those with Langerhans's APC deficiencies. Acute lymphoblastic leukaemia (specifically acute T-cell leukaemia) and T-cell lymphoma are associated with human T-lymphotropic virus 1 (HTLV-1).

Further Reading

Dojcinov SD, Fend F, Quintanilla-Martinez L. EBV-positive lymphoproliferations of B- T- and NK-cell derivation in non-immunocompromised hosts. *Pathogens*. 2018;7(1):28.

A6.4   Answer B: Oral aciclovir

Varicella zoster causes a vesicular ("dew drop on rose petal") rash that in primary infection appears mainly on the torso. Typically in temperate regions, including the United Kingdom, primary varicella infection is a childhood infection and a significant proportion of the population is seropositive for this virus by adolescence. However, natural acquisition is less prevalent in more equatorial regions, and those who are seronegative who come into contact with children with varicella or are exposed to shingles from older individuals, may develop primary varicella as an adult. Childhood varicella is self-limiting with few acute sequelae. Chronic dormancy in the trigeminal and dorsal root (afferent/sensory) ganglia is the norm, later recurring as a dermatomal vesicular infectious zoster rash. Adult primary varicella, however, can have serious acute sequelae including varicella pneumonia and should be treated with aciclovir; oral in non-severe infection, and intravenous where there are respiratory symptoms, neurological changes or a haemorrhagic rash. Respiratory and circulatory support may be needed in some cases. Zoster, as a distinct entity from adult varicella, can also be treated with acyclovir, which may reduce the severity and duration of the attack but does not reliably prevent post-herpetic neuralgia.

Further Reading

Tunbridge AJ, Breuer J, Jeffery KJM. Chickenpox in adults – clinical management. *J Infect*. 2008;57:95–102.

A6.5   Answer D: Oral valganciclovir for 6 months

The baby has been infected with CMV, which is most likely vertically transmitted from the mother. Primary infection occurred during pregnancy confirmed by the maternal serology. This is a case of congenital cytomegalovirus infection. Foetal diagnosis can be made from either antenatal amniotic fluid PCR or post-natal PCR of saliva or urine. Saliva sample is best taken 1 hour after breastfeeding to avoid maternal contamination. Congenital CMV infection can range from asymptomatic to severe neurological disease or death. The most common development disability is unilateral or bilateral hearing loss. Current treatment recommendations state if the baby has moderate-to-severe symptomatic congenital cytomegalovirus disease, then oral valganciclovir for 6 months within the first month of life should be given. Mild or asymptomatic cases should not be treated which include isolated sensorineural hearing loss.

Moderate-to-severe criteria include thrombocytopenia, petechiae, hepatomegaly, splenomegaly, hepatitis or central nervous system involvement (microcephaly, ventriculomegaly, intracerebral calcifications, periventricular echogenicity, cerebellar malformations) or chorioretinitis and abnormal cerebrospinal fluid.

Further Reading

Rawlinson WD, Boppana SB, Fowler KB, Kimberlin DW, Lazzarotto T, Alain S, Daly K, Doutré S, Gibson L, Giles ML, Greenlee J, Hamilton ST, Harrison GJ, Hui L, Jones CA, Palasanthiran P, Schleiss MR, Shand AW, van Zuylen WJ. Congenital cytomegalovirus infection in pregnancy and the neonate: consensus recommendations for prevention, diagnosis, and therapy. *Lancet Infect Dis.* 2017;17(6):177–188.

A6.6 Answer C: Lansoprazole

The proton-pump inhibitor (lansoprazole) would be the beneficial drug to withhold as acid suppressants are associated with both the acquisition and recurrence of *C. difficile* infection. Gastric acid suppression increases risk due to the loss of the protective gastric acid and/or changes in the gut microbiota. A meta-analysis in 2017 of 16 studies comprising 7,703 patients showed that the use of gastric acid suppressants was associated with a significantly increased risk of recurrent *C. difficile* infection. Subgroup analyses of studies with potential confounders confirmed an increased risk of recurrent *C. difficile* infection.

Further Reading

Tariq R, Singh S, Gupta A, Pardi DS, Khanna S. Association of gastric acid suppression with recurrent *Clostridium difficile* infection. A systematic review and meta-analysis. *JAMA Intern Med.* 2017;177 (6):784–791.

A6.7 Answer A: *Pseudomonas aeruginosa*

In the initial stage, common bacteria such as *S. aureus* and *H. influenzae* colonise and infect the lungs. Eventually, however, *P. aeruginosa* (and sometimes *B. cepacia*) dominates. The bacterium *P. aeruginosa* permanently colonises cystic fibrosis lungs and probably exists as biofilms coordinated by quorum sensing – structured communities of bacteria encased in a self-produced polymeric matrix. A study cited the causes of CF infections to be *P. aeruginosa* (40–58%), *S. aureus* (24–63%), *B. cepacia* (5–13%), *Stenotrophomonas maltophilia* (8%) and *Achromobacter xyloxidans* (3%). *B. cepacia* infection follows a variable clinical course but often leads to an accelerated rate of lung function decline and can lead to a necrotising pneumonia – "Cepacia syndrome." This is particularly associated with genovar III.

Anti-staphylococcal antibiotic prophylaxis is recommended until 3 years old. Samples of respiratory secretions are taken, and on initial isolation of *P. aeruginosa*, an eradication programme is recommended to try and stop permanent colonisation of the organism. Systemic and nebulised anti-pseudomonal antibiotics are first line. Chronically infected patients with *Pseudomonas* should be on prophylactic nebulised antibiotics.

Further Reading

Report of the UK Cystic Fibrosis Trust Antibiotic Working Group. Antibiotic Treatment for Cystic Fibrosis. Third Edition. May 2009. Available at: www.cysticfibrosis.org.uk/~/media/documents/ the-work-we-do/care/consensus-docs-with-new-address/anitbiotic-treatment.ashx?la=en

A6.8 Answer B: Erythema chronicum migrans

The classic sign of early local infection with Lyme disease is a circular, outwardly expanding rash called erythema chronicum migrans, which occurs 3–30 days after a tick bite. The rash is red and may be warm, but is generally painless. Classically, the innermost portion remains dark red and becomes indurated, the outer edge remains red, and the portion in between clears, giving the appearance of a bull's-eye. Erythema migrans is thought to occur in anywhere from 30% to 80% of infected patients.

Erythema marginatum is a pink rash, involving the trunk and sometimes limbs (but not face) and is associated with acute rheumatic fever. Erythema multiforme is an acute, immune-mediated condition which is associated with target-like lesions on the skin, usually involving other sites such as the oral cavity and genital area. Erythema multiforme is usually induced by infection, especially herpes simplex, and is self-limiting. Erythema nodosum is a delayed-type hypersensitivity reaction that most often presents with tender, erythematous, raised nodules on the anterior aspect of the lower limbs. Lesions on palms and soles can be non-specific but associated with syphilis, viruses such as Enterovirus/ Coxsackie (hand, foot and mouth disease) and drug eruptions.

Further Reading

Moore A, Nelson C, Molins C, Mead P, Schriefer M. Current guidelines, common clinical pitfalls, and future directions for laboratory diagnosis of Lyme disease, United States. *Emerg Infect Dis.* 2016;22(7):1169–1177.

A6.9 Answer B: *Streptococcus pyogenes*

This patient does not have cellulitis but instead is presenting with erythema nodosum. Erythema nodosum is a common delayed-type hypersensitivity reaction to various antigens, many of which are infective in origin. It most often presents with tender, erythematous, nodules which most commonly appear on the anterior aspect of the lower limbs but can also appear on the thighs, calves and buttocks. Biopsy of these lesions would demonstrate a septal panniculitis but no signs of vasculitis. Common triggers for erythema nodosum include infection (a quarter to a half of cases), sarcoidosis (up to a quarter of cases), drugs (up to 10% of cases), pregnancy (a few percent) or inflammatory bowel disease (a few percent). Among the infective causes, streptococcal pharyngitis is the most common cause, with erythema nodosum typically appearing 2–3 weeks after the pharyngitis resolves. Other infective causes include *Mycoplasma* spp., *Chlamydia* spp., *Yersinia* spp. and *Mycobacterium* spp. In other areas of the world, it can be associated with systemic mycoses as well, including *Histoplasma* spp. and *Coccidioides* spp. Erythema nodosum usually resolves without intervention, but should very much be used to initiate investigations for the underlying aetiology.

Further Reading

Chowaniec M, Starba A, Wiland P. Erythema nodosum – review of the literature. *Reumatologia.* 2016;54(2):79–82.

A6.10 Answer A: Kikuchi's disease

Kikuchi–Fujimoto Disease (KFD) is a rare, benign, self-limiting illness characterised by fever and predominantly cervical lymphadenopathy. It was first described almost simultaneously by Kikuchi and Fujimoto in 1972 in Japan. Traditionally, KFD was thought to affect predominantly younger adult females of South East Asian origin but it is a worldwide disease that affects males and females equally. The pathogenesis is unknown but is associated with a wide variety of viral and bacterial triggers. Histology shows classic appearances of necrosis and a histiocytic infiltration. The condition is self-limiting, but can take a few months to resolve symptoms. Lymphoma and autoimmune disease are the major associations and these patients need long-term follow-up.

Further Reading

Dumas G, Prendki V, Haroche J Amoura Z, Cacoub P, Galicier L, Meyer O, Rapp C, Deligny C, Godeau B, Aslangul E, Lambotte O, Papo T, Pouchot J, Hamidou M, Bachmeyer C, Hachulla E, Carmoi T, Dhote R, Gerin M, Mekinian A, Stirnemann J, Charlotte F, Farge D, Molina T, Fain O. Kikuchi-Fujimoto disease: retrospective study of 91 cases and review of the literature. *Medicine (Baltimore)*. 2014;93(24):372–382.

Shirakusa T, Eimoto T, Kikuchi M. Histiocytic necrotizing lymphadenitis. *Postgrad Med J*. 1988;64 (748):107–109.

A6.11 Answer C: Histoplasmosis

Histoplasmosis is an endemic mycosis in the United States and worldwide. Most infections are asymptomatic, but some individuals develop acute pulmonary infections and disseminated disease. Dissemination probably occurs in most individuals, but normal cellular immunity should lead to control of the infection. Altered immunity and extremes of age are risk factors. Histoplasma capsulatum is a dimorphic fungus and a Category 3 pathogen in the laboratory. Disease is usually either acute (infants and immunocompromised) or chronic (older adults in men greater than women). Chronic infection often presents with pancytopenia, hepatosplenomegaly, oropharyngeal or gastrointestinal lesions. Other sites include the skin, brain and adrenal glands.

Further Reading

Wheat LJ, Freifeld AG, Kleiman MB, Baddley JW, McKinsey DS, Loyd JE, Kauffman CA. Clinical practice guidelines for the management of patients with histoplasmosis: 2007 update by the Infectious Diseases Society of America. *Clin Infect Dis*. 2007;45(7):807–825.

A6.12 Answer B: Dirofilariasis

Dirofilariasis is a zoonotic filarial infection with humans as dead-end hosts. It is caused by filarial nematodes of genus *Dirofilaria*. There are 40 species but only 6 have caused disease in humans. Mosquitoes are the vectors of transmission. The natural hosts are domestic and wild animals such as dogs and foxes. *Dirofilaria repens* is the most widely reported cause with cases across Europe and Central Asia. Italy has a particularly high prevalence, and the Piedmont region in Northern Italy has a large reported number of cases. *D. repens* typically manifests as either subcutaneous nodules and most commonly involves face, conjunctiva, chest wall, upper arms, thighs and male genitalia. *Dirofilaria immitis* is usually found in the United States and causes pulmonary disease. Usually, these are picked up accidentally as coin-shaped lesions that are resected due to concern regarding malignancy. Those with pulmonary symptoms report chest pain, fever and cough.

Further Reading

Pampiglione S, Rivasi F, Angeli G, Boldorini R, Incensati RM, Pastormerlo M, Pavesi M, Ramponi A. Dirofilariasis due to Dirofilaria repens in Italy, an emergent zoonosis: report of 60 new cases. *Histopathology*. 2001;38(4):344–354.

Reddy M. Human dirofilariasis: an emerging zoonosis. *Trop Parasitol*. 2013;3(1):2–3.

A6.13 Answer A: Primary amoebic meningoencephalitis

The most likely answer is primary amoebic encephalitis caused by *Naegleria fowleri*. This is a thermophilic protozoan parasite that is globally distributed in water. It is associated with fresh and warm water sources rather than sea water. Activities that increase the risk of disease relate to inhalation or facial contact of infested water. Jumping and diving into water will increase the risk including white water rafting. It has a very high mortality and causes rapid decline. It is an acute haemorrhagic encephalitis, CT findings are non-specific but motile trophozoites can be found in the CSF. Amphotericin B deoxycholate may be the best therapy but no studies on outcome have shown optimum treatment due to the high mortality. Granulomatous amoebic meningoencephalitis caused by species of *Acanthomoeba* and *Balamuthia* are more insidious in onset with lower mortality rates.

Further Reading

Grace E, Asbill S, Virga K. *Naegleria fowleri*: pathogenesis, diagnosis, and treatment options. *Antimicrob Agents Chemother*. 2015;59(11):6677–6681.

A6.14 Answer C: *Cryptococcus neoformans*

The most likely diagnosis is cryptoccocal meningitis in the context of a patient with profound immunosuppression. While cryptococcal meningitis is typically described in the context of human immunodeficiency virus, it can occur following other cases of immunocompromise. While a Gram stain would be negative, performing a cryptococcal antigen on blood and cerebrospinal fluid is a useful diagnostic tool. On occasion *Cryptococcus* spp. can be visualised by performing an India ink stain on cerebrospinal fluid (Figure 6.14), but this is less common.

Figure 6.14 India ink stain of cerebrospinal fluid.

S. capitis is a coagulase-negative staphylococcal species, and although associated with central line-related infections, it would not cause a meningitis outside of the neonatal period. *C. auris* is a rare but important *Candida* spp. which is associated with outbreaks and antifungal resistance. *Candida* spp. are important causes of line infections but rarely cause meningoencephalitis. *Nocardia* spp. would most likely present with a respiratory illness and infection of the central nervous system will often reveal a lesion on CT scanning. *M. tuberculosis* is an important cause of meningitis but usually has a significantly raised CSF protein level and a more indolent course.

Further Reading
Schmalzie SA, Buchwald UK, Gilliam BL, Riedel DJ. *Cryptococcus neoformans* infection in malignancy. *Mycoses*. 2016;59(9):542–552.

A6.15 Answer C: Hidradenitis suppurativa
Hidradenitis suppurativa (HS) is an inflammatory skin disease with a characteristic clinical presentation of recurrent painful or suppurating lesions in apocrine gland-bearing regions.

HS is a disease of the hair follicles with lymphocytic infiltrate and sebaceous gland loss. Early lesions have normal bacterial flora suggesting infection is secondary to the inflammation. As inflammation progresses, so does tissue damage. Hurley classification separates the disease into three stages. Treatment is in stages and weight loss is important for overweight patients. Systemic antibiotics are the usual first treatment but this is not based on good quality evidence but clinical experience. Adalimumab was the first biologic licensed for treatment but there are more being used such as anakinra and ustekinumab. Newer surgical approaches include skin tissue sparing excision with electrosurgical peeling (STEEP) and carbon dioxide laser evaporation.

Further Reading
Saunte D, Jemec G. Hidradenitis suppurativa: advances in diagnosis and treatment. *JAMA*. 2017;318(20):2019–2032.

A6.16 Answer E: *Corynebacterium pseudodiphtheriticum*
Early prosthetic valve endocarditis (PVE) is defined as the diagnosis of PVE within 60 days of implantation. The cumulative hazard of developing PVE was highest within the initial 12 months after valve replacement surgery, influenced by an increased incidence of *Staphylococcus aureus* and coagulase-negative staphylococcal infection both from 0 to 2 months and from 2 to 12 months after valve implantation. Early PVE is probably due to greater exposure to health care contact and lack of complete endothelialisation of the prosthetic valve early after implantation. With regards to Gram-positive bacilli, incidence in PVE is low. Of all *Corynebacterium* species, only *C. pseudodiphtheriticum* showed a predilection for prosthetic versus native valves. Associations with native infective endocarditis of nosocomial origin are found for *C. striatum*, *C. jeikeium* and *A. haemolyticum*.

Further Reading
Belmares J, Detterline S, Pak JB, Parada JP. *Corynebacterium endocarditis* species-specific risk factor and outcomes. *BMC Infect Dis*. 2007;7:4.

A6.17   **Answer B: Bartonella neuroretinitis and encephalitis**

This case highlights the difficulty in diagnosing a rare condition when multiple tests are positive needing careful interpretation. *B. henselae* (cat scratch disease) is an uncommon cause of lymphadenopathy in children but can cause ophthalmic and neurological sequelae. The presence of antibodies, especially prior to IVIG, would make this the most likely diagnosis. Borrelia testing, especially C6 EIA and IgM P41 antigen, often cross-react with *Bartonella*. The ASOT is weakly positive and not relevant, and the diagnosis of PANDAS does not fit with the presentation. Herpes simplex virus is the most common cause of encephalitis and an important differential due to improvement if acyclovir is given early in the disease. The negative HSV PCR in CSF does not rule out this diagnosis as the lumbar puncture was undertaken early into the illness and should be repeated if clinical suspicion is high. The MRI findings are not in keeping with HSV.

Further Reading

Angelakis E, Raoult D. Pathogenicity and treatment of *Bartonella* infections. *Int J Antimicrob Agents.* 2014;44(1):16–25.

A6.18   **Answer A: Anthrax**

Anthrax is one of the oldest diseases of grazing animals and was responsible for the deaths of hundreds and thousands of livestock prior to the twentieth century when effective veterinary and human public health programs brought it under control. Robert Koch first identified the bacteria that causes anthrax in 1875 and his experiments with this microbe helped elucidate the role of microbes in causing illness. Anthrax associated with injection of heroin use does not manifest like classic anthrax (cutaneous, inhalational or gastrointestinal) Anthrax produces a toxin comprising three components: protective antigen (PA), lethal factor (LF) and oedema factor (OF). The PA combines with the OF that leads to significant oedema. Early recognition is vital as it progresses rapidly and has a high mortality. Anthrax spores survive for long periods of time in the environment after release, hence appropriate disposal of contaminated tissue, equipment and clothes is vital, as is the handling of biological samples. Person-to-person spread of anthrax has not been reported. There was an outbreak of injectional anthrax in the United Kingdom from 2009 to 2010 with a high case fatality.

Further Reading

Berger T, Kassirer M, Aran AA. Injectional anthrax – new presentation of an old disease. *Euro Surveill.* 2014;19(32):pii:20877.

A6.19   **Answer D: Hepatitis E virus**

Hepatitis E virus (HEV) infection usually causes an acute self-limiting illness, which requires no therapy. However, numerous studies from low- and middle-income countries have demonstrated an excess mortality among expectant mothers who acquire the infection. Mortality can be as high as 20–25%, particularly if it occurs in the third trimester. While the pathophysiology remains unclear, the most common modes of death are haemorrhage or eclampsia or development of fulminant hepatic failure. Stillbirths can occur, as can vertical transmission. A chronic form of HEV can also occur among immunocompromised patients, including those with solid organ transplants, haematological malignancies and people living with HIV. In these individuals, it results in rapidly progressive cirrhosis. HEV has also been associated with extrahepatic manifestations, including renal injury and several neurological syndromes. Chronic infection should be treated by reducing immunosuppression where possible and antiviral therapy may on occasion be indicated.

CMV and EBV may both cause an infectious mononucleosis-like syndrome and when acquired in adults may cause a mild-to-moderate transaminitis, but not in the range of this patient. CMV has prognostic implications for the foetus, but the long-term implications for the mother from this virus, or from EBV, are not marked. Similarly, rubella virus can cause a mild transaminitis and has implications for the foetus, but the prognosis for the mother is not poor. Hepatitis A virus causes an acute self-limiting hepatitis, with full recovery being the norm. While mortality from fulminant liver failure in HAV does increase with age, it is still overall low. Vertical transmission of HAV is rare. Management of HAV in pregnancy is supportive, and no specific management is needed in pregnant women.

Further Reading

Kamar N, Dalton HR, Abravanel F, Izopet J. Hepatitis E virus infection. *Clin Microbiol Rev.* 2014;27(1):116–138.

A6.20 Answer C: Parainfluenza virus 1

Laryngotracheobronchitis (croup) can be caused by both bacterial and viral pathogens, but is most commonly caused by parainfluenza virus (usually type 1 or 3). It can also less frequently be caused by influenza, respiratory syncytial virus, human metapneumovirus, coronavirus and rhinovirus. It usually presents in children between 6 months of age and 3 years, but can on occasion occur in older children. It is characterised with a usually rapid-onset barking cough, stridor and fever. This arises from inflammation of the upper airway mucosa, particularly in the subglottic region. Symptoms are often worse at night and can also be exacerbated when the child is agitated. Symptoms usually last only 2–3 days. Management is supportive, with steroids being indicated in mild, moderate and severe disease, with the addition of nebulised adrenaline in the latter group. Patients with mild disease may then be discharged, but those with moderate or severe disease need a period of observation. Delineating the cause of the croup is particularly relevant during winter peaks of this disease, where side room availability may be breached and cohorting may be necessary. In these cases, only children with the same viral pathogen should be cohorted together.

Further Reading

Bjornson CL, Johnson DW. Croup in children. *Canadian Med Assoc J.* 2013;185(15):1317–1323.

Cherry JD. Croup. *N Engl J Med.* 2008;358:384–391.

A6.21 Answer D: Coxsackie virus B

Coxsackie viruses are RNA viruses and form part of the genus enterovirus, along with echovirus and polio. Coxsackie virus is divided into group A and group B viruses. At least 23 serotypes (1–22, 24) of group A and 6 serotypes (1–6) of group B are recognised. Coxsackie A viruses frequently infect and cause inflammation in mucous membranes, causing herpangina, conjunctivitis and hand-foot-and-mouth disease. Coxsackie B viruses tend to infect and cause inflammation in viscera, including the pancreas and liver in the abdomen, and the heart and pleura in the thorax. Both Coxsackie A and B viruses can cause non-specific febrile illnesses, rashes, upper respiratory tract disease and aseptic meningitis. Adenovirus most commonly causes illness of the respiratory system, gastroenteritis, kerato-conjunctivitis, cystitis and rash illness. ECHO (Enteric Cytopathic Human Orphan) viruses are also from the genus enterovirus, and while most infections cause only a mild self-limiting rash, echovirus can cause a myocarditis or aseptic meningitis.

Further Reading
Imazio M, Gaita F, LeWinter M. Evaluation and treatment of pericarditis: a systematic review. *JAMA.* 2015;314(14):1498–1506.

A6.22   Answer E: 40% of foetuses become infected with cytomegalovirus
Cytomegalovirus (CMV) primary infection is usually asymptomatic but can produce a spectrum of diseases ranging from mild fever, through an infectious mononucleosis-like syndrome, through to an adenopathy/hepatitis presentation. CMV in the immunocompromised can be much more severe, and can occur as either a new primary acquisition or as a re-activation. CMV in pregnancy leads to approximately 40% of foetuses becoming infected, 10% of these show symptoms of congenital CMV infections at birth which can be multisystem. Long-term effects may include sensorineural hearing loss, developmental delay and visual impairment. Of the remaining 90% ostensibly asymptomatic, 5–15% are at risk of developing long-term effects including sensorineural deafness. The most common infectious cause of congenital cataracts is rubella, although other herpesviridae have been associated with them less frequently, as have syphilis and toxoplasmosis. Parvovirus is most frequently associated with hydrops foetalis.

Further Reading
Naing ZW, Scott GM, Shand A, Hamilton ST, van Zuylen WJ, Basha J, Hall B, Craig ME, Rawlinson WD. Congenital cytomegalovirus infection in pregnancy: a review of prevalence, clinical features, diagnosis and prevention. *Aust N Z J Obstet Gynaecol.* 2016;56(1):9–18.

A6.23   Answer B: *Vibrio vulnificus*
V. vulnificus causes an infection often incurred after eating seafood, although bacteria can also enter the body through open wounds when swimming or wading in infected waters or via puncture wounds from the spines of fish such as tilapia. Patients with liver diseases appear particularly vulnerable to severe infection. Symptoms include vomiting, diarrhoea and a blistering dermatitis that is sometimes mistaken for pemphigus or pemphigoid. *V. parahaemolyticum* is acquired through ingestion of raw or undercooked seafood and causes acute gastroenteritis. Wound infections can occur but are less common than seafood-borne disease.

S. minus is associated with rat-bite fever. Skin lesions produced by *M. marinum* infections are often multiple with clusters of superficial painful or painless nodules or papules particularly over cooler parts of the body such as the extremities. Lesions appear after an incubation period of about 2–4 weeks. *E. rhusiopathiae* is a Gram-positive bacillus, which most commonly presents as mild cutaneous erysipeloid, although it can cause an indolent cellulitis, more commonly in individuals who handle fish and raw meat and often gains entry through abrasions on the hand.

Further Reading

Daniels NA. *Vibrio vulnificus* oysters: pearls and perils. *Clin Infect Dis.* 2011;52(6):788–792.

A6.24 Answer A: *Bartonella hensleae*

B. henselae and *B. clarridgeiae* are rod-shaped, Gram-negative bacteria spread by kittens with fleas (*Ctenocephalides felis*) serving as the vector. Classic cat scratch disease presents as tender and swollen regional lymph nodes. There may be a papule at the site of initial infection. While some patients have fever and other systemic symptoms, many do not. Incubation is typically 7–14 days but can be as long as 2 months. Most cases are benign and self-limiting, but lymphadenopathy may persist for several months. The prognosis is generally favourable but complications include Perniaud's syndrome (a granulomatous conjunctivitis) and optic neuritis. Azithromycin, ciprofloxacin and doxycycline have been used successfully. *B. bacilliformis* is the etiologic agent of the sand flea spread Carrion's disease or Oroya fever and Verruga peruana or Peruvian wart. *B. rochalimae* causes a similar disease in South America. *B. quintana* is the cause of the louse-borne Trench Fever. *S. moniliformis* along with *S. minus* is a cause of rat-bite fever.

Further Reading

Mazur-Melewska K, Mania A, Kemnitz P, Figlerowicz M, Służewski W. Cat-scratch disease: a wide spectrum of clinical pictures. *Postepy Dematol Alergol.* 2015;32(3):216–220.

A6.25 Answer A: *Capnocytophagia canimorsus*

The two most likely organisms from this case are *C. canimorsus* and *P. multocida* due to the severity of sepsis. *B. fragilis* would be unusual to cause severe sepsis but implicated in abscesses. *S. pyogenes* is Gram-positive. *P. multocida* often grows well on blood agar, but *C. canimorsus* is difficult to grow and often appears first on chocolate agar 48–72 hours incubation enriched with carbon dioxide. It is oxidase and catalase positive. Originally called dysgonic fermenter-2 (DF-2), it is normal flora of dogs and cats. *C. canimorsus* can cause cellulitis, endocarditis and meningitis associated with severe sepsis. Most cases are associated with underlying immune dysfunction such as splenectomy or liver disease. As with *P. multocida* it responds well to beta-lactam-beta-lactamase combination antibiotics such as co-amoxiclav, which is the treatment of choice. Flucloxacillin is inappropriate for treatment of dog and cat bites. Other active antibiotics include clindamycin, linezolid, doxycycline, carbapenems and chloramphenicol.

Further Reading

Oehler RL, Velez AP, Mizrachi M, Lamarche J, Gompf S. Bite-related and septic syndromes caused by cats and dogs. *Lancet Infect Dis.* 2009;9:439–447.

A6.26 Answer D: Permethrin 5% cream

The condition is classical scabies. It is likely that the patient acquired the disease through casual sexual contact. The differential diagnosis would include dermatitis, psoriasis, folliculitis and secondary syphilis. Cutaneous larva migrans can present with itching and wavy elevations but the lesions occur mainly on areas that have had contact with the beach, and genital lesions are rare. Scabies is caused by the human mite Sarcoptes scabiei var hominis. They burrow into the skin and lay eggs before dying. This causes the classic signs of burrows or tracks which are intensely itchy and worse at night. Often these are found in the interdigital spaces. First-line treatment for immunocompetent individuals is permethrin 5% cream, which is carefully applied to the whole body. Benyzl benzoate is no longer recommended as it is not as effective as permethrin. Crusted (Norwegian) scabies is a severe form of scabies in the immunosuppressed, and secondary bacterial infection is common. Crusted scabies should be treated with a combination of permethrin cream and oral ivermectin.

Further Reading
Salavastru CM, Chosidow O, Boffa MJ, Janier M, Tiplica GS. European guideline for the management of scabies. *J Eur Acad Dermatol Venereol.* 2017;31(8):1248–1253.

A6.27 Answer C: Erythromycin orally
Vertical transmission of *C. trachomatis* can occur via direct contact with the infected maternal genital tract. Common manifestations are opthalmia neonatorum and pneumonia. Infection may be asymptomatic. Conjunctivitis generally develops 5–12 days after birth but pneumonia occurs weeks later. Diagnosis is usually clinical and gonorrhoea must be ruled out. Although NAAT for this indication is unvalidated, it is often undertaken. The swab should be taken from the everted eyes to try and obtain conjunctival cells and not exudate alone. Treatment should be oral erythromycin for 14 days but azithromycin may be an effective alternative. Doxycycline should not be administered to neonates and ceftriaxone would be suitable for a gonococcal infection.

Further Reading
Nwokolo NC, Dragovic B, Patel S, Tong CY, Barker G, Radcliffe K. 2015 UK national guidelines for the management of infection with *Chlamydia trachomatis. Int J STD AIDS.* 2016;27 (4):251–267.

A6.28 Answer D: *Trichomonas vaginalis*
T. vaginalis (TV) is a flagellated protozoon. Transmission is sexual and up to 50% of female and male infections are asymptomatic. Vaginal and penile discharge can occur. Complications in pregnancy include preterm labour and low birth weight. Microscopy from swabs can detect motile trichomonads by light microscopy, which is best read within 10 minutes of sampling by wet prep. Point-of-care tests and NAATs are available for diagnosis. Treatment should be with a nitroimidazole and the partner should be treated simultaneously. Metronidazole is first-line therapy and should be used in pregnancy.

Further Reading
Sherrard J, Ison C, Moody J. United Kingdom National Guideline on the management of *Trichomonas vaginalis* 2014. *Int J STD AIDS.* 2014;25(8):541–549.

A6.29 Answer B: Treat mother with benzathine penicillin intramuscularly and baby with intravenous benzylpenicillin
Although it is difficult to ascertain the exact timing of the acquisition of syphilis, the treatment of choice for an adult with either primary, secondary or early late syphilis is benzathine penicillin G 2.4 million units once intramuscularly. This is preferred to procaine penicillin which is a good alternative. In penicillin allergy, doxycycline, ceftriaxone or azithromycin are recommended.

Infants born to mothers who have untreated syphilis, even if clinically normal, should be treated. If the mothers had inadequate treatment (including treatment within 30 days) or syphilis that was treated with non-penicillin regimens, it is recommended to treat the baby with either intravenous benzylpenicillin 100,000–150,000 U/kg/day for 10–15 days or procaine penicillin 50,000 U/kg/day single dose intramuscularly for 10–15 days.

Further Reading

WHO Guidelines Approved by the Guidelines Review Committee. WHO Guidelines for the Treatment of *Treponema pallidum* (Syphilis). Geneva: World Health Organisations. 2016. Available at: www.who.int/reproductivehealth/publications/rtis/syphilis-treatment-guidelines/en/

A6.30   Answer C: Oral suppressive therapy with acyclovir 400 mg twice daily

It is recommended that all episodes of genital herpes infection should be treated. Aciclovir is the preferred choice of agent over valaciclovir or famciclovir due to cost.

For adults with recurrent clinical episodes that are frequent, severe or cause distress, it is suggested to choose suppression therapy rather than episodic therapy with review at 1 year. Frequency of 4–6 times a year or more should warrant suppression. This is the same for individuals living with HIV or immunocompromised. The evidence for suppressive therapy compared to episodic therapy (treatment within 24 hours of symptoms starting) for HSV infection is of moderate quality for acyclovir and valaciclovir but low quality for famciclovir.

Further Reading

WHO Guidelines Approved by the Guidelines Review Committee. WHO Guidelines for the Treatment of *Genital Herpes Simplex Virus*. Geneva: World Health Organisations. 2016. Available at: www.who.int/reproductivehealth/publications/rtis/genital-HSV-treatment-guidelines/en/

A6.31   Answer C: Toxoplasma

Microcephaly can be caused by genetic abnormalities or by infection during gestation. Several infections have been implicated in causing microcephaly, including rubella, cytomegalovirus, *T. gondii*, Herpes simplex virus and Zika virus. Cases are more severe when acquired during the first trimester. While rubella vaccination is part of the UK childhood vaccination schedule, the others currently have no effective vaccine available. Most women, particularly in low- and middle-income countries have already been exposed to cytomegalovirus and *T. gondii* during adolescence, but this is not universal. In this case the CMV serology represents previously acquired infection, and the negative PCR demonstrates she has not reactivated her CMV at this stage of her pregnancy.

Pregnant women infected with *T. gondii* generally do not have clinical manifestations. However, infection can lead to intrauterine growth restriction, premature birth, hepatosplenomegaly and neurological abnormalities, including microcephaly and hydrocephalus as well as chorioretinitis. Interpreting serology for toxoplasmosis is complicated by prolonged persistence of IgM. Toxoplasma IgG becomes positive within 2–3 weeks of infection, but remains positive lifelong. The avidity of the toxoplasma IgG can be tested, however, and helps indicate whether the infection was acquired less than, or greater than, 12–16 weeks ago. Toxoplasma IgM can persist in the chronic stage of infections and have been documented up to 12 years after infection. Limited data suggest that treatment of infected women during pregnancy may be beneficial to the foetus.

Spiramycin has been used to prevent materno-foetal transmission but once foetal disease is established, as in this case, treatment will not reverse the established disease process.

Further Reading

Devakumar D, Bamford A, Ferreira MU, Broad J, Rosch RE, Groce N, Breuer J, Cardoso MA, Copp AJ, Alexandre P, Rodrigues LC, Abubakar I. Infectious causes of microcephaly: epidemiology, pathogenesis, diagnosis, and management. *Lancet Infect Dis*. 2018;18(1):1–13.

A6.32   Answer D: *Treponema pallidum*

Primary syphilis is typically acquired via direct sexual contact with infectious lesions on mucous membranes (including genital, rectal or oral). Typically, incubation is between 1 and 4 weeks, although dome lesions have been documented to occur up to 3 months after exposure. Primary syphilis is characterised by a single painless ulcer (chancre), but on occasion there may be multiple lesions apparent. Adenopathy can occur, but does not ulcerate. The ulcers usually resolve by 4–6 weeks. If primary syphilis remains untreated, the characteristic rash of secondary syphilis may then occur 2 weeks to 2 months later. The rash is maculopapular and may affect any or all of the body, including the palms and soles, but is not pruritic. There may be associated fever and disseminated adenopathy.

The main differential for a painless genital ulcer is Donovanosis (or granuloma inguinale). This is caused by *Klebsiella granulomatis*. It is characterised by one or more small, painless nodules on the genitals 1 week to 1 month after sexual contact. Unlike in syphilis, however, these nodules may burst leaving oozing lesions, as may local lymph nodes. Lymphogranuloma venereum (LGV) is a sexually transmitted disease caused by invasive serovars (L1, L2 or L3) of *Chlamydia trachomatis*. Primary LGV may also present as a self-limited painless genital ulcer that occurs at the contact site several days and up to 2 weeks after sexual contact. The ulcer is frequently asymptomatic and there is infrequent adenopathy. This primary ulcer usually heals after a few days. There may be associated erythema nodosum. Chancroid (caused by *H. ducreyi*) and herpes simplex infection cause painful ulcers and gonorrhoea causes a discharge.

Further Reading

WHO Guidelines Approved by the Guidelines Review Committee. WHO Guidelines for the Treatment of *Treponema pallidum* (Syphilis). Geneva: World Health Organisations. 2016. Available at: www.who.int/reproductivehealth/publications/rtis/syphilis-treatment-guidelines/en/

A6.33   Answer A: *Fusobacterium necrophorum*

F. necrophorum is the causative agent of Lemierre's syndrome. Infection occurs primarily in the head and neck region in 85–90% of cases but it can also start as otitis, mastoiditis, sinusitis or parotitis. During the primary infection, *F. necrophorum* colonises the infection site and the infection spreads to the parapharyngeal space. The bacteria then invades the peritonsillar blood vessels where they can spread to the internal jugular vein causing a thrombus, and subsequent embolisation. disease then spreads frequently to the lungs (causing cavitating lesions and effusion), followed by the joints (knee, hip, sternoclavicular joint, shoulder and elbow). Production of lipopolysaccharide can lead to marked inflammation while hemagglutinin causes platelet aggregation that can lead to diffuse intravascular coagulation and thrombocytopenia. *F. necrophorum* is a fusiform, Gram-negative anaerobe that is usually sensitive to penicillin and metronidazole. *Streptococcus pyogenes* remains highly sensitive to penicillin, therefore, high dose benzylpenicillin still remains a suitable choice for patients presenting with sore throat and sepsis.

Further Reading

Kuppalli K, Livorsi D, Talati NJ, Osborn M. Lemierre's syndrome due to *Fusobacterium necrophorum*. *Lancet Infect Dis.* 2012;12(10):808–815.

Riordan T. Human infection with *Fusobacterium necrophorum* (Necrobacillosis), with a focus on Lemierre's syndrome. *Clin Microbiol Rev.* 2007;20(4):622–659.

A6.34   Answer D: Benzylpenicillin and gentamicin

Current NICE guidance for empirical antibiotic therapy for suspected early-onset sepsis in a neonate recommends intravenous benzylpenicillin with gentamicin, unless local bacterial resistance data indicates a different regime. Antibiotics should then be tailored to isolated pathogens. Lumbar puncture should be performed in all neonates with signs of sepsis. Duration of antibiotic treatment with a positive blood culture or negative cultures should be 7 days unless the baby is not fully recovered or an identified organism needs longer treatment. Shortest possible antibiotic courses are advised due to the increased risk of necrotising enterocolitis with antibiotic exposure.

Further Reading

National Institute for Health and Care Excellence. Neonatal infection: antibiotics for prevention and treatment NICE guidance. 2012. Available at: www.nice.org.uk/guidance/cg149

A6.35   Answer A: No need to screen partner

The venereal disease reference laboratory (VDRL) test and the rapid plasma regain (RPR) test can both be positive in the absence of syphilis. Specifically, these tests can be indicative of a false positive VDRL in infectious mononucleosis, systemic lupus erythematosus, antiphospholipid antibody syndrome, acute viral hepatitis and as a result of pregnancy itself.

If the treponemal fluorescent antibody test is positive, or if a *Treponema pallidum* haemagglutination (TPHA) is positive, then the positive VDRL test would be indicative of active syphilis. Syphilis can be transmitted from the mother to the foetus in the primary, secondary or early latent phase of infection, but usually occurs after the 18th week of pregnancy. However, the majority of pregnant women with syphilis are asymptomatic and are diagnosed through routine antenatal screening. Infection during pregnancy can result in miscarriage, foetal growth restriction, preterm labour or congenital syphilis of the new-born. The most common feature of congenital syphilis is interstitial keratitis, although it can also manifest with hepatosplenomegaly, musculoskeletal abnormalities, such as periostitis or osteochondritis, ascites or hydrops.

Further Reading

Peeling RW, Mabey D, Kamb ML, Chen XS, Radolf JD, Benzaken AS. Syphilis. *Nat Rev Dis Primers.* 2017;3:17073.

A6.36   Answer A: Culture on Lowenstein-Jensen at 30°C

The most likely diagnosis in this case is fish tank granuloma, a dermatological infection caused by *Mycobacterium marinum*. Although the infection is usually limited to the periphery of limbs, in addition to the red/violaceous nodules or plaques which characterise the cutaneous lesions of this disease, it can also cause a tenosynovitis, osteomyelitis or arthritis in the affected area. Biopsies of infected areas will demonstrate necrotising granulomas on histopathological examination. Microbiological confirmation will only be possible, however, if the culture conditions are facilitated. On primary isolation, *M. marinum* grows on Lowenstein-Jensen sloped culture medium at 30–33°C in 7–21 days. Unlike *M. tuberculosis*, most strains of *M. marinum* will not grow at the usual incubation temperature of 37°C. *M. marinum* colonies are cream in colour but are photochromogenic, meaning they change colour on exposure to light, in the case of *M. marinum* to yellow. There is no universally accepted treatment regime, but trimethoprim-sulfamethoxazole, minocycline, rifampicin or ciprofloxacin-based regimes have been demonstrated to work in small series of patients. While surgery should be avoided, local hyperthermic therapy and photodynamic therapy have been tried and found to improve cutaneous lesions.

Further Reading

Gonzalez-Santiago TM, MD, Drage LA. Nontuberculous mycobacteria skin and soft tissue infections. *Dermat Clin.* 2015;33(3):563–577.

Public Health England. UK Standards for Microbiology Investigations B 40: Investigation of Specimens for *Mycobacterium* species. 2014. Available at: www.gov.uk/government/publications/smi-b-40-investigation-of-specimens-for-mycobacterium-species

A6.37   Answer A: *Bordetella pertussis*

B. pertussis is a Gram-negative cocco-bacillus which causes whooping cough, and despite being vaccine preventable, has been having a resurgence in many regions since 2012. The clinical case definition describes a syndrome of paroxysms of coughing, often with an inspiratory whoop, which lasts for at least 2 weeks. This is often preceded by a more general catarrhal phase which lasts for a week or more. There may be vomiting after the coughing episodes. There should be no other identifiable causes. In infants, there is often a lack of a fever, but there may be a lymphocytosis, particularly at the end of the catarrhal phase. Diagnosis is predominantly through PCR for *B. pertussis*, which can be on an upper respiratory tract sample. Culture can be undertaken for *B. pertussis* from a variety of samples including pernasal swabs, nasopharyngeal aspirates, as well as from nasopharyngeal swabs (preferably with a rayon swab). Samples should be collected in the first 2 weeks of the cough or the sensitivity of the test decreases markedly as viable bacteria become significantly fewer. Samples should be inoculated onto a charcoal blood agar with cephalexin and incubated aerobically for 7 days.

Further Reading

Hartzell JD, Blaylock JM. Whooping cough in 2014 and beyond: an update and review. *Chest.* 2014;146(1):205–214.

A6.38 Answer A: Amoxicillin should be given for dental prophylaxis in patients with metallic valves

Antibiotic prophylaxis for infective endocarditis was developed on observations and animal studies, suggesting bacteria adhere to the endocardium following procedures that may result in transient bacteraemia. This led to recommendations for widespread prophylaxis for patients with underlying cardiac conditions. Increasing understanding of the pathogenesis of endocarditis led to restriction of prophylaxis based on risk-benefit analyses. Most case–control studies did not report association, and risk is low with dental procedures, transient bacteraemias occur on daily activities, such as teeth brushing, antibiotic administration carries risk of allergy and resistance. NICE guidelines took these principles and recommended no antibiotic prophylaxis for any circumstances. The European guidelines retain antibiotic prophylaxis for high-risk procedures such as dental surgery for high-risk patients. Patients deemed at high risk include patients with any prosthetic valve; patients with a previous episode of IE; patients with congenital heart disease (cyanotic disease or where prosthetic material placed). Amoxicillin is the recommended antibiotic unless penicillin allergic where clindamycin is advocated.

Further Reading

Habib G Lancellotti P, Antunes MJ, Bongiorni MG, Casalta JP, Del Zotti F, Dulgheru R, El Khoury G, Erba PA, Iung B, Miro JM, Mulder BJ, Plonska-Gosciniak E, Price S, Roos-Hesselink J, Snygg-Martin U, Thuny F, Tornos Mas P, Vilacosta I, Zamorano JL and the ESC Scientific Document Group. 2015 ESC guidelines for the management of infective endocarditis: The Task Force for the Management of Infective Endocarditis of the European Society of Cardiology (ESC). *Eur Heart J.* 2015;36(44):3075–3128.

A6.39 Answer E: *Staphylococcus epidermidis* in three different samples

Prosthetic joints can cause pain for mechanical reasons, as well as from infection. Where they are infected, this can be either in the acute phase or more chronic. Early infections usually arise from inoculation of organisms during surgery. Late infections can also arise from inoculation (usually of indolent organisms) during surgery or can seed into the prosthetic joint during bacteraemias from another cause.

Semi-quantitative white cell counts on joint fluid is a useful test for differentiating inflammatory from non-inflammatory arthritidies and has been suggested to have a specificity of 93%; however, it is not diagnostic. Furthermore, the organisms that cause prosthetic joint infections are frequently the same as those that contaminate microbiological samples. This can make interpretation difficult when only one or two samples are submitted for culture. It is, therefore, recommended that at least five samples are recommended, and that these samples are collected using separate surgical instruments and not pooled in the laboratory, but instead cultured separately. Growth of an indistinguishable organism from two samples is reported as having a 71% sensitivity and a 97% specificity, while three samples with growth of an indistinguishable organism (as in this case) has a 66% sensitivity and a 99.6% specificity.

Further Reading

Public Health England. UK Standards for Microbiology Investigations B 44: Investigation of orthopaedic implant associated infections. 2016. Available at: www.gov.uk/government/publications/smi-b-44-investigation-of-prosthetic-joint-infection-samples

Qu X, Zhai Z, Liu X, Li H, Wu C, Li Y, Li H, Zhu Z, Qin A, Dai K. Evaluation of white cell count and differential in synovial fluid for diagnosing infections after total hip or knee arthroplasty. *PLoS ONE.* 2014;9(1):e84751.

A6.40 Answer C: Legionella urinary antigen should be undertaken on all severely ill patients

British thoracic society guidelines state investigations for legionella infection are recommended for all patients with severe community acquired pneumonia (CAP), for other patients with specific risk factors and for all patients with CAP during outbreaks. Rapid testing and reporting for legionella urine antigen should be available in at least one laboratory per region. Legionella culture should be specifically requested by clinicians on laboratory request forms from patients with severe CAP or where legionella infection is suspected on epidemiological grounds. Legionella cultures should be routinely performed on invasive respiratory samples (e.g. obtained by bronchoscopy) from patients with CAP (on buffered charcoal yeast extract (BCYE) agar). *Chlamydophila* antigen or PCR detection tests should be available for invasive respiratory samples from patients with severe CAP or where there is a strong suspicion of psittacosis. Recommendations in the BTS guideline overlap with a more recent NICE guideline. Of the 36 recommendations that overlap, only 5 differ but this includes legionella urinary antigen testing. The NICE guidelines recommend to consider legionella urinary antigen testing for patients with moderate as well as high severity CAP.

Further Reading

Lim WS, Baudouin SV, George RC, Hill AT, Jamieson C, Le Jeune I, Macfarlane JT, Read RC, Roberts HJ, Levy ML, Wani M, Woodhead MA. BTS guidelines for the management of community acquired pneumonia in adults: update 2009. *Thorax.* 2009;64(S3):iii1–55.

National Institute for Health and Care Excellence. Pneumonia (including community acquired pneumonia). 2014. Available at: www.nice.org.uk/guidance/cg191

A6.41 Answer C: *Escherichia coli*

Although it varies a little by region and by patient age, *E. coli* remains the most frequent bacterial cause of lower urinary tract infection, and in the community-acquired case in this question, *E. coli* is likely to be the causative organism on 70–90% of occasions. In healthcare-associated urinary tract infections, *E. coli* is also the single most common cause, but accounts for only approximately 50% of cases. *E. coli* is a Gram-negative rod which is indole positive, which enables relatively easy presumptive identification in the laboratory, but other biochemical aspects of *E. coli* have also been utilised to enable rapid identification, including beta-D-glucoronidase.

S. saprophyticus can cause cystitis (and on occasion pyelonephritis) and is thought to account for 5–15% of cases in young women. It is particularly associated with women who are sexually active. *S. saprophyticus* can be distinguished from other coagulase-negative staphylococci (which are usually contaminants) as it is novobicin resistant. The other Enterobacteriales, including *Klebsiella* spp., *Proteus* spp. and *Enterobacter* spp., are more common in healthcare-associated and catheter-associated urinary tract infections. *Enterococcus* spp. is a frequent contaminant of urine specimens, but is acknowledged to cause cystitis in a small number of cases.

Further Reading

Gupta K, Grigoryan L, Trautner B. Urinary tract infection. *Ann Intern Med.* 2017;167(7):ITC49–ITC64.

A6.42   **Answer A: *Staphylococcus aureus***

S. aureus is a rare cause of UTI (0.5%–1% of positive urine cultures), and it can be a contaminant or a colonising bacteria of urinary catheterisation. If there is no obvious urinary source, then it is important to rule out *S. aureus* bacteraemia with spill over into the urine and blood cultures should be considered. *S. Typhi* and *M. tuberculosis* would be very unusual to isolate from urine. *S. saprophyticus* and *E. coli* are common uropathogens but are considerably more likely to cause urinary tract infections through ascending the urethra than from haematological dissemination.

Further Reading

Tong SY, Davis JS, Eichenberger E, Holland TL, Fowler VG Jr. *Staphylococcus aureus* infections: epidemiology, pathophysiology, clinical manifestations, and management. *Clin Microbiol Rev.* 2015;28(3):603–661.

A6.43   **Answer B: Urethral distance is shorter in women**

Females are more likely to have urinary tract infections than males because their urethra is shorter, enabling easier ascent of bacteria into the bladder. The risk is higher still among sexually active women, and particularly those who use diaphragms as a method of birth control and those who have undergone menopause. Vulvo-vaginal conditions do propagate bacterial growth, but this is usually (over 90%) *Lactobacillus* spp., which produces hydrogen peroxide and is likely to suppress *E. coli* vaginal colonisation. Post-coital micturition decreases the likelihood of getting urinary tract infections among those who are sexually active, and should be advocated to those who have had an episode already.

Further Reading

Stapleton AE. The vaginal microbiota and urinary tract infection. 2016;4(6):10.1128.

A6.44   **Answer A: Use of a spermicidal gel**

The interaction between specific bacteria causing urinary tract infections and the uroendothelium characteristics underlies the pathogenesis of this disease. Pathogen-related characteristics which increase the frequency of urinary tract infections include *E. coli* virulence factors (such as outer membrane vesicles). Host characteristics which increase the frequency of urinary tract infections include behavioural risk factors (such as frequent sexual intercourse, use of only oral contraceptive without a condom and use of spermicides).

Avoiding anal sex, always using a condom and post-coital micturition can all decrease the frequency of urinary tract infections among those with recurrent disease. Cranberry juice consumption has long been considered to decrease the frequency of urinary tract infections, but this has not been borne out in a Cochrane review, but neither was there evidence that it increased the frequency of urinary tract infections.

Further Reading

Flores-Mireles AL, Walker JN, Caparon M, Hultgren SJ. Urinary tract infections: epidemiology, mechanisms of infection and treatment options. *Nat Rev Microbiol.* 2015;13(5):269–284.

Jepson R, Craig J, Williams G. Cranberry products and prevention of urinary tract infections. *JAMA.* 2013;310(13):1395–1396.

A6.45   **Answer A: Urethral catheterisation**

In older males without a catheter, residual urine volumes of up to 20 mL can be present, in which bacteria can proliferate. Asymptomatic bacteriuria among older males varies between 10% and 40%. This does not necessitate antimicrobial treatment. Catheters are not uncommon among older males, usually inserted because of urinary retention or symptoms of bladder outlet obstruction arising from change in prostatic size – usually enlargement from benign prostatic hyperplasia. All urinary catheters increase the frequency of urinary tract infections, but urethral catheters are typically associated with a higher rate of infection than suprapubic catheters. In older males with catheters, colonisation of the catheter is almost universal within several days of insertion. While this colonisation does not necessarily represent infection, it may precede it.

Prostatic secretions usually inhibit bacterial growth, but secretions may be reduced in older men. Vesico-ureteric reflux is associated with more frequent urinary tract infections in children and adolescents, but is not usually a feature among older men.

Further Reading

Schaeffer AJ, Nicolle LE. Urinary tract infections in older men. *N Eng J Med.* 2016;374:562–571.

A6.46   **Answer A: Catheter-associated urinary tract infections account for up to 40% nosocomial infections**

Catheter-associated urinary tract infections represent a significant burden on healthcare, manifesting as dysuria, pyuria or discomfort, through to overt sepsis with resultant bacteraemias. Within several days of a catheter being inserted, it becomes colonised with organisms, and this is commonly polymicrobial. Cather stream urines, therefore, are frequently reported as culturing mixed growth, but in the absence of symptoms does not necessarily warrant antimicrobial treatment. While initial insertion of a urethral catheter may warrant peri-insertion antimicrobial prophylaxis in some cases, ongoing antimicrobials for those with indwelling urinary catheters is not indicated as a matter of course.

Further Reading

Schaeffer AJ, Nicolle LE. Urinary tract infections in older men. *N Eng J Med.* 2016;374:562–571.

A6.47   **Answer C: Cognitive decline**

Long-term memory problems, including dementia and cognitive decline, can make diagnosing urinary tract infections in older individuals difficult. While asymptomatic bacteriuria in older individuals does not warrant antimicrobial therapy, sometimes the only symptom can be increased confusion. In those who have a baseline of chronic confusion, this can, therefore, leave diagnostic complexity around whether to treat fluctuations in the level of confusion in the context of a positive urine dipstick. In these cases other causes of fluctuating confusion should be ruled out before empiric antimicrobials are commenced. It must also be noted, however, that cognitive decline itself is a risk factor for urinary tract infections.

Vaginal lactobacilli have been suggested to be protective against urinary tract infections, and it is decreased commensal lactobacilli which is associated with more frequent urinary tract infections. Hormone replacement therapy is associated with decreased rates of urinary tract infections. Vesicoureteric reflux is a risk factor for urinary tract infections in children and young adults. Although proteinuria may be associated with urinary tract infections, the relationship between these two findings is not clearly defined.

Further Reading

Mody L, Juthani-Mehta M. Urinary tract infections in older women: a clinical review. *JAMA*. 2014;311(8):844–854.

Ninan S, Walton C, Barlow G. Investigation of suspected urinary tract infection in older people. *BMJ*. 2014;349:g4070.

A6.48   Answer B: Asymptomatic bacteriuria is diagnosed with a bacterial count higher than 10^5 CFU/mL

Pregnancy distorts the pelvic anatomy, including the bladder, and this alters the significance of asymptomatic bacteriuria compared to non-pregnant individuals. The prevalence of asymptomatic bacteriuria is approximately 2–10%, but those in whom this is detected have a 20- to 30-fold increased risk of going on to develop an upper urinary tract infection compared to pregnant women without bacteriuria. Furthermore, pregnant women with asymptomatic bacteriuria are more likely to deliver low-birth-weight or premature babies.

However, because of the potential for vulvo-vaginal contamination of mid-stream urine samples, it is recommended that a second urine culture be used to confirm the presence of true asymptomatic bacteriuria before treatment is commenced. Where treatment is indicated, amoxicillin or nitrofurantoin are the preferred choices, although cephalexin and in some cases trimethoprim (the latter usually only in the third trimester) can be used.

Further Reading

Smaill FM, Vazquez JC. Antibiotics for asymptomatic bacteriuria in pregnancy. *Cochrane Database Syst Rev*. 2015;(8):CD000490.

A6.49   Answer E: *Staphylococcus saprophyticus* urinary tract infection

Sterile pyuria can be detected after urine examination in either patients symptomatic of a urinary tract infection or from screening urine samples when investigating more systemic conditions. Cases of sterile pyuria may be infective or non-infective. Infective causes include recent (within last 2 weeks) treated UTI, a UTI with fastidious organism (including *N. gonorrhoea*), renal tract tuberculosis, *C. trachomatis* urethritis or prostatitis. Non-infective causes include interstitial nephritis, interstitial cystitis, sarcoidosis (although the pyuria in this case is lymphocytic rather than a neutrophilia), urolithiasis, renal papillary necrosis (in turn resulting from sickle-cell disease, analgesic abuse or diabetes) or a renal tract malignancy. False positives in sterile pyuria results can also arise, usually from contamination with vaginal leucocytes or from aseptic suppressing bacterial growth.

S. saprophyticus is a common cause of urinary tract infections among those who are sexually active and is easily identifiable in a urine culture. It can be distinguished from other coagulase-negative staphylococci as it is resistant to novobicin, whereas *S. epidermidis* is typically susceptible.

Further Reading

Glen P, Prashar A, Hawary A. Sterile pyuria: a practical management guide. *Br J Gen Pract*. 2016;66(644):e225–e227.

A6.50   Answer D: *Vibrio vulnificus*

V. vulnificus is a curved Gram-negative rod which is common in coastal waters, and as such can be found in some shellfish, including oysters as in this case. It can cause three main syndromes; an acute enteritis in immunocompetent patients who consume contaminated shell fish, an acute skin and skin structure infection which can present with large blisters and become necrotic in limbs (usually with pre-existing lacerations) exposed to contaminated water and then among immunocompromised patients (particularly those with liver disease) ingestion or cutaneous inoculation can lead to a fulminant septicaemia.

B. cereus is a Gram-positive rod which can cause a toxin-mediated enteritis, typically characterised by nausea and vomiting but also diarrhoea in some cases, and is associated with improperly cooled and re-heated cooked rice. Symptoms typically begin a few hours after ingestion. Non-Typhi *Salmonella* spp., such as *Salmonella* Heidelberg, are common zoonotic causes of enteritis. In particular, *Salmonella* Heidelberg has been associated with outbreaks of poultry-associated enteritis, with symptoms usually beginning several hours to several days after inoculation. Cyclosporiasis can cause an enteritis, which typically presents as diarrhoea and abdominal cramps, and is most often acquired through (human) faecal contamination of raw fruit and vegetables.

Further Reading

Horseman MA, Surani S. A comprehensive review of *Vibrio vulnificus*: an important cause of severe sepsis and skin and soft-tissue infection. *Int J Infect Dis*. 2011;15(3):157–166.

A6.51   Answer D: *Salmonella* Arizonae

Salmonella enterica subsp. *Arizonae* and *Salmonella enterica* subsp. Poona are both non-Typhi *Salmonella* spp., which have been particularly associated with reptiles, including turtles, which can shed these *Salmonella* spp. for prolonged periods (frequently over 6 months). They typically cause an enteritis, as with other non-Typhi *Salmonella* spp., and this is typically self-limiting in nature. Rarely, it can cause more serious complications including meningitis and septic arthritis.

P. shigelloides has been also been isolated from amphibians (as well as mammals and aquatic life) and can cause enteritis and lead to bacteraemia in immunocompromised patients. Of note, in laboratory diagnosis, some *P. shigelloides* share antigens with *Shigella sonnei*, and mis-diagnosis due to cross-reaction antisera to *Shigella* spp. can occur. To distinguish these two organisms biochemically, *P. shigelloides* is oxidase positive, whereas *Shigella* spp. are not. Zoonotic transmission of *Strongyloides stercoralis* has been reported (predominantly from mammals including cats and dogs) but direct transmission from soil is more common.

Further Reading

Lee YC, Hung MC, Hung SC, Wang HP, Cho HL, Lai MC, Wang JT. *Salmonella enterica* subspecies Arizonae infection of adult patients in Southern Taiwan: a case series in a non-endemic area and literature review. *BMC Infect Dis*. 2016;16:746.

A6.52 Answer A: *Shigella* spp.

Shigellosis typically presents with low-volume bloody/mucus diarrhoea, as in this case. *Shigella sonnei* is the most frequent *Shigella* spp. identified globally, and has been well documented as a cause of outbreaks among children at nursery and pre-school. It typically causes self-limiting disease and no antimicrobial treatment is usually indicated.

Enterotoxigenic *Escherichia coli* is the most common cause of travellers' diarrhoea and can cause outbreaks among children in low- and middle-income countries. It usually presents as a non-inflammatory watery diarrhoea, however, and per-rectal blood and mucus would be unusual. Norovirus and rotavirus can cause outbreaks in schools and nurseries, but usually present with short-lived nausea and vomiting, the latter may be projectile in nature, however. Treatment for both is supportive. Giardiasis usually occurs in those who have travelled to low- and middle-income countries and typically presents with offensive diarrhoea and excess eructation and flatulence. Treatment for giardiasis is usually needed and tinidazole or metronidazole are typically used.

Further Reading

Kotloff KL, Riddle MS, Platts-Mills JA, Pavlinac P, Zaidi AKM. Shigellosis. *Lancet*. 2018;391 (10122):801–812.

A6.53 Answer D: *Yersinia enterocolitica*

Y. enterocolitica is a Gram-negative bacillus, which causes a zoonotic enterocolitis, and can progress to causing a mesenteric adenitis and terminal ileitis. These latter two presentations typically present in older children, and can be misconstrued as an appendicitis, leading to unnecessary appendectomies. Yersiniosis has also been associated with several post-infectious syndromes, including a reactive arthropathy, uveitis or glomerulonephritis. Erythema nodosum post *Yersinia* spp. infection has also been reported. Yersiniosis is transmitted by faecal–oral transmission, usually from handling the carcasses of contaminated animals or from undercooked meat, such as the chitterlings in this case.

Shigellosis is not particularly associated with eating undercooked pork, and when it occurs usually causes an inflammatory diarrhoea. *Campylobacter* spp. enteritis is associated with animals and frequently presents with abdominal discomfort and bloating, but usually takes less than 5 days to present and is not usually associated with fever among immunocompetent individuals. *V. parahaemolyticus* typically enteritis after un- or under-cooked seafood.

Further Reading

Drummond N, Murphy BP, Ringwood T, Prentice MB, Buckley JF, Fanning S. *Yersinia enterocolitica*: a brief review of the issues relating to the zoonotic pathogen, public health challenges, and the pork production chain. *Foodborne Pathog Dis*. 2012;9(3):179–189.

A6.54 Answer B: *Listeria monocytogenes*

L. monocytogenes is a Gram-positive rod which usually displays haemolytic activity on blood agar (unlike most other *Listeria* spp.) and demonstrates tumbling motility at room temperature (but not at 37°C). *L. monocytogenes* is present in many dairy products, including some unpasteurised soft cheeses. In immunocompetent individuals *L. monocytogenes* ingestion in large quantities can cause a mild enteritis. However, in immunocompromised individuals, ingestion can be significantly more problematic and bacteraemia or meningitis can ensue. In early pregnancy there is a high risk of *L. monocytogenes* acquisition causing miscarriage, while after 20 weeks acquisition is associated with pre-term labour. Neonates born to mothers with *L. monocytogenes* puerperal infection may then develop neonatal sepsis and meningitis. *L. monocytogenes* is not susceptible to cephalosporins, and where infection is suspected or confirmed, amoxicillin (or ampicillin) is indicated.

Non-Typhi *Salmonella* spp. infection during pregnancy may lead to more severe maternal disease, including chorioamnionitis, and can cause trans-placental infection of the foetus. This is less likely than with *L. monocytogenes* infection. A similar disease process can arise from *P. shigelloides* acquisition during pregnancy. Tapeworm (*T. saginata* from beef, *T. solium* from pork *and Diphyllobothrium latum* from fish) infection during pregnancy does not usually present with diarrhoea and fever and does not usually present a risk for the pregnancy. Treatment with praziquantel for tapeworms must be undertaken only with caution during pregnancy, and more often treatment is delayed until the post-partum period.

Further Reading

Madjunkov M, Chaudhry S, Ito S. Listeriosis during pregnancy. *Arch Gynecol Obstet.* 2017;296(2):143–152.

A6.55   **Answer B: *Ureaplasma urealyticum***
Premature rupture of membranes can lead to chorioamnionitis and foetal (and subsequent neonatal) infection. The most common infective agent associated with preterm premature rupture of membranes is *U. urealyticum*, and it is also the most common organism associated with spontaneous preterm labour with intact membranes, although *Mycoplasma hominis, G. vaginalis, Peptostreptococcus* spp. and *Bacteroides* spp. have also been implicated. Following rupture of the membranes, the bacteria most frequently found as the cause of chorioamnionitis and foetal infection are *S. agalactiae* and *E. coli.*

Women with clinical signs of active infection (such as chorioamnionitis) should receive systemic antimicrobials likely to cover *S. agalactiae* and *E. coli.* Women with spontaneous preterm labour but who have intact membranes and who do not have signs of active infection should not routinely receive antimicrobials, as there is evidence that antimicrobials in these cases may increase the risk of functional impairment and cerebral palsy. It is currently recommended that those mothers who have preterm premature rupture of membranes do receive antimicrobials, but that this should not be co-amoxiclav (which has been associated with increased risk of necrotising enterocolitis); erythromycin is frequently given as an alternative.

Further Reading

Kenyon S, Boulvain M, Neilson J. Antibiotics for preterm rupture of membranes. *Cochrane Database Syst Rev.* 2013;(12):CD001058.

Kwak DW, Hwang HS, Kwon JY, Park YW, Kim YH. Co-infection with vaginal *Ureaplasma urealyticum* and *Mycoplasma hominis* increases adverse pregnancy outcomes in patients with preterm labour or preterm premature rupture of membranes. *J Maternal-Fetal Neonatal Med.* 2014;27(4):333–337.

A6.56   **Answer C: Treatment with amoxicillin and gentamicin is optimal even where there is low-level gentamicin resistance**

Older males (typically over 65 years of age) are the more commonly affected cohort to develop enterococcal endocarditis. It may follow enterococcal bacteraemia from a urinary source (including associated with catheters) or from a hepatobiliary infection. Young women may be affected, but frequently this is in the context of immunocompromise or pregnancy. Treatment of native-valve enterococcal endocarditis is with 4–6 weeks of intravenous antimicrobials, with beta-lactam susceptible strains preferably treated with amoxicillin plus gentamicin where there is some degree of gentamicin susceptibility retained in the strain. For those cases where there is high-level gentamicin resistance (i.e. MIC > 500 mg/L) amoxicillin plus ceftriaxone may be used (for 6 weeks). Enterococci have acquired many different genes encoding aminoglycoside-modifying enzymes, but almost all are resistant to amikacin and tobramycin, and testing is therefore not warranted. Streptomycin may be tested, and if found susceptible, some treatment algorithms advocated considering its use in conjunction with amoxicillin.

In cases of *Enterococcus faecium* endocarditis, vancomycin plus gentamicin may be used. Where there is multi-drug resistance to beta-lactams, aminoglycosides and glycopeptides, linezolid, daptomycin or quinupristin-dalfopristin may be tested for susceptibility and considered often in combination with beta-lactams. The *van* glycopeptide resistance genes confer resistance to glycopeptides among *Enterococcus* spp. with *vanA* and *vanB* conferring vancomycin high-level resistance, but while *vanA* isolates are also teicoplanin resistant, *vanB* isolates are teicoplanin susceptible. *VanC* isolates have low-level resistance to vancomycin.

Further Reading

Habib G, Lancellotti P, Antunes MJ Bongiorni MG, Casalta JP, Del Zotti F, Dulgheru R, El Khoury G, Erba PA, Iung B, Miro JM, Mulder BJ, Plonska-Gosciniak E, Price S, Roos-Hesselink J, Snygg-Martin U, Thuny F, Tornos Mas P, Vilacosta I, Zamorano JL and the ESC Scientific Document Group. 2015 ESC guidelines for the management of infective endocarditis: The Task Force for the Management of Infective Endocarditis of the European Society of Cardiology (ESC). Endorsed by: European Association for Cardio-Thoracic Surgery (EACTS), the European Association of Nuclear Medicine (EANM). *Eur Heart J*. 2015;36(44):3075–3128.

Yim J, Smith JR, Rybak MJ. Role of combination antimicrobial therapy for vancomycin-resistant *Enterococcus faecium* infections: review of the current evidence. *Pharmacotherapy*. 2017;37(5):579–592.

A6.57   Answer B: *Staphylococcus aureus*

Acute cavitating pneumonia is frequently caused by *S. aureus*, but can also be caused by *Klebsiella*, *Pseudomonas* and *Proteus* which are important healthcare-associated, Gram-negative pathogens. *S. aureus* can be isolated in respiratory samples as colonising flora; however, it can also cause devastating fulminant pneumonia. Massive polymorphonuclear leucocyte infiltration into the lungs with abscess formation is typical in severe *S. aureus* infection. Panton–Valentine leucocidin (PVL) producing *S. aureus* is commonly thought to be implicated but the minority of isolates produce PVL and another pore forming toxin called alpha-haemolysin may be more important.

Further Reading

Tong SY, Davis JS, Eichenberger E, Holland TL, Fowler VG Jr. *Staphylococcus aureus* infections: epidemiology, pathophysiology, clinical manifestations, and management. *Clin Microbiol Rev*. 2015;28(3):603–661.

A6.58 Answer B: Meropenem

The important aspect in this question is the clinical context of the patient. Fever and hypotension imply the patient is bacteraemic with severe sepsis who may be developing septic shock. An antibiotic must, therefore, be chosen which can be given by the intravenous route, which rules out nitrofurantoin. A beta-lactam antibiotic would be preferable but the resistance pattern including cefoxitin and cefuroxime suggest presence of a beta-lactamase enzyme which may include an ESBL or AmpC enzyme. Antibiotics containing beta-lactamase inhibitors such as co-amoxiclav and piperacillin-tazobactam may be used if sensitive in vitro, but this practice is controversial especially in patients with severe sepsis. The safest choice is a carbapenem such as meropenem and then de-escalating the antibiotic therapy when full sensitivities are available.

Further Reading

Wagenlehner FM, Pilatz A, Weidner W, Naber KG. Urosepsis: overview of the diagnostic and treatment challenges. *Microbiol Spectr*. 2015;3(5).

A6.59 Answer C: Co-trimoxazole

S. maltophilia is naturally resistant to many broad-spectrum antibiotics (including all carbapenems). Many strains of *S. maltophilia* are sensitive to co-trimoxazole and ticarcillin, though resistance has been increasing. It is not usually sensitive to piperacillin, and sensitivity to ceftazidime is variable. The preferred agent is co-trimoxazole, but studies have shown synergistic action with tigecycline, ceftazidime and fluoroquinolones. Aerosolised antibiotics such as colistin, doxycycline and levofloxacin have been used.

Further Reading

Brooke JS. *Stenotrophomonas maltophilia*: an emerging global opportunistic pathogen. *Clin Microbiol Rev*. 2012;25(1):2–41.

A6.60 Answer D: Septicaemia

Diphtheria is an acute disease caused by *Corynebacterium diphtheria*. It is highly infectious but due to effective vaccination is now extremely rare in resource rich countries. The bacterium grows locally in the pharynx forming a pseudomembrane and systemic dissemination of toxin causes disease of distant organs causing myopathy and neuropathy rather than bacteraemia. Cervical lymph nodes can be involved causing severe adenitis and a "bull neck" appearance.

Further Reading

Hadfield TL, McEvoy P, Polotsky Y, Tzinserling VA, Yakovlev AA. The pathology of diphtheria. *J Infect Dis*. 2000;181(S1):S116–S120.

A6.61 Answer D: Treated syphilis

This patient is presenting with a clinical syndrome most likely to be consistent with gonorrhoea or possibly chlamydia or other causes of non-specific urethritis. Primary syphilis would likely have presented with a painless ulcer (chancre) at a site of sexual activity (genitalia, anorectal, oral), with secondary syphilis presenting several weeks (usually 2–8) after the initial lesion with an all over (including palms and soles) non-pruritic rash. Secondary syphilis, if not treated, is followed by a period of latency which may last many years before complications start to arise. Tertiary syphilis may be characterised by destructive gummas, meningitis (which in late disease may progress to generalised paresis or tabes dorsalis) or aortitis with aneurysm formation. In all forms of syphilis, from primary through to tertiary, the majority of cases would have a positive TPHA and VDRL results. In this case, the serology is suggestive of the patient having had previous syphilis (positive TPHA) which has been treated (negative RPR).

T. pallidum ssp. pertenue is the cause of yaws, which presents with chronic relapsing lesions on the skin and mucous membranes. Deeper destruction of underlying bone structures can also occur where treatment with penicillin is not undertaken. Serological tests for syphilis are currently unable to differentiate between T. pallidum ssp. Pertenue (yaws) and T. pallidum ssp. pallidum (venereal syphilis).

Further Reading

Tipple C, Taylor GP. Syphilis testing, typing, and treatment follow-up: a new era for an old disease. Curr Opin Infect Dis. 2015;28(1):53–60.

A6.62   **Answer B: Urethral stricture**
Among male patients untreated gonorrhoea can lead to epididymitis, prostatitis, or urethral strictures, with the latter the most frequent. Among female patients the most common sequelae of untreated gonorrhoea is pelvic inflammatory disease, while less frequent complications include perihepatitis (Fitz-Hugh-Curtis syndrome), infertility, and among those who are pregnant, chorioamnionitis and neonatal conjunctivitis. Septic arthritis (usually monoarticular) can occur as part of the syndrome of disseminated gonococcal infection, as can a bacteraemia (the latter may be associated with a polyarticular migratory arthralgia).

Treatment of gonorrhoea in the United Kingdom is currently is currently with dual antimicrobial therapy because of concerns over resistance. Intramuscular ceftriaxone is used along with oral azithromycin. Alternate regimes include pairing cefixime or spectinomycin with azithromycin. Disseminated gonococcal infection is treated with daily parenteral ceftriaxone for 7 days. A test of cure is recommended in all cases of gonorrhoea, with samples taken at least 72 hours after completing therapy (if still symptomatic) but preferable after 2 weeks (if asymptomatic after therapy).

Further Reading

Bignell C, Fitzgerald M; Guideline Development Group; British Association for Sexual Health and HIV UK. UK national guideline for the management of gonorrhoea in adults, 2011. Int J STD AIDS. 2011;22(10):541–547.

A6.63   **Answer B: *Ancylostoma braziliense***
This patient presents with cutaneous larva migrans indicative of infection from a zoonotic hookworm, caused by the A. braziliense whose usual lifecycle involves cats or dogs. A. braziliense eggs are deposited in cat and dog faeces, where they then develop through larval stages, before penetrating the skin of mammals which subsequently walk over the infested ground. In the case of humans, these hookworms cannot penetrate beyond the superficial skin layers and migrate in the immediate subcutaneous tissue, causing a pruritic and unsightly rash, but not otherwise causing wider issues. The rash in cutaneous larva migrans advances slowly over a period of several weeks. Treatment can either be with topical thiabendazole or where there is more extensive disease (which can affect any area of the

body in contact with faecal contaminated ground) oral ivermectin may be used. Secondary bacterial infection can occur and should be managed with appropriate antibacterials.

S. stercoralis is the cause of larva currens, a fast moving pruritic rash. N. americanus is one of the human hookworms, and although this helminth also penetrates through skin contact, it migrates through deep structures and around the body before ending up in the intestine. The rash in Lyme disease, caused by B. burgdorferi is erythema migrans, a target-shaped lesion. C. perfringens can cause infections of the feet, but causes gas gangrene when it invades into deep tissue.

Further Reading

Lupi O, Downing C, Lee M, Bravo F, Giglio P, Woc-Colburn L, Tyring SK. Mucocutaneous manifestations of helminth infections: trematodes and cestodes. *J Am Acad Dermatol.* 2015;73(6):947–957.

A6.64   **Answer C: *Clostridium sordellii***

The computerised tomograph in this case depicts a markedly oedematous right thigh, with fluid dispersed through muscle and fat layers widely distributed in both medial and lateral compartments. The Gram stain demonstrates Gram-positive rods, and the causative organism here is *C. sordellii*. *C. sordellii* is commonly found in soil and the intestines of animals, and has been seen as a commensal in a small number of human intestines. *C. sordellii* infection has been documented to cause materno-foetal infection, including septic abortion and gynaecological infections, but also significantly skin and skin structure infections among patients who misuse intravenous drugs. Among patients with *C. sordellii* infection, significant amounts of oedema in affected tissues is a particular feature, mediated through clostridia exotoxins, which are a feature of many *Clostridium* species. Similarly the markedly raised white cell count is a feature of clostridial infections, and the combination of a leukaemoid reaction and oedema together is strongly suggestive.

Spore forming Gram positive organisms (*C. sordellii*, *Clostridium novyii* type A, and *B. anthracis*) can cause particular problems in drug users, contaminating the illicit substances during their production and transport. *B. anthracis* can cause cutaneous anthrax, presenting as a suppurating abscess which then develops a central eschar, or if inhaled it can present as a rapid onset pulmonary syndrome which includes a haemorrhagic mediasteinitis. If *B. anthracis* infected meat is consumed, a severe enteritis can also ensue. *S. aureus* and *S. pyogenes* can both cause a type II (monomicrobial) necrotising fasciitis, including in those who are intravenous drug users. However, both are Gram-positive cocci, rather than the rods seen in this case. *C. perfringens* is a cause of gas gangrene. While the Gram stain here could be indicative of *C. perfringens*, the tissue appearances in gas gangrene are usually characteristic and differ from this case.

Further Reading

Aldape MJ, Bryant AE, Stevens DL. *Clostridium sordellii* infection: epidemiology, clinical findings, and current perspectives on diagnosis and treatment. *Clin Infect Dis.* 2006;43(11):1436–1446.

Ascough S, Altmann DM. Anthrax in injecting drug users: the need for increased vigilance in the clinic. *Expert Rev Anti-infect Ther.* 2015;13(6):681–684.

A6.65   **Answer D: Mastoiditis**

This patient has clinical and radiographic features of a right-sided mastoiditis. This often presents with pain, swelling and tenderness in the post-auricular area, and headaches are common. Less frequent are cranial neuropathies, but the proximity of the route of cranial nerve VII and VI in particular means there can be nerve palsies at presentation for some patients. Chronic sinusitis can give headaches, but cranial neuropathies are very unusual, and the imaging in this case does not fit. Meningitis can occur as a sequelae in some cases of sinusitis and mastoiditis, but does not fit with the examination in this case. Similarly, cerebral abscesses can develop secondary to pyogenic infections of the skull bones, and can give cranial neuropathies (most commonly in the form of a false localising cranial nerve VI palsy), but the imaging here does not support that diagnosis.

Otitis externa, also known as swimmers ear, is a relatively benign condition caused by inflammation limited to the external auditory canal which presents with pain and often discharge. It is most commonly caused by *Pseudomonas aeruginosa* or *Staphylococcus aureus*, but fungi (particularly *Aspergillus* spp.) can also be causative. It rarely causes headache and is not associated with cranial neuropathies. Malignant otitis externa is a much more aggressive pyogenic process around the auditory canal and into the skull base (particularly the temporal bone), which may cause multiple cranial neuropathies. It most commonly occurs in those with a degree of immunocompromised, such as diabetes, and is also most commonly caused by *P. aeruginosa* or *S. aureus*.

Further Reading

Karaman E, Yilmaz M, Ibrahimov M, Haciyev Y, Enver O. Malignant otitis externa. *J Craniofac Surg*. 2012;23(6):1748–1751.

A6.66   Answer C: Refer to ear nose and throat specialists for tonsillectomy

Children frequently present with upper respiratory tract infections, most commonly caused by viruses, and less frequently by bacteria (predominantly Group A streptococci or Group C/G streptococci, although other organisms including *Staphylococcus aureus* and anaerobes can also play a role). The majority of upper respiratory tract infections, including tonsillitis, are self-limiting. In adults, the same spread of potential microbiological causes is apparent, but infections are typically much less frequent, usually because of adequate self-hygiene. Some patients do, however, have recurrent episodes and this can place a significant burden on their daily activities and the health service. In these cases, three approaches are available: watch and wait, recurrent courses of antimicrobials or referral for consideration for tonsillectomy. Antimicrobials for recurrent tonsillitis do reduce the duration of symptoms and the risk of subsequent development of peritonsillar abscesses, but adverse events from the antimicrobials do occur. Tonsillectomy does reduce the frequency of episodes of tonsillitis and improves quality of life measures, but is costly and has a risk of surgical complications. Indicators to refer patients to ear nose and throat specialists to consider tonsillectomy in adults include:

- Seven or more episodes of clinically significant adequately treated sore throats in the preceding year (or five episodes a year for each of the last 2 years)
- The episodes of sore throat are disabling and prevent normal function
- The episodes of sore throat are due to acute tonsillitis

Further Reading

Powell J, O'Hara J, Carrie S, Wilson JA. Is tonsillectomy recommended in adults with recurrent tonsillitis? *BMJ*. 2017;357:j1450.

A6.67   **Answer C: *Neisseria meningitidis***

Brain abscesses can arise from either haematogenous seeding or from direct extension, either from penetrating trauma or from infected mastoid air cells or other sinuses. The microbiological cause of cerebral abscesses, therefore, reflect these two routes of entry. The organisms most frequently associated with cerebral abscesses include streptococci (both aerobic from emboli from infective endocarditis or anaerobic from other foci of infection) and staphylococci (either *S. aureus* or coagulase-negative staphylococci depending on the route of entry and the presence of implantable medical devices), although Gram-negative organisms are increasing in frequency. Among neonates, the most frequently found organisms include the Enterobacteriales (such as *Citrobacter*, *Proteus* and *Serratia* spp.) and *Pseudomonas aeruginosa,* as well as *S. aureus.* Among neonates cerebral abscesses are often large and have poorly formed abscess wall.

Less frequently other organisms may cause cerebral abscesses, including *Mycobacterium tuberculosis*, non-tuberculous *Mycobacteria* spp., fungi, parasites and *Actinomyces* and *Nocardia* species. *Nocardia* spp. are Gram-positive branching (filamentous) rods which are strict aerobes. *Actinomyces* spp. are Gram-positive branching (filamentous) rods which are facultative or strict anaerobes. Focal intracranial collections due to *Salmonella* spp. are rare, and cerebral abscesses due to *N. meningitidis* are even more so.

Further Reading

Brouwer MC, van de Beek D. Epidemiology, diagnosis, and treatment of brain abscesses. *Curr Opin Infect Dis.* 2017;30(1):129–134.

A6.68   **Answer C: Colistin and tigecycline**

The patient is in septic shock and, therefore, optimum antimicrobial therapy should be initiated as soon as possible. Nitrofurantoin is a urinary antiseptic and should not be used in septic patients. Fosfomycin has not been tested and is more reliable for use in *Escherichia coli*. PHE recommend dual antibiotic therapy for treatment of severe infection by carbapenemase-producing Enterobacteriaceae. Meropenem is an option where the meropenem minimum inhibitory concentration is less than 8 mg/L, but in this case tigecycline has shown to be in vitro sensitive. The Food Drug Agency (FDA) established five categories to indicate potential of a drug to cause birth defects if used during pregnancy. Tigecycline is FDA Category D meaning its potential benefit in a critically ill patient outweighs the foetal risk.

Further Reading

Gutiérrez-Gutiérrez B, Salamanca E, de Cueto M, Hsueh PR, Viale P, Paño-Pardo JR, Venditti M, Tumbarello M, Daikos G, Cantón R, Doi Y, Tuon FF, Karaiskos I, Pérez-Nadales E, Schwaber MJ, Azap ÖK, Souli M, Roilides E, Pournaras S, Akova M, Pérez F, Bermejo J, Oliver A, Almela M, Lowman W, Almirante B, Bonomo RA, Carmeli Y, Paterson DL, Pascual A, Rodríguez-Baño J. Effect of appropriate combination therapy on mortality of patients with bloodstream infections due to carbapenemase-producing Enterobacteriaceae (INCREMENT): a retrospective cohort study. *Lancet Infect Dis.* 2017;17(7):726–734.

Public Health England. Acute trust toolkit for the early detection, management and control of carbapenemase-producing Enterobacteriaceae. 2014. Available at: www.gov.uk/government/publications/carbapenemase-producing-enterobacteriaceae-early-detection-management-and-control-toolkit-for-acute-trusts

A6.69 **Answer E: *Giardia lamblia***

Reactive arthritis is an arthritis that occurs following an infection and is a form of spondyloarthritis. It can be caused by a wide range of infective agents. Reiter's syndrome (a now defunct term) is a subset of reactive arthritis and is defined by the classical triad of arthritis, urethritis and conjunctivitis and mostly affects men in their third decade of life. Pathogens commonly associated with this condition are *Shigella*, *Salmonella*, *Yersinia*, *Campylobacter*, *Amoeba* and *Chlamydia*. Reactive arthritis often has an interval ranging from several days to weeks between the infection and arthritis. It is typically mono or oligoarticular pattern of arthritis involving the lower extremities. In a 2013 systematic review from the United States found the incidence of reactive arthritis following infection with *Campylobacter*, *Salmonella* and *Shigella* was estimated as 9, 12 and 12 per 1,000 patients, respectively.

Further Reading

Ajene AN, Fischer Walker CL, Black RF. Enteric pathogens and reactive arthritis: a systematic review of *Campylobacter*, *Salmonella* and *Shigella*-associated reactive arthritis. *J Health Popul Nutr.* 2013;31(3):299–307.

A6.70 **Answer D: Respiratory rate, altered mentation, hypotension**

In 1991, a consensus conference developed definitions of sepsis focussed on the view that sepsis resulted from a host's systemic inflammatory response syndrome to infection. In 2001 the diagnostic criteria were expanded but changed little in the definition. In 2016, a task force set to redefine sepsis in light of new evidence and an up-to-date examination of the pathobiology. Sepsis was redefined as "life-threatening organ dysfunction caused by a dysregulated host response to infection." Organ dysfunction can be identified as an acute change in total SOFA (Sequential Organ Failure Assessment) score ≥ 2 points consequent to the infection. This would reflect an overall mortality risk of approximately 10% in a general hospital population. Due to the complexity of the SOFA score a qSOFA score was developed to identify patients with infection that are likely to have poor outcomes and, therefore, need escalation of care. The qSOFA consists of altered mentation (GCS < 15), systolic blood pressure <100 mmHg and respiratory rate of 22/min or greater.

Further Reading

Singer M, Deutschman CS, Seymour CW, Shankar-Hari M, Annane D, Bauer M, Bellomo R, Bernard GR, Chiche JD, Coopersmith CM, Hotchkiss RS, Levy MM, Marshall JC, Martin GS, Opal SM, Rubenfeld GD, van der Poll T, Vincent JL, Angus DC. The third international consensus definitions for sepsis and septic shock (sepsis-3). *JAMA.* 2016;315(8):801–810.

Understanding the Use of Antimicrobial Agents

A basic understanding of the mechanism of action and indication for antimicrobials is held by most prescribers. The key properties of different classes of antimicrobials, their anticipated side effects and the spectrum of activity against different pathogens is inherent in most undergraduate and post-graduate medical curricula. Practitioners in the fields of infectious diseases, microbiology and virology must have a firm grasp of this knowledge, and should be able to apply it to patients with bacterial, viral, fungal or parasitic infections. They must be able to integrate this knowledge with the pharmacokinetic properties of the antimicrobials, and should be able to adapt this in differing patient populations including those with renal impairment or on renal replacement therapy and those with allergies or other host factors.

Practitioners in infectious diseases, microbiology and virology must be able to construct and adhere to guidelines based upon evidence, and have an awareness of new developments in the field of antimicrobials, as well as understand how and where these agents fit into the armamentarium. There should be an understanding of the duration of antimicrobials needed for various infective conditions and the appropriate dosing strategies for these infections.

Practitioners must be able to use the least toxic regime wherever possible, and be able to use antimicrobials safely in pregnant women, children and neonates. Where therapeutic drug monitoring is available and advocated, practitioners must be able to advise on when this should be conducted, and how to interpret the laboratory results. Practitioners should also have a core understanding of the concepts of antimicrobial stewardship, and be able to integrate these programmes into their healthcare setting in an effective manner.

Questions

Q7.1 A 21-year-old au pair from Columbia who is 21 weeks pregnant presents with a morbiliform rash, conjunctivitis and fever. She develops a pneumonitis. Which specific therapy is advocated for this patient?

A. Ribavarin

B. Aciclovir

C. Palivizumab monoclonal antibody

D. Measles-specific immunoglobulin

E. Human normal immunoglobulin

Q7.2 A 26-year-old female presents 16 weeks pregnant with fever and upper respiratory tract symptoms. A viral swab is sent and is positive for influenza A and she is started on oseltamivir. What is the mechanism of action of oseltamivir?

A. Inhibits neuraminidase cleavage of budding virions

B. Inhibits haemagglutinin binding to epithelia sialic acid

C. Inhibits dissociation of viral ribonuclearproteins

D. Inhibits neuraminidase preventing virion epithelial entry

E. Inhibits epithelial endosome fusion with the viral membrane

Q7.3 A 22-year-old presents with a high fever and a viral cause is suspected. Which of the following antiviral agents is not used for clinical therapy against the corresponding wildtype virus?

A. Lamivudine and human immunodeficiency virus

B. Lamivudine and hepatitis B virus

C. Amantadine and influenza B virus

D. Ribavirin and respiratory syncytial virus

E. Acyclovir and herpes simplex virus

Q7.4 A 63-year-old female presented with a discharging sinus over her left hip. She had a prosthetic left hip placed for osteoarthritis 2 years previously. MRSA was grown from deep tissue samples, but due to her anaesthetic risk, she was not deemed fit for surgical replacement. A strategy of oral suppression therapy was chosen including doxycycline and fusidic acid. What is the mechanism of action of fusidic acid?

A. Binding to ribosomes and dissociation of peptide-tRNA

B. Inhibition of topoisomerase IV

C. Inhibition of protein synthesis at the 30S subunit

D. Interference with penicillin binding protein activity

E. Binding with elongation factor G and interference with protein synthesis

Q7.5 A sample of pus taken from a discharging wound following an animal bite grows meticillin-sensitive *Staphylococcus aureus*. The antibiogram shows resistance to penicillin, fusidic acid and gentamicin. What is the main mechanism of staphylococcal resistance to aminoglycoside therapy?

A. Ribosomal binding site alteration

B. Aminoglycoside degrading enzyme production

C. Loss of porin channels

D. Up-escalation of efflux mechanisms

E. Alteration of cell wall d-ala-d-ala cross linkage

Q7.6 A 65-year-old patient is admitted with urosepsis and commenced on gentamicin monotherapy due to a significant penicillin allergy and a high risk of *Clostridioides difficile*-associated diarrhoea. What is the mechanism of aminoglycoside post-dose effect?

A. Prevention of cross-linking of peptide chains

B. Inhibition of cell wall synthesis

C. Binding to protein G and inhibition of protein synthesis

D. Inhibition of ribosomal function

E. Inhibition of topoisomerase IV

Q7.7 A 33-year-old patient who is 20 weeks pregnant attends with a productive cough and fever following 5 days of cold and flu-like symptoms. On auscultation, crepitations were elicited over the right lung base. You diagnose a lower respiratory tract infection following a viral upper respiratory tract infection and prescribe a 7-day course of oral amoxicillin. The patient asks whether this drug is safe to use in pregnancy. Which pregnancy safety category is amoxicillin classed under?
   A. Category A
   B. Category B
   C. Category C
   D. Category D
   E. Category X

Q7.8 A 45-year-old Vietnamese male attended the emergency room with a gradual onset headache, confusion and difficulty walking. MRI with gadolinium showed basal leptomeningeal enhancement and a subsequent lumbar puncture revealed an increase in protein with a mononuclear pleocytosis. Tuberculous meningitis was suspected and commenced on anti-tuberculous chemotherapy. In *Mycobacterium tuberculosis* meningitis, which drug is the best for crossing the blood–brain barrier?
   A. Rifampicin
   B. Isoniazid
   C. Ethambutol
   D. Streptomycin
   E. Pyrazinamide

Q7.9 A 34-year-old male patient is diagnosed with drug-susceptible tuberculosis and commenced on standard quadruple therapy. He was still smear positive for acid-fast bacilli 2 months into treatment. Therapeutic drug monitoring showed low levels of some of the anti-mycobacterials. Genetic testing showed that he was a "fast acetylator." Which anti-tuberculous drug is affected by this genetic mechanism?
   A. Isoniazid
   B. Rifampicin
   C. Pyrazinamide
   D. Ethambutol
   E. Moxifloxacin

Q7.10 A 40-year-old female attended her general practitioner with respiratory tract symptoms. She was not systemically unwell and was given erythromycin due to a penicillin allergy. After 1 week of therapy since she had not improved, therapy was changed to oral doxycycline, where she made a good recovery. What is the mechanism through which *Streptococcus pneumoniae* displays phenotypic resistance to both erythromycin and clindamycin?
   A. Efflux pump
   B. Enzymatic degradation
   C. Porin loss
   D. Target alteration
   E. Impermeability

Q7.11 A 55-year-old male attends his general practice complaining of pain on passing urine and on examination has a painful prostate. He is diagnosed with prostatitis and given a 4-week prescription for ciprofloxacin. At which site do the fluoroquinolone class of antimicrobials act?
A. Cell wall synthesis
B. DNA-dependent RNA polymerase
C. RNA-dependent DNA polymerase
D. Topoisomerase IV
E. Ribosomal protein synthesis

Q7.12 A 34-year-old female with an infection of spinal metalwork underwent deep tissue sampling without removal of metalwork. Tissue samples grew meticillin-sensitive *Staphylococcus aureus* and she receives flucloxacillin intravenously. Due to the presence of metalwork, rifampicin was added into therapy. What is the mechanism of action of rifampicin?
A. Cell wall inhibitor
B. DNA gyrase inhibitor
C. DNA-dependent RNA polymerase inhibitor
D. DNA-dependent DNA polymerase inhibitor
E. Folate inhibition

Q7.13 A 34-year-old female with an infection of spinal metalwork underwent deep tissue sampling without removal of metalwork. Tissue samples grew meticillin-sensitive *Staphylococcus aureus* and she receives flucloxacillin intravenously. Due to the presence of metalwork, rifampicin was added into therapy. What is the main side effect of rifampicin therapy?
A. Eighth nerve toxicity
B. Optic neuritis
C. Hepatitis
D. Dental discolouration
E. Pulmonary fibrosis

Q7.14 A 23-year-old female presents with enteritis and *Campylobacter jejuni* is detected in stool by PCR. What would be a suitable antimicrobial therapy?
A. Amoxicillin
B. Ciprofloxacin
C. Tetracycline
D. Azithromycin
E. Ceftriaxone

Q7.15 A 65-year-old patient is diagnosed with paucibacilliary leprosy. What is an essential component of the treatment regime?
A. Isoniazid
B. Moxifloxacin
C. Dapsone

    D. Clarithromycin
    E. Clofazimine

Q7.16 A 65-year-old patient is diagnosed with paucibacilliary leprosy and is commenced on dapsone and rifampicin. He develops a rash and fever and has the below full blood count.

    Haemoglobin: 115 g/L
    White cell count: 8.3×10^9/L
    Neutrophils: 2.5×10^9/L
    Lymphocytes: 1.9×10^9/L
    Eosinophils: 2.8×10^9/L
    Platelets: 190×10^9/L

What is the most likely diagnosis?
    A. Agranulocytosis
    B. Allergic dermatitis
    C. Stevens–Johnson syndrome
    D. Toxic epidermal necrolysis
    E. Dapsone syndrome

Q7.17 A 65-year-old lady with poorly controlled diabetes is diagnosed with *Staphylococcus aureus* osteomyelitis of her foot and is prescribed linezolid. What monitoring should be undertaken?
    A. Monitoring therapeutic drug levels
    B. Monitoring full blood count
    C. Monitoring colour vision
    D. Monitoring liver function tests
    E. Monitoring clotting parameters

Q7.18 A 65-year-old lady with poorly controlled diabetes is diagnosed with *Staphylococcus aureus* osteomyelitis of her foot and is prescribed linezolid. Which other medications may significantly interact with this antimicrobial?
    A. Venlafaxine
    B. Propranolol
    C. Salbutamol
    D. Nifedipine
    E. Sodium valproate

Q7.19 A 6-day-old male has meningitis. What is a frequent adverse event arising from chloramphenicol usage in neonates?
    A. Optic neuritis
    B. Isolated thrombocytopaenia
    C. Agranulocytosis
    D. Gray baby syndrome
    E. Aplastic anaemia

Q7.20 A 6-day-old male has meningitis. The mother was noted to be colonised with Group B *Streptococcus* on a puerperal vaginal swab. The mother has previously had a rash with penicillin. What should be the empiric therapy for the neonate?
A. Ceftriaxone
B. Benzylpenicillin
C. Chloramphenicol
D. Amoxicillin
E. Vancomycin

Q7.21 A 6-day-old male has meningitis. A blood culture grows an *Escherichia coli*. What should be the empiric therapy for the neonate?
A. Ceftriaxone
B. Cefotaxime
C. Amoxicillin
D. Meropenem
E. Benzylpenicillin

Q7.22 A 54-year-old man has a meticillin-susceptible *Staphylococcus aureus* bacteraemia. What treatment regime should be used?
A. Flucloxacillin
B. Flucloxacillin and rifampicin
C. Flucloxacillin and gentamicin
D. Vancomycin
E. Vancomycin and rifampicin

Q7.23 A 54-year-old man has a meticillin-susceptible *Staphylococcus aureus* bacteraemia. He is found to have prosthetic mitral valve endocarditis. What treatment regime should be used?
A. Flucloxacillin
B. Flucloxacillin and rifampicin
C. Flucloxacillin, rifampicin and gentamicin
D. Vancomycin and rifampicin
E. Vancomycin, rifampicin and gentamicin

Q7.24 A 65-year-old male has been commenced on standard quadruple therapy for suspected tuberculosis. He has an extensive past medical history and is taking a number of other medications. Which drug is most likely to have a clinically significant interaction with rifampicin?
A. Penicillin
B. Ibuprofen
C. Lansoprazole
D. Furosemide
E. Warfarin

Q7.25 A 75-year-old female presents with urosepsis and is prescribed an aminoglyco-side. What is the bactericidal mode of action of aminoglycosides?
   A. Disruption of cytoplasmic membrane function
   B. Inhibition of bacterial cell wall synthesis
   C. Inhibition of bacterial DNA gyrase
   D. Inhibition tRNA binding at ribosomal active site
   E. Interference with bacterial folic acid metabolism

Q7.26 A 75-year-old female presents with urosepsis and is prescribed an aminoglyco-side. What is the most frequent adverse event from this agent?
   A. Low-frequency hearing loss
   B. High-frequency hearing loss
   C. Interstitial tubular nephritis
   D. Focal segmental glomerulonephritis
   E. Nephrotic syndrome

Q7.27 A 51-year-old male with a meticillin-resistant *Staphylococcus aureus* compli-cated skin and soft tissue infection is started on intravenous daptomycin. What monitoring must be undertaken?
   A. Creatinine clearance
   B. Creatine phosphokinase
   C. Platelet count
   D. Alanine transaminase
   E. Alkaline phosphatase

Q7.28 A 14-year-old female with cerebral palsy is diagnosed with sepsis secondary to an extended-spectrum beta-lactamase producing *Escherichia coli* urinary tract infection. Meropenem is commenced. What medication might this antimicrobial significantly interact with?
   A. Levetiracetam
   B. Baclofen
   C. Valproate
   D. Phenytoin
   E. Gabapentin

Q7.29 A 45-year-old female has a sputum which grows a *Pseudomonas aeruginosa* phenotypically resistant to ceftazidime, piperacillin-tazobactam and meropenem. The computerised tomograph of her chest is undertaken (Figure 7.1).

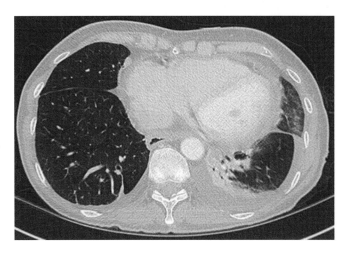

Figure 7.1 Mid thoracic high-resolution computerised tomograph, axial plane.

Which drug is most likely to be effective as treatment for this patient?
A. Ceftobiprole
B. Ceftaroline
C. Ceftolozone-tazobactam
D. Ceftazidime-avibactam
E. Cefotaxime

Q7.30 A patient undergoing a haemopoietic stem cell transplantation developed cellulitis 5 days prior to stem cell infusion. He was commenced on aciclovir, voriconazole and ciprofloxacin prophylaxis and given intravenous flucloxacillin and oral fusidic acid for the treatment or localised cellulitis in a patient who was non-neutropenic.

The clinical team wanted a more effective anti-staphylococcal antimicrobial as concerns were raised due to impending neutropenia. The team decided to change fusidic acid to rifampicin orally but had concerns regarding potential drug interactions. Which agent must rifampicin not be co-prescribed with?
A. Fusidic acid
B. Flucloxacillin
C. Voriconazole
D. Aciclovir
E. Ciprofloxacin

Q7.31 A 64-year-old male with a disseminated fungal infection is commenced on anti-fungal therapy. Which antifungal agent requires therapeutic drug monitoring?
A. Amphotericin B
B. Micafungin
C. Flucytosine
D. Caspofungin
E. Anidulofungin

Q7.32 A 15-year-old male is diagnosed with tinea capitis and a *Microsporum* spp. is grown. Which antifungal treatment is appropriate for this fungal infection of the hair shaft?
A. Topical terbinafine
B. Topical ketoconazole
C. Oral ketoconazole
D. Oral voriconazole
E. Oral griseofulvin

Q7.33 A 37-year-old female neutropenic patient is on the ward and there is building work going on in the next ward. Which antifungal is not indicated for prophylaxis?
A. Liposomal amphotericin (e.g. ambisome)
B. Amphotericin B deoxycholate
C. Posaconaozle
D. Voriconazole
E. Fluconazole

Q7.34 A patient undergoing haemopoietic stem cell transplantation showed widespread diffused infiltrates on chest radiograph with hypoxia during the neutropenic phase of transplantation. Upper respiratory tract samples were positive on PCR for *Pneumocystis jirovecii*. Which antifungal agent is not effective against *P. jirovecii* pneumonia (PJP)?
A. Caspofungin
B. Voriconazole
C. Pentamidine
D. Dapsone
E. Co-trimoxazole

Q7.35 Future use of antibacterials are threatened by increasing drug resistance and lack of incentive for pharmaceutical companies to invest in future drug development. A small company is designing an alternative to traditional antibiotics which work to increase the expression of anti-inflammatory chemokines and cytokines and reduce the expression of pro-inflammatory cytokines. In which class of antiinfective would this agent be described?
A. Antimicrobial peptide
B. Innate defence peptide
C. Engineered bacteriophage
D. Probiotic
E. Metal chelation

Answers

A7.1 Answer E: Human normal immunoglobulin

The classical symptoms of measles include 4-day fevers, the three Cs – cough, coryza (runny nose) and conjunctivitis (red eyes) and a generalised maculopapular rash that starts at the head. It is spread by respiratory droplets and is highly contagious. Complications with measles are relatively common – more so in infected adults, ranging from diarrhoea, to pneumonia and encephalitis (subacute sclerosing pan-encephalitis) and to corneal ulceration leading to scarring. Human normal immunoglobulin may be used to prevent or attenuate an attack in immunocompromised patients, pregnant women or infants under the age of 9 months. MMR vaccine is effective and is part of the UK vaccination schedule.

Further Reading

Department of Health, UK Government. Measles: post-exposure prophylaxis. 2009;5. Available at: www.gov.uk/government/publications/measles-post-exposure-prophylaxis

A7.2   Answer A: Inhibits neuraminidase cleavage of budding virions

Oseltamivir is a pro-drug which is hepatically metabolised to its active form. This then acts competitively to inhibit viral neuraminidase, preventing the cleaving of new budding virions from their binding to sialic acid. Amantadine and rimantidine act on influenza A through interfering with the viral M2 proton channel. Normally, this channel allows acidification of the virus which in turn enables dis-association of ribonuclear proteins. Influenza binds to sialic acid on host epithelia through haemagglutinin and then gains cell entry through endosome fusion with the viral membrane, although there are as yet no licenced antivirals that inhibit this part of the infective process for influenza.

Further Reading

Davies BE. Pharmacokinetics of oseltamivir: an oral antiviral for the treatment and prophylaxis of influenza in diverse populations. *J Antimicrob Chemother*. 2010;65(S2):5–10.

A7.3   Answer C: Amantadine and influenza B virus

Lamivudine (a cytidine analogue, 3TC) is phosphorylated to its triphosphate form inhibiting reverse transcriptase as well as cellular DNA polymerase; this agent can be used for human retroviruses, including HIV and hepatitis B virus. Amantadine interferes with the M2 ion channel in influenza virions, preventing influenza A viral un-coating, however, resistance develops quickly, and in addition this agent is not active against influenza B because of M2 structural differences. Nebulised ribavirin, a prodrug which when metabolised resembles purine RNA nucleotides (adenine or guanine), causes mutations when incorporated in RNA viruses, and in its phosphorylated form can inhibit RNA-dependent RNA polymerases in ss (−) RNA viruses. In DNA viruses, ribavirin acts through inhibiting inosine monophosphate dehydrogenase, thus depleting intracellular GTP and may also switch immune response from T_H2 to T_H1, although the evidence for this is less clear. Aciclovir is a guanosine analogue that is phosphorylated (to become around 3,000 more times active) by viral thymidine kinase allowing subsequent inhibition of DNA polymerase.

Further Reading

NICE Technology Appraisal Guidance [TA168]. Amantadine, oseltamivir and zanamivir for the treatment of influenza. 2009. Available at: www.nice.org.uk/guidance/ta168

A7.4   Answer E: Binding with elongation factor G and interference with protein synthesis

Fusidic acid is a bacterial protein synthesis inhibitor which acts through preventing the turnover of elongation factor G (EF-G) from the ribosome. Fusidic acid is only effective on Gram-positive bacteria. It is bacteriostatic, highly protein-bound with good oral bioavailability. The use of fusidic acid in topical creams has led to an increase in community *Staphylococcus aureus* isolates. Fusidic acid should not be co-prescribed with statins due to the risk of myotoxicity, with case reports of fatal outcome.

Further Reading

Wang JL, Tang HJ, Hsieh PH, Chiu FY, Chen YH, Chang MC, Huang CT, Liu CP, Lau YJ, Hwang KP, Ko WC, Wang CT, Liu CY, Liu CL, Hsueh PR. Fusidic acid for the treatment of bone and joint infections caused by meticillin-resistant *Staphylococcus aureus*. *Int J Antimicrob Agents*. 2012;40(2):103–107.

A7.5   Answer B: Aminoglycoside degrading enzyme production

There are three mechanisms of aminoglycoside resistance among bacteria: reduced uptake/decreased cell permeability, alterations at the ribosomal binding sites or production of aminoglycoside modifying enzymes. Reduced uptake or decreased cell permeability is common in *Pseudomonas aeruginosa* and other Gram-negative bacilli through a chromosomally mediated mechanism and results in cross-reactivity to all aminoglycosides but usually induces intermediate susceptibility. Altered ribosome binding sites usually induce resistance to streptomycin as this agent binds to a single site on the 30S subunit. Resistance to the other aminoglycosides by this mechanism is uncommon since they bind to multiple sites on both ribosomal subunits, and high-level resistance cannot be selected by a single step. Enzymatic modification is the most common type of aminoglycoside resistance with over 50 different enzymes identified. Enzymatic modification usually results in high-level resistance, with genes encoding for this usually found on plasmids and transposons. Most enzyme-mediated resistance in Gram-negative bacilli is due to multiple genes. There are three types of aminoglycoside modifying enzymes: *N*-acetyltransferases (AAC), O-adenyltransferases (ANT) and O-phosphotransferases (APH).

Further Reading

Jackson J, Chen C, Buising K. Aminoglycosides: how should we use them in the 21st century? *Curr Opin Infect Dis*. 2013;26(6):516–525.

A7.6   Answer D: Inhibition of ribosomal function

Traditionally, aminoglycosides were believed to act through inhibition of bacterial protein synthesis by irreversible binding to the 30S bacterial ribosome. Newer evidence points to rapid and marked bactericidal activity being attributable to the cationic antibiotic molecules creating fissures in the outer cell membrane. This results in leakage of intracellular contents and enhanced antibiotic uptake and probably accounts for most of the bactericidal activity. These agents exhibit a post-antibiotic effect which is due to strong, irreversible binding to the ribosome. This allows a prolonged dosage interval. The microbiologic activity is pH-dependent, and as a result the antibiotic effect may be reduced in low pH environments including abscesses and bronchial secretions.

Further Reading

Jackson J, Chen C, Buising K. Aminoglycosides: how should we use them in the 21st century? *Curr Opin Infect Dis*. 2013;26(6):516–525.

A7.7 Answer B: Category B

The Food and Drug Administration (FDA) established five categories to indicate potential of a drug to cause birth defects if used during pregnancy. Amoxicillin is under Category B. Although there is extensive experience with penicillin-based antibiotics, no well-controlled studies in pregnant women exist.

Table 9 Food and Drug Administration categorisation of risk for drugs in pregnancy.

Category A	Adequate and well-controlled studies fail to demonstrate a risk in the first trimester
Category B	Animal reproduction studies have failed to demonstrate foetal risk, and there are no adequate and well-controlled studies in pregnant women
Category C	Animal reproduction studies have failed to demonstrate foetal risk and there are no adequate and well-controlled studies in pregnant women, but potential benefits may warrant use of the drug despite risks
Category D	There is positive evidence of human foetal risk based on adverse reaction data from investigational experience or studies in humans, but potential benefits may warrant use of the drug despite potential risks
Category X	Studies in animals or humans have demonstrated foetal abnormalities and/or there is positive evidence of human foetal risk based on adverse reaction data from investigational experience, and risks clearly outweigh the benefits

Modified from Bookstaver et al. (2015).

Further Reading

Bookstaver PB, Bland CM, Griffin B, Stover KR, Eiland LS, McLaughlin M. A review of antibiotic use in pregnancy. *Pharmacotherapy*. 2015;35(11):1052–1062.

A7.8 Answer B: Isoniazid

The best antimicrobial agents in the treatment of *M. tuberculosis* meningitis include isoniazid, rifampicin, pyrazinamide and streptomycin, all of which enter CSF readily in the presence of meningeal inflammation. Ethambutol is less effective in meningeal disease unless used in high doses. Isoniazid and rifampicin are active against both intra and extracellular *M. tuberculosis*. Pyrazinamide is active only against intracellular *M. tuberculosis* and streptomycin only against extracellular organisms.

Isoniazid is bactericidal against replicating bacteria. Ethambutol is bacteriostatic at low doses, but is used in tuberculosis treatment at higher, bactericidal doses. Rifampicin is bactericidal and has a sterilising effect. Pyrazinamide is only weakly bactericidal, but is very effective against bacteria located in acidic environments, inside macrophages or in areas of acute inflammation.

Fluoroquinolones penetrate well into the CSF but the inclusion of moxifloxacin at standard and higher doses have so far failed to show clinical benefit. A large randomised trial using an intensified regime including high-dose oral rifampicin and inclusion of levofloxacin showed no survival benefit to the overall 28% mortality.

Further Reading

Donald OR. Chemotherapy for tuberculous meningitis. *N Engl J Med*. 2016;374:179–181.

Donald PR. Cerebrospinal fluid concentrations of antituberculosis agents in adults and children. *Tuberculosis (Edinb)*. 2010;90(5):279–292.

A7.9 Answer A: Isoniazid

Poor clinical responses in patients can be a result of inadequate serum levels of antituberculous medication. Isoniazid, pyrazinamide and rifampicin levels are decreased when taken with food. Rifapentine absorption is increased with a high fat meal. Moxifloxacin levels are lower when concomitant antacids are given. Metabolic pathways can influence serum drug levels, *N*-acetyltransferase is an enzyme involved in isoniazid clearance, and genetic variation encoding *N*-acetyltransferase can lead to underexposure ("fast acetylators") or elevated risk of liver toxicity ("slow acetylators"). The slow-acetylator genotype is present in more than 50% of white persons.

Further Reading

Horsburg R, Barry CE, Lange C. Treatment of tuberculosis. *N Engl J Med*. 2015;373:2149–2160.

A7.10 Answer D: Target alteration

Macrolides (erythromycin) and lincosamides (clindamycin) insert into the 23S subunit of the 50S ribosome-blocking protein assembly, which is bactericidal for *S. pneumoniae* but bacteriostatic for *Staphylococcus aureus*. Resistance to macrolides is encoded by two genes, *ermB* and *mefA*, but only *ermB* causes target alteration leading to resistance to both macrolides and lincosamides.

ermB encodes methylation of a base in domain V of the 23S rRNA. This alters the site of attachment such that the macrolide no longer binds to the ribosome. This causes high-level resistance.

mefA encodes an efflux pump that expels macrolides but does not affect lincosamides. This resistance is at a lower level, which could be overcome by high antibiotic concentrations.

Further Reading

Reinert RR. The antimicrobial resistance profile of *Streptococcus pneumoniae*. *Clin Microbiol Infect*. 2009;15(S3):7–11.

A7.11 Answer D: Topoisomerase IV

Quinolones act on Gram-negative bacteria DNA gyrase, whereas topoisomerase IV is the target for many Gram-positive bacteria. Conversion of DNA gyrase and topoisomerase IV into toxic enzymes causes fragmentation of the bacterial chromosome and cell death. Rifampicin acts through inhibition of DNA-dependent RNA polymerase. The NRTIs act on RNA-dependent DNA polymerase in HIV.

Further Reading

Aldred KJ, Kerns RJ, Osheroff N. Mechanism of quinolone action and resistance. *Biochemistry*. 2014;53(10):1565–1574.

A7.12 Answer C: DNA dependent RNA polymerase inhibitor

Rifampicin is a rifamycin derivative first isolated from *Streptomyces mediterranei* in 1957. It is bactericidal. Rifampicin resistance is caused by alterations in the *rpoB* which encodes the beta-subunit of the RNA polymerase enzyme. Rifampicin resistance is common when used as monotherapy, and therefore its role in treatment is nearly always in combination. Rifampicin has excellent oral bioavailability and penetrates tissue and CSF well.

Rifampicin penetrates into cells and biofilms to treat infections and is supported by strong clinical data. The exact timing of introducing rifampicin into treatment of biofilm infections is controversial but should be considered when the bioburden is low in order to reduce the chance of inducing resistance.

Further Reading

Forrest GN, Tamura K. Rifampicin combination therapy for non-mycobacterial infections. *Clin Microbiol Rev.* 2010;23(1):14–34.

A7.13 Answer C: Hepatitis

Rifampicin therapy frequently causes a transient abnormality in liver function tests. This may manifest as transient elevations in bilirubin, serum transaminases or alkaline phosphatase. Other possible adverse events from rifampicin therapy include thrombocytopaenia (and more rarely leukopaenia or haemolytic anaemia), dermatological manifestations (from pruritic rash through to erythema multiforme including Stevens–Johnson, and Drug Reaction with Eosinophilia and Systemic Symptoms (DRESS) syndrome), and more general side effects such as gastrointestinal upset and headaches and lethargy.

When rifampicin is used for other indications, including as part of quadruple therapy for tuberculosis, there are more defined risks of adverse events. Overall, there is an 8.6% risk that a patient having standard 6-month tuberculosis therapy will need to have an alteration to their drug therapy because of drug side-effects. Those patients most at risk include those over 60 years of age, females, people living with HIV and those with Asian ancestry. As part of tuberculosis quadruple therapy, drug-related hepatitis is a frequent adverse event, with pyrazinamide perhaps being the most frequent cause, followed by rifampicin and isoniazid.

Optic neuropathy can be caused by ethambutol or linezolid. Peripheral neuropathy can also be caused by linezolid or isoniazid. Dental discolouration typically follows tetracycline prescription, although it has also been reported after prescription of beta-lactam agents. Pulmonary fibrosis has been reported after long-term nitrofurantoin prescription.

Further Reading

Forrest GN, Tamura K. Rifampicin combination therapy for non-mycobacterial infections. *Clin Microbiol Rev.* 2010;23(1):14–34.

A7.14 Answer D: Azithromycin

Almost all cases of *Campylobacter* spp. enteritis recover without any antimicrobial therapy needed and with appropriate fluid rehydration. However, in more severe cases, effective antimicrobial options include either macrolides (azithromycin or erythromycin) or a fluoroquinolone. In the United Kingdom, the causative organism is predominantly *C. jejuni* (91%), but with less frequency *C. coli* (8%), *C. lari*, *C. upsaliensis*, *C. fetus* and

C. hyointestinalis (all less than 1%) are identified. In the United Kingdom, the overall rate of quinolone resistance among *Campylobacter* spp. is approximately 22%, with the rate in *C. jejuni* being lower than in *C. coli*. In imported cases of *Campylobacter* spp. infection, rates of quinolone resistance are even higher, and rates of over 50% have been documented. For azithromycin and erythromycin, resistance rates are much lower and approximately 1% overall, although again *C. coli* has a higher rate at approximately 7%.

Globally, rates of tetracycline resistance vary markedly (usually reflecting variable use of tetracyclines in animal food production) and have reached up to 95% in some settings. Similarly, rates of resistance to amoxicillin are high, and many *Campylobacter* spp. produce a beta-lactamase. Almost all are resistant to first-generation cephalosporins, and susceptibility to third-generation cephalosporins is variable.

Further Reading

Shane AL, Mody RK, Crump JA, Tarr PI, Steiner TS, Kotloff K, Langley JM, Wanke C, Warren CA, Cheng AC, Cantey J, Pickering LK. 2017 Infectious Diseases Society of America Clinical Practice Guidelines for the Diagnosis and Management of Infectious Diarrhoea. *Clin Infect Dis.* 2017;65 (12):1963–1973.

A7.15   Answer C: Dapsone

Leprosy can be recognised as either "paucibacillary" (lepromatous; typically one or more anaesthetic hypopigmented skin macules) and "multibacillary" (tuberculoid; typically symmetric skin nodules or plaques with a thickened dermis and with frequent nasal mucosal involvement) based upon the proliferation of bacteria. Treatment of paucibacilliary leprosy is with dapsone and rifampicin for 6 months. Multibacilliary leprosy treatment involves daily dapsone, clofazimine and rifampicin for 2 years. Dapsone (diaminodiphenyl sulfone or DDS) acts against bacteria by inhibiting synthesis of dihydrofolic acid through competition for the active site of dihydropteroate synthase (similar to the mode of action of sulphonamide antibacterials). In addition to its use in leprosy, dapsone has been used as second-line therapy for *Pneumocystis jirovecii* pneumoniae and in toxoplasmosis. Dapsone also has an anti-inflammatory role through inhibition of myeloperoxidase. Because of this property it has been used in the treatment of acne, dermatitis herpetiformis and several other skin conditions.

During treatment for multibacillary leprosy, patients may experience either a type I (reversal) reaction or a type II (erythema nodosum leprosum) reaction. In a reversal reaction neuropathic pain or weakness can indicate the onset of permanent nerve damage and steroids should be prescribed. In erythema nodosum leprosum, mild reactions may respond to aspirin but severe reactions may require steroids or thalidomide.

Further Reading

Rodrigues LC, Lockwood DN. Leprosy now: epidemiology, progress, challenges, and research gaps. *Lancet Infect Dis.* 2011;11(6):464–470.

A7.16   Answer E: Dapsone syndrome

At the dose used in leprosy, dapsone is usually well tolerated, with the most frequent side effects being headaches or nausea. More serious adverse events are associated with effects on blood cell lines or skin.

Haematological side effects include methaemoglobinaemia (which can present with a bluish tinge to the lips or fingertips), agranulocytosis (which can present with fever and rigors and a sore throat, and is characterised by neutropaenia) or haemolytic anaemia (particularly in those with glucose-6-phosphate dehydrogenase (G6PD) deficiency; which should be tested for before commencing dapsone). Dermatological side effects can range from allergic dermatitis through to Stevens–Johnson syndrome (which presents with fever, blistering and peeling of the skin and mucous membranes, and haemodynamic instability) and toxic epidermal necrolysis (the severe end of the Stevens–Johnson spectrum, typically classified as when more than 30% of the skin is affected).

Dapsone syndrome is a hypersensitivity which is infrequent but does occur more commonly in patients receiving multiple drugs. It typically presents as a rash with fever and eosinophilia and jaundice. Dapsone syndrome can be considered to be on the spectrum of "Drug Reaction with Eosinophilia and Systemic Symptoms" (DRESS syndrome). There is a clear relationship between those who have the HLA-B*13:01 human leukocyte antigen type and dapsone hypersensitivity syndrome. It typically happens within the first few weeks of commencing dapsone therapy, and may be improved with discontinuation of therapy and prednisolone.

Further Reading

Zhang FR, Liu H, Irwanto A, Fu XA, Li Y, Yu GQ, Yu YX, Chen MF, Low HQ, Li JH, Bao FF, Foo JN, Bei JX, Jia XM, Liu J, Liany H, Wang N, Niu GY, Wang ZZ, Shi BQ, Tian HQ, Liu HX, Ma SS, Zhou Y, You JB, Yang Q, Wang C, Chu TS, Liu DC, Yu XL, Sun YH, Ning Y, Wei ZH, Chen SL, Chen XC, Zhang ZX, Liu YX, Pulit SL, Wu WB, Zheng ZY, Yang RD, Long H, Liu ZS, Wang JQ, Li M, Zhang LH, Wang H, Wang LM, Xiao P, Li JL, Huang ZM, Huang JX, Li Z, Liu J, Xiong L, Yang J, Wang XD, Yu DB, Lu XM, Zhou GZ, Yan LB, Shen JP, Zhang GC, Zeng YX, de Bakker PI, Chen SM, Liu JJ. HLA-B*13:01 and the dapsone hypersensitivity syndrome. *N Engl J Med.* 2013;369:1620–1628.

A7.17   Answer B: Monitoring full blood count

Linezolid is an oxazolidinone which provides broad-spectrum anti-Gram-positive activity. It is indicated in pneumonia and complicated skin and skin structure infections, although it is used for wider indications than this for resistant pathogens (such as meticillin resistant *S. aureus* or glycopeptide-resistant enterococci). Use for over 10–14 days of therapy may be associated with myelosuppression, which is most frequently heralded by thrombocytopaenia (but on occasion leukopaenia or anaemia can occur first). Myelosuppression is uncommon among patients who receive linezolid for less than 14 days, but it is more frequent in the context of renal failure.

Prolonged therapy (typically beyond 28 days) can also lead to severe optic neuropathy, and patients should be warned to report any change in vision, including blurring, loss of visual fields or changes to acuity or colour vision. Formal visual function monitoring should be regularly undertaken if treatment is continued for more than 28 days, and should include visual field, acuity and colour.

Further Reading

Douros A, Grabowski K, Stahlmann R. Drug-drug interactions and safety of linezolid, tedizolid, and other oxazolidinones. *Expert Opin Drug Metab Toxicol.* 2015;11(12):1849–1859.

Dryden MS. Linezolid pharmacokinetics and pharmacodynamics in clinical treatment. *J Antimicrob Chemother*. 2011;66(S4):7–15.

A7.18 Answer A: Venlafaxine

Linezolid is a weak non-selective inhibitor of monoamine oxidase A and B. It may, therefore, interact with certain other medications to produce a serotonergic effect, and to a lesser extent adrenergic interactions. The typical time to onset is from 1 to 20 days, but this effect is reversible and often resolves within 1–5 days of discontinuing the agent. Serotonergic agents likely to have appreciable interaction with linezolid include antidepressants such as selective serotonin re-uptake inhibitors (SSRI) including citalopram (and escitalopram), fluoxetine, paroxetine, sertraline and the serotonin-norepinephrine re-uptake inhibitors (SNRI), including venlafaxine, and the tricyclic antidepressants such as amitriptyline. It can also interact with Parkinson's medications such as levodopa, medications to treat migraine such as sumatriptan and several medications used as diet pills and stimulants. Some analgesics can also interact to a lesser degree, including notable tramadol.

There is also some interaction with some dietary components, particularly those rich in tyramine. These include mature cheeses, yeast extract and some alcoholic beverages.

Further Reading

Ramsey TD, Lau TT, Ensom MH. Serotonergic and adrenergic drug interactions associated with linezolid: a critical review and practical management approach. *Ann Pharmacother*. 2013;47 (4):543–560.

A7.19 Answer D: Gray baby syndrome

Chloramphenicol binds to the 23S rRNA component of the 50S ribosomal subunit, thereby preventing peptide elongation. It has particularly good pharmacokinetic properties enabling effective penetration into all tissues including the brain. It has a broad spectrum of activity against most bacteria, with the biggest exception perhaps being *Pseudomonas aeruginosa*. Despite these attributes, it is infrequently used predominantly because of its adverse-event profile.

The most serious side effects of chloramphenicol therapy are haematological. The most serious of these is bone marrow suppression leading to dose-related blood dyscrasia (hypoplastic anaemia, thrombocytopenia and agranulocytosis). In addition, there is an idiosyncratic dose-independent risk (cited as 1:24,000–1:40,000) of aplastic anaemia. This may occur weeks or months after chloramphenicol therapy has ceased. Because of this propensity for blood dyscrasia, a full blood count should be regularly monitored during chloramphenicol therapy.

In neonates, intravenous chloramphenicol may cause Gray baby syndrome. This occurs in neonates due to a relative deficiency in fully developed liver enzymes (specifically UDP-glucuronic transferase). This leads to high un-metabolised chloramphenicol concentrations, which cause hypotension and cyanosis.

Further Reading

Dinos GP, Athanassopoulos CM, Missiri DA, Giannopoulou PC, Vlachogiannis IA, Papadopoulos GE, Papaioannou D, Kalpaxis DL. Chloramphenicol derivatives as antibacterial and anticancer agents: historic problems and current solutions. *Antibiotics*. 2016;5(2):20.

A7.20   Answer B: Benzylpenicillin

Group B *Streptococcus* colonisation in the maternal birth canal can lead to colonisation of neonates with Group B *Streptococcus*. In a small proportion of cases, this is associated with either early-onset (6 days or less) or late-onset (7 days or greater) disease in the neonate, including bacteraemia and meningitis. Blood cultures should be taken, a lumbar puncture should be considered and treatment should be commenced with benzylpenicillin and gentamicin. A maternal history of a rash with penicillin is not predictive of any neonatal allergy to similar agents and should not preclude administration of a beta-lactam agent to the child.

Further Reading

Russell NJ, Seale AC, O'Sullivan C, Le Doare K, Heath PT, Lawn JE, Bartlett L, Cutland C, Gravett M, Ip M, Madhi SA, Rubens CE, Saha SK, Schrag S, Sobanjo-Ter Meulen A, Vekemans J, Baker CJ. Risk of early-onset neonatal group B streptococcal disease with maternal colonization worldwide: systematic review and meta-analyses. *Clin Infect Dis.* 2017;65(S2):S152–S159.

A7.21   Answer B: Cefotaxime

Third-generation cephalosporins can be used in neonatal meningitis where there is a suspected or confirmed Gram-negative component. The favourable pharmacokinetics (specifically concentration in the cerebrospinal fluid) and lower minimum inhibitory concentrations for Enterobacteriales compared to aminoglycosides make the third-generation cephalosporins particularly favourable in the context of inflamed meninges. However, among the third-generation cephalosporins, ceftriaxone should not be used in neonates because it competes with bilirubin in binding to serum albumin, which can contribute to hyperbilirubinemia. This is not a feature of cefotaxime use, however, and can be used if there is a concern over *E. coli* meningitis. Amoxicillin is only needed if there is a concern over listeriosis.

Further Reading

Simonsen KA, Anderson-Berry AL, Delair SF, Davies HD. Early-onset neonatal sepsis. *Clin Microbiol Rev.* 2014;27(1):21–47.

A7.22   Answer A: Flucloxacillin

Morbidity and mortality from *S. aureus* bacteraemia remains high. Beta-lactam agents remain the preferred option, and treatment with glycopeptides for meticillin susceptible *S. aureus* has been demonstrated to have higher mortality.

Combinations of beta-lactam agents (specifically flucloxacillin) with gentamicin have been investigated in several studies, and have demonstrated no improvement in mortality but increase in adverse events, particularly in relation to renal function. This combination should, therefore, be avoided.

Combination of beta-lactam agents (predominantly flucloxacillin) with rifampicin has been investigated in a large prospective randomised controlled trial. This demonstrated no benefit over monotherapy, although there were no excess serious adverse events in the rifampicin group.

Further Reading

Gudiol C, Cuervo G, Shaw E, Pujol M, Carratalà J. Pharmacotherapeutic options for treating *Staphylococcus aureus* bacteremia. *Expert Opin Pharmacother.* 2017;18(18):1947–1963.

McDanel JS, Perencevich EN, Diekema DJ, Herwaldt LA, Smith TC, Chrischilles EA, Dawson JD, Jiang L, Goto M, Schweizer ML. Comparative effectiveness of beta-lactams versus vancomycin for treatment of methicillin-susceptible *Staphylococcus aureus* bloodstream infections among 122 hospitals. *Clin Infect Dis.* 2015;61(3):361–367.

Thwaites GE, Scarborough M, Szubert A, Nsutebu E, Tilley R, Greig J, Wyllie SA, Wilson P, Auckland C, Cairns J, Ward D, Lal P, Guleri A, Jenkins N, Sutton J, Wiselka M, Armando GR, Graham C, Chadwick PR, Barlow G, Gordon NC, Young B, Meisner S, McWhinney P, Price DA, Harvey D, Nayar D, Jeyaratnam D, Planche T, Minton J, Hudson F, Hopkins S, Williams J, Török ME, Llewelyn MJ, Edgeworth JD, Walker AS. Adjunctive rifampicin for *Staphylococcus aureus* bacteraemia (ARREST): a multicentre, randomised, double-blind, placebo-controlled trial. *Lancet.* 2018;391(10121):668–678.

A7.23 Answer C: Flucloxacillin and rifampicin and gentamicin

Flucloxacillin monotherapy remains the regime of choice for native-valve meticillin susceptible *S. aureus* endocarditis, and where there is a contraindication to flucloxacillin such as allergy, either vancomycin monotherapy (in the context of anaphylaxis) or cefazolin or cefotaxime (if the allergy is not anaphylactic) are acceptable therapies. For meticillin resistant *S. aureus* native-valve endocarditis, vancomycin monotherapy is the regime of choice, with alternatives including daptomycin or co-trimoxazole plus clindamycin.

Where there is an infected prosthetic valve, as in this case, meticillin susceptible *S. aureus* endocarditis should be treated with flucloxacillin, rifampicin and gentamicin. If the causative organism is meticillin resistant, vancomycin, rifampicin and gentamicin should be used.

Further Reading

Habib G, Lancellotti P, Antunes MJ, Bongiorni MG, Casalta JP, Del Zotti F, Dulgheru R, El Khoury G, Erba PA, Lung B, Miro JM, Mulder BJ, Plonska-Gosciniak E, Price S, Roos-Hesselink J, Snygg-Martin U, Thuny F, Tornos Mas P, Vilacosta I, Zamorano JL. 2015 ESC guidelines for the management of infective endocarditis: The Task Force for the Management of Infective Endocarditis of the European Society of Cardiology (ESC). *Eur Heart J.* 2015;36(44):3075–3128.

A7.24 Answer E: Warfarin

Significant interactions occur with the following group of drugs: oral contraceptives, glucocorticoids, cyclosporine, statins, tacrolimus, warfarin, azole antifungals, oral sulfonylurea hypoglycaemics, antiretrovirals such as protease inhibitors and integrase inhibitors.

Rifampicin's significant effect on warfarin via CYP3A4 and CYP2C9 metabolism has been known since the mid-1970s. The rate of clearance of warfarin is increased in the presence of rifampicin leading to reduced serum levels. Warfarin levels should be closely monitored and adjusted accordingly during and after rifampicin therapy.

Further Reading

Baciewicz AM, Chrisman CR, Finch CK, Self TH. Update on rifampicin, rifabutin, and rifapentine drug interactions. *Curr Med Res Opin.* 2013;29(1):1–12.

A7.25 Answer A: Disruption of cytoplasmic membrane function

Gentamicin was developed from *Micromonospora purpurea* (unlike other aminoglycosides which end with "-mycin" such as neomycin and streptomycin which were developed from

Streptomyces spp.). Most aminoglycosides are relatively broad-spectrum antimicrobials which have two main mechanisms of action. The first is through binding to bacterial 30S ribosomal subunits, thereby inhibiting protein synthesis through interfering with formation of the initiation complex and causing ribosomes to separate from mRNA. This mode of action provides a significant post-dose effect against bacteria. The second mechanism of action is concentration-dependent killing related to membrane disruption, and it is this effect that is thought to generate the potent bactericidal effects seen with aminoglycosides.

Entry of aminoglycosides into bacterial cells is via an aerobic energy-dependent electron transport system across the inner cytoplasmic membrane. This does not occur in anaerobic organisms. There may be synergistic activity between aminoglycoside mechanisms of action and that of β-lactams against both Gram-negative and Gram-positive organisms.

Further Reading

Garneau-Tsodikovaa S, Labby KJ. Mechanisms of resistance to aminoglycoside antibiotics: overview and perspectives. *Med Chem Comm.* 2016;7(1):11–27.

Hanberger H, Edlund C, Furebring M, G Giske C, Melhus A, Nilsson LE, Petersson J, Sjölin J, Ternhag A, Werner M, Eliasson E. Rational use of aminoglycosides – review and recommendations by the Swedish Reference Group for Antibiotics (SRGA). *Scand J Infect Dis.* 2013;45(3):161–175.

A7.26 Answer B: High-frequency hearing loss

Aminoglycoside toxicity predominantly affects the renal and cochleovestibular systems. Aminoglycoside cochlear toxicity may lead to high-frequency hearing loss from irreversible destruction of the auditory hair cells in the organ of Corti.

Aminoglycoside ototoxicity occurs more frequently with larger doses and longer durations of therapy. It also occurs with increased frequency among older patients, those with impaired renal function, those with existing hearing impairment and where there is concomitant prescription of loop diuretics or other medications which may impact hearing.

The nephrotoxicity arising from aminoglycosides occurs through effects on the proximal tubule cells and through causing a degree of vasoconstriction. Aminoglycosides are taken up by the proximal tubule epithelial cells after glomerular filtration where they alter the metabolism of phospholipids. This can lead to acute tubular necrosis (rather than interstitial tubular nephritis). Prolonging the interval between aminoglycoside doses (i.e. once daily rather than multi-dose per day) is effective for reducing the incidence of nephrotoxicity. However, transient rises in creatinine clearance is seen even with a single dose of aminoglycosides.

Further Reading

Hayward RS, Harding J, Molloy R, Land L, Longcroft-Neal K, Moore D, Ross JDC. Adverse effects of a single dose of gentamicin in adults: a systematic review. *Br J Clin Pharmacol.* 2018;84 (2):223–238.

Huth ME, Ricci AJ, Cheng AG. Mechanisms of aminoglycoside ototoxicity and targets of hair cell protection. *Int J Otolaryngol.* 2011;937861.

A7.27   Answer B: Creatine phosphokinase

Daptomycin is a lipopeptide antibiotic which is active against Gram-positive organisms. It acts through disrupting cell membrane function leading to the formation of pores, which leak ions leading to cell death. It is indicated in complicated skin and skin structure infections, in right-sided endocarditis and in *S. aureus* bacteremia associated with either of these indications. It may also be used for *Enterococcus* spp. infections, but higher doses are likely to be needed. It should not be used to treat Gram-positive pneumonia as it is inactivated by lung surfactant.

It should only be prescribed in patients with renal impairment with caution and where other options have been explored. All patients should have their creatine phosphokinase monitored, preferably weekly, to detect any incipient myositis. Patients should also be counselled to notify the prescriber if they experience any myalgia. The initial trials looking at daptomycin use cited rates of raised creatine phosphokinase at 1.9% compared to 0.5% among the comparator antimicrobials.

Among those who have suboptimal renal function, creatinine clearance should also be monitored closely throughout the course of therapy. In addition, those with impaired renal function should have their creatine phosphokinase monitored more frequently; preferably every 2–3 days. Patients on other medications with the potential to cause myositis, such as fibrates, ciclosporin or 3-hydroxy-3-methyl-glutaryl-coenzyme A (HMG-CoA) reductase agents (also known as "statins") should also have their creatine phosphokinase monitored more closely if co-prescription is truly felt necessary. Liver function disturbance is not a common facet of daptomycin prescription, and it can be prescribed in those with mild-to-moderate liver impairment without dose adjustment.

Further Reading

Gonzalez-Ruiz A, Seaton RA, Hamed K. Daptomycin: an evidence-based review of its role in the treatment of Gram-positive infections. *Infect Drug Resist*. 2016;9:47–58.

A7.28   Answer C: Valproate

All beta-lactam antimicrobials may reduce the seizure threshold. Among the carbapenems, imipenem, in particular, is associated with seizure activity, with some studies citing seizure rates of 3–33%, compared to less than 1% for the other carbapenems. Use of high doses of beta-lactams, or use in the context of renal impairment, or in those with a predisposition to seizures or where there is structural brain disease, increases the risk of drug-induced seizure activity.

Specific to the carbapenems, there is an acknowledged interaction with valproate, whereby carbapenems cause a decrease in the serum concentration of valproate which can lead to seizure activity in patients with pre-existing epilepsy. Therefore, this drug combination should be avoided where possible or if use of a carbapenem is necessary in someone established on valproate, an alternative antiepileptic (such as Levetiracetam) may need to be introduced for the duration of the antimicrobial therapy.

Further Reading

Miller AD, Ball AM, Brandon Bookstaver P, Dornblaser EK, Bennett CL. Epileptogenic potential of carbapenem agents: mechanism of action, seizure rates, and clinical considerations. *Pharmacotherapy*. 2011;31(4):408–423.

A7.29 Answer C: Ceftolozane-tazobactam

In patients with structural lung disease, such as the focal area of bronchiectasis seen with this patient, treatment of *P. aeruginosa* in a sputum sample may be appropriate. *P. aeruginosa* may be resistant to beta-lactam antimicrobials through production of beta-lactamases, porin loss or upregulation of efflux pumps. Loss of carbapenem susceptibility is often through porin loss (although some isolates of *P. aeruginosa* have acquired metal-beta-lactamases). Loss of ceftazidime susceptibility is often through a combination of upregulation of AmpC betalactamase production and increased efflux. Loss of piperacillin-tazobactam susceptibility may be due to AmpC upregulation, acquired penicillinases and/or increased efflux. Ceftolozane-tazobactam usually retains susceptibility against *P. aeruginosa* isolates, which have become resistant to ceftazidime, piperacillin-tazobactam and meropenem through these mechanisms. In the United Kingdom, among *P. aeruginosa* isolates referred to the national reference laboratory with similar resistance patterns to the isolate in this question, over 94% were still susceptible to ceftolozane-tazobactam.

Some *P. aeruginosa* strains have acquired extended-spectrum beta-lactamases, which are usually VEB rather than CTX-M, TEM- or SHV- ESBLs. These VEB ESBL *P. aeruginosa* isolates, and those which have acquired a metallo-beta-lactamase, are almost universally resistant to ceftolozane-tazobactam. Ceftobiprole is a fifth-generation cephalosporin with broad-spectrum activity against both Gram-positive (including meticillin resistant *Staphylococcus aureus*) and Gram-negative (including Enterobacteriales and *P. aeruginosa*) organisms. The cover for *P. aeruginosa* isolates is comparable to that of ceftazidime. Ceftaroline is also a fifth-generation cephalosporin, with a predominantly Gram-positive spectrum of activity (including MRSA).

Further Reading

Farrell DJ, Flamm RK, Sader HS, Jones RN. Ceftobiprole activity against over 60,000 clinical bacterial pathogens isolated in Europe, Turkey, and Israel from 2005 to 2010. *Antimicrob Agents Chemother.* 2014;58(7):3882–3888.

Livermore DM, Mushtaq S, Meunier D, Hopkins KL, Hill R, Adkin R, Chaudhry A, Pike R, Staves P, Woodford N. Activity of ceftolozane/tazobactam against surveillance and 'problem' Enterobacteriaceae, *Pseudomonas aeruginosa* and non-fermenters from the British Isles. *J Antimicrob Chemother.* 2017;72(8):2278–2289.

A7.30 Answer C: Voriconazole

Rifampicin is an effective inducer of both the hepatic and intestinal cytochrome P-450 (CYP) enzyme system and P-glycoprotein (P-gp) transport system. Rifampicin markedly alters the metabolism of azoles and should be avoided in those on voriconazole. Significant interactions occur with the following group of drugs: oral contraceptives, glucocorticoids, cyclosporine, statins, tacrolimus, warfarin, azole antifungals, oral sulfonylurea hypoglycaemics, antiretrovirals such as protease inhibitors and integrase inhibitors.

Further Reading

Baciewicz AM, Chrisman CR, Finch CK, Self TH. Update on rifampin, rifabutin, and rifapentine drug interactions. *Curr Med Res Opin.* 2013;29(1):1–12.

A7.31   **Answer C: Flucytosine**
The five predominant classes of antifungal agents are the polyenes (such as amphotericin, nystatin), the triazoles (such as fluconazole, itraconazole, voriconazole, posaconazole), the echinocandins (such as caspofungin, anidulofungin, micafungin), the pyrimidine analogues (such as flucytosine (5-fluorocytosine)) and the allylamines (such as terbinafine).

The polyenes have one of the broadest spectra of activity against both yeasts and filamentous fungi. The triazoles spectrum of activity varies between agents, with fluconazole limited to some *Candida* spp. (mainly *Candida albicans*), voriconazole and itraconazole covering a broader range of yeasts and additionally covering *Aspergillus* spp., and posaconazole offering an even broader spectrum including the mucoraceous moulds. The echinocandins offer a predominant spectrum of activity against *Candida* spp., with some activity against *Pneumocystis jirovecii*. Flucytosine is active against *Cryptococcus neoformans* and the majority of *Candida* spp. Flucytosine has been associated with myelosuppression, deranged liver function and rash.

Therapeutic drug monitoring for antifungals is advocated for flucytosine, and for several of the triazoles including itraconazole, voriconazole and posaconazole. There is no evidence or indication at the current time to support the routine use of TDM for polyenes (amphotericin B deoxycholate, liposomal amphotericin B and amphotericin B lipid complex) or the echinocandins (micafungin, caspofungin and anidulofungin).

Further Reading
Ashbee HR, Barnes RA, Johnson EM, Richardson MD, Gorton R, Hope WW. Therapeutic drug monitoring (TDM) of antifungal agents: guidelines from the British Society for Medical Mycology. *J Antimicrob Chemother*. 2014;69(5):1162–1176.

A7.32   **Answer E: Oral griseofulvin**
Tinea capitis (or scalp ringworm) is predominantly caused by the dermatophytes *Trichophyton* spp. or *Microsporum* spp. These fungi invade the hair shaft, making topical therapy suboptimal (unlike in dermatophyte infection of other areas of the skin), and systemic (oral) antifungal therapy the mainstay. Griseofulvin has long been the preferred option for treatment of tinea capitis, particularly for *Trichophyton* spp. tinea capitis. However, there is now growing data that terbinafine, itraconazole or fluconazole may be as effective for *Microsporum* spp. infection, and have shorter treatment durations, and fewer adverse events than griseofulvin.

Other oral antifungals, including triazoles such as voriconazole and posaconazole, have not been demonstrated to have a role in this disease.

Further Reading
Hay RJ. Tinea capitis: current status. *Mycopathologia*. 2017;182(1):87–93.

A7.33   **Answer D: Fluconazole**
Studies comparing regimens that included azoles (fluconazole, itraconazole, ketoconazole and miconazole) or polyenes (intravenous low-dose amphotericin B deoxycholate or lipid-based formulations of amphotericin B) in neutropaenic prophylaxis confirmed reduced morbidity, superficial fungal infection, invasive fungal infection and fungal infection-related

mortality. Specifically regarding immunocompromised patients during building work, *Aspergillus* sp. needs to be considered. Therefore, the appropriate prophylactic agent will need to have activity against *Aspergillus* spp., which all do except fluconazole.

Further Reading

Fleming S, Yannakou CK, Haeusler GM, Clark J, Grigg A, Heath CH, Bajel A, van Hal SJ, Chen SC, Milliken ST, Morrissey CO, Tam CS, Szer J, Weinkove R, Slavin MA. Consensus guidelines for antifungal prophylaxis in haematological malignancy and haematopoietic stem cell transplantation, 2014. *Intern Med J.* 2014;44(12b):1283–1297.

Table 10 Expected antifungal susceptibility of common medically important fungi.

	Amphotericin B	Fluconazole	Itraconazole	Voriconazole	Caspofungin
Candida spp.	Yes	Variable	Variable	Yes	Yes
Aspergillus spp.	Yes	No	Yes	Yes	Yes
Fusarium spp.	Yes	No	No	Yes	No
Mucor spp.	Yes	No	No	No	No
Cryptococcus spp.	Yes	Yes	Yes	Yes	No

Robenshtok E, Gafter-Gvilli A, Goldberg E, Weinberger M, Yeshurun M, Leibovici L, Paul M. Antifungal prophylaxis in cancer patients after chemotherapy or haematopoietic stem cell transplantation: systematic review and meta-analysis. *J Clin Oncol.* 2007;25(34):5471–5489.

A7.34   Answer B: Voriconazole

Co-trimoxazole is the recommended first-line antimicrobial for both prophylaxis and treatment of PJP. Second-line regimes including primaquine plus clindamycin, pentamidine, dapsone plus trimethoprim and atovaquone. Caspofungin is a third-line regime and should only be used as salvage therapy. It is routine practice to administer corticosteroids for moderate or severe PJP infection in HIV-infected individuals but the data is conflicted in non-HIV-infected patients. Although not recommended in consensus guidance for non-HIV infected patients, it may be appropriate to co-administer corticosteroids at doses used in HIV-positive patients on a case by case basis.

Further Reading

Cooley L, Dendle C, Wolf J, The BW, Chen SC, Boutlis C, Thurskey KA. Consensus guidelines for diagnosis, prophylaxis and management of *Pneumocystis jirovecii* pneumonia in patients with haematological and solid malignancies, 2014. *Intern Med J.* 2014;44(12b):1350–1363.

A7.35   Answer B: Innate defence peptide

Host defence peptides (small, natural peptides) and innate defence regulators (small, synthetic peptides) have indirect antimicrobials effects. They act by increasing expression of anti-inflammatory cytokines and reducing the expression of pro-inflammatory cytokines. These should work as adjuvants to other therapies and should be useful against both Gram-positive and

Gram-negative organisms. Probiotics are live microorganisms, which can rebalance a host's microflora leading to a health benefit, and have been explored in treatment and prevention of *Clostridium difficile* disease. Bacteriophages can either be wild-type or manufactured, and are bacteria-specific viruses that kill specific bacteria. Metal chelation involves blocked bacterium from utilising metal ions such as zinc, manganese and iron, which they need to fully express their pathogenicity, virulence, biofilm or essential enzymatic processes.

Further Reading

Czaplewski L, Bax R, Martha C, Clokie M, Dawson M, Fairhead H, Fischetti VA, Foster S, Gilmore BF, Hancock RE, Harper D, Henderson IR, Hilpert K, Jones BV, Kadioglu A, Knowles D, Ólafsdóttir S, Payne D, Projan S, Shaunak S, Silverman J, Thomas CM, Trust TJ, Warn P, Rex JH. Alternatives to antibiotics – a pipeline portfolio review. *Lancet Infect Dis.* 2016;16:239–251.

Vaccination

Practitioners in the field of infectious diseases, microbiology and virology must be proficient in advising on vaccination against communicable diseases. Practitioners must have a working knowledge of World Health Organisation's (WHO) childhood vaccination schedules, occupationally indicated vaccinations and the use and timing of post-exposure vaccinations. Practitioners should also be aware of adverse event profiles of vaccines and of the contraindications to certain vaccine preparations in certain patient cohorts.

Practitioners in the field of infection should also be able to select and interpret tests to delineate immunity and to use passive immunisation (such as immunoglobulin therapy) when they are clinically indicated. There should also be an understanding of the public health principles underlying immunisation, including heard immunity, and of the microbial and immunological principles, which can make vaccine protection suboptimal or time limited.

Questions

Q8.1 An 18-year-old intravenous drug user presents with a soft tissue infection. His serology for blood-borne viruses is negative and hepatitis B vaccine is considered. What type of vaccine is hepatitis B vaccine?
A. Killed virus
B. Live attenuated virus
C. Subunit
D. Toxoid
E. Conjugate

Q8.2 A 65-year-old male who had a successful renal transplant 18 months ago presents for pre-travel vaccinations. Which of the following vaccines is safe to administer in this patient?
A. Influenza A virus
B. Measles virus
C. Rubella virus
D. Yellow fever virus
E. Varicella zoster virus

Q8.3 A 68-year-old male with pulmonary fibrosis and non-tuberculous mycobacterial infection attends clinic and receives an annual influenza vaccine. Why do influenza vaccines need to be given annually?
A. Influenza antigenic shift
B. Influenza antigenic drift

C. Suboptimal B-cell response

D. Suboptimal T-cell response

E. Recipient relative immune paresis

Q8.4 A 54-year-old healthcare professional is found to be varicella zoster virus IgG negative on occupational health screening and is subsequently assessed for varicella zoster vaccination. Which of the following is a contraindication to receiving this vaccination?

A. HIV with a CD4 count of 550

B. Radiotherapy 12 months ago

C. 1 week of 40 mg prednisolone 1 month ago

D. Azathioprine 12 months ago

E. Weber–Christian disease

Q8.5 Patients with which of the following conditions should be recommended to receive pneumococcal vaccine?

A. Hepatitis C-induced liver cirrhosis

B. β Thalassaemia minor

C. Asthma

D. Recurrent otitis media

E. Those recovered from acute malaria

Q8.6 Which vaccine is given at 12–15 months of age to avoid inhibition by maternal antibodies?

A. Haemophilus influenzae B

B. Measles, mumps and rubella

C. Bacille Calmette–Guerin

D. Diphtheria, pertussis and tetanus

E. Meningococcus C

Q8.7 Which of the following food-borne pathogens can be prevented by vaccination?

A. *Campylobacter jejuni*

B. *Giardia intestinalis*

C. *Shigella* spp.

D. *Vibrio cholerae*

E. *Salmonella* Enteriditis

Q8.8 A 23-year-old female is 20 weeks pregnant and presents for pre-travel medical advice. She is travelling to Nigeria to visit friends and relatives, is leaving in 2 months and staying there for 1 month. She has no past medical history of note, and her obstetric history has been normal so far. She is up to date with her childhood vaccinations, but has not previously received any travel vaccines. What advice should be given to this patient regarding yellow fever vaccination?

A. Yellow fever vaccination is contraindicated and should not be given

B. Yellow fever vaccination should be given and is likely to confer at least 35 years of protection

C. Yellow fever vaccination should be given and is likely to confer lifelong protection

    D. Yellow fever vaccination should be given and early re-vaccination considered

    E. Yellow fever antivirals should be prescribed as chemoprophylaxis

Q8.9 A 47-year-old male presents for pre-travel medicine advice prior to a Latin American cruise which includes sailing up the Amazon to Manaus. He has no past medical history of note, and thinks he has previously had yellow fever vaccination but it would have been more than 15 years ago and has lost his certificate. What advice should be given to this patient regarding yellow fever vaccination?

    A. Yellow fever vaccination is contraindicated and should not be given

    B. He is protected from yellow fever and a replacement certificate should be issued

    C. He is not protected from yellow fever and should be re-vaccinated

    D. He is not protected from yellow fever and should have a medical exemption issued

    E. He is not at risk of yellow fever and neither vaccination nor certificate is required

Answers

A8.1 Answer C: Subunit

Intravenous drug use and needle sharing puts users at risk of many infections, including all blood-borne viruses – hepatitis C, hepatitis B and HIV. Recreational drug users who present for medical care should be offered screening for blood-borne viruses where available. Where there is no evidence of current or previous infection with hepatitis B, vaccination should be considered. In the United Kingdom, national guidelines suggest vaccination should be considered for all current intravenous drug users as a high priority, those who inject intermittently, those who are likely to "progress" to injecting (including those who are heavily dependent amphetamine users or who are currently smoking heroin or crack cocaine), and the sexual partners, co-inhabitants and children of intravenous drug users. Hepatitis B vaccine is a genetically engineered single-antigen (i.e. subunit) vaccine, which in its administered form contains hepatitis B surface antigen epitopes, yeast and two adjuvants – aluminium and thimerosal. There is limited data suggesting that administration of this vaccine may rarely be associated with autoimmune diseases, but the benefits of this vaccine far outweigh any potential risks.

Further Reading

Geier MR, Geier DA, Zahalsky AC. A review of hepatitis B vaccination. *Expert Opin Drug Saf.* 2003;2(2):113–122.

Salisbury D, Ramsay M, Noakes K. Chapter 18. Immunisation against infectious disease (the 'Green Book'). 2006. Available at: www.gov.uk/government/collections/immunisation-against-infectious-disease-the-green-book

A8.2 Answer A: Influenza A virus

In some immunosuppressed individuals live vaccines can cause severe or even fatal infections, and are therefore contraindicated, except in consultation with an appropriate specialist. Killed, toxoid, subunit and conjugate vaccines are all safe to administer to immunocompromised individuals (as long as no other contraindication exists), although a lower immunological response may be elicited.

Table 11 Categorisation of common vaccines against infectious diseases.

Killed	Attenuated	Toxoid	Subunit	Conjugate
Influenza	Yellow fever	Tetanus	Hepatitis B	Haemophilus influenzae B
Cholera (O1)	Cholera (O1)	Diphtheria	Papilloma virus	Pneumococcal
Yersinia pestis	Measles			
Polio (IPV)	Polio (OPV)			
Hepatitis A	Rubella			
Rabies	Mumps			
	BCG			
	Varicella zoster virus			

Further Reading

Salisbury D, Ramsay M, Noakes K. Chapter 1. Immunisation against infectious disease (the 'Green Book'). 2006. Available at: www.gov.uk/government/collections/immunisation-against-infectious-disease-the-green-book

A8.3   Answer A: Influenza antigenic drift

Influenza viruses make up three of the five genera of the family Orthomyxoviridae (influenza A, B, C and isavirus and thogotovirus). The influenza A genome contains 11 genes on 8 pieces of ss(−) RNA. Mutations can cause small changes in the haemagglutinin and neuraminidase antigens on the surface of the virus; this is antigenic drift. In contrast, when influenza viruses re-assort, including for example in re-assortment between avian strains and human strains, they acquire completely new antigens; this is antigenic shift. Due to continual antigenic drift, a particular influenza vaccine which may imbue protection to only the three or four most common circulating strains at any one time usually confers protection for no more than a few years.

Further Reading

Treanor J. Influenza vaccine – outmanoeuvring antigenic shift and drift. *N Engl J Med*. 2004;350:218–220.

A8.4   Answer C: 1 week of 40 mg prednisolone 1 month ago

Not all forms of immunocompromise make live vaccinations contraindicated. Patients with the following conditions or receiving the following treatments should not receive live vaccinations:

- Severe primary immunodeficiencies, such as Wiskott–Aldrich syndrome and other combined immunodeficiency syndromes.
- Current or recent immunosuppressive chemotherapy or radiotherapy until at least 6 months after treatment.
- Solid organ transplant with continuing immunosuppressive therapy.

- Bone marrow transplant until at least 12 months after immunosuppressive therapy has stopped (longer if there was graft versus host disease).
- High-dose steroids (at least 40 mg of prednisolone per day for a week) until at least 3 months after treatment.
- Other immunosuppressive agents, including cyclophosphamide, methotrexate, cyclosporine, azathioprine, until at least 6 months after treatment.
- HIV, although while BCG and yellow fever are contraindicated, MMR and VZV vaccines can be considered unless they have severe immunosuppression (CD4 counts <200).
- Weber–Christian disease is a cutaneous condition also known as idiopathic relapsing febrile non-supperative panniculitis; there is no know associated immunocompromise with this condition.

Further Reading

Salisbury D, Ramsay M, Noakes K. Immunisation against infectious disease (the 'Green Book'). Chapter 6 'Contraindications and special considerations'. 2006. Available at: www.gov.uk/government/collections/immunisation-against-infectious-disease-the-green-book

A8.5   Answer A: Hepatitis C-induced liver cirrhosis

Pneumococcal vaccination is dependent upon inducing an immunological response to the capsule of *Streptococcus pneumoniae* (acapsular pneumococci are not usually pathogenic). Unfortunately, the *S. pneumoniae* capsule is particularly variable, and over 90 capsular serotypes have been identified. Among these, however, invasive pneumococcal disease can be attributed to a much smaller number of capsular variants in the majority of cases.

There are three types of pneumococcal vaccine in widespread use; the 23 valent polysaccharide vaccine, the 13 valent conjugate vaccine and the 10 valent conjugate vaccine. These vaccines are all inactivated. For the polysaccharide vaccine, children under 2 years of age do not demonstrate a good immunological response, but among adults it provides a good level of response protecting against pneumococcal bacteraemia (but not otitis media or non-bacteraemic pneumonia) and covers 96% of circulating serotypes in the United Kingdom. The polysaccharide vaccine is indicated for all adults over the age of 65 years and for those between 2 years and 65 years if they are in an at-risk group; asplenia or dysfunction of the spleen, chronic respiratory disease (but not asthma unless requiring constant or frequent steroids), chronic heart disease, chronic renal disease, chronic liver disease, diabetes, immunosuppression, individuals with cochlear implants or cerebrospinal fluid leaks. The 10 valent and 13 valent conjugate vaccine provide improved immunogenicity for children, and is indicated in the infant immunisation schedule at 2 months and 4 months of age.

Further Reading

Cafiero-Fonseca ET, Stawasz A, Johnson ST, Sato R, Bloom DE. The full benefits of adult pneumococcal vaccination: a systematic review. *PLoS ONE*. 2017;12(10):e0186903.

Salisbury D, Ramsay M, Noakes K. Immunisation against infectious disease (the 'Green Book'). Chapter 25 'Pneumococcal vaccination'. 2006. Available at: https://assets.publishing.service.gov.uk/government/uploads/system/uploads/attachment_data/file/674074/GB_Chapter_25_Pneumococcal_V7_0.pdf

A8.6   Answer B: Measles, mumps and rubella

Childhood vaccination schedules should be timed so as to allow maternal passive immunity (from antepartum transmission of maternal antibodies) to have dissipated, while ensuring that the periods of highest risk of the illness are preempted. For measles, maternal antibodies have been demonstrated to be extremely low by 9 months of age. Maternal antibodies to mumps and rubella persist for some time longer, however, up to 12 months. Depending upon prevailing immunity levels, measles, mumps and rubella can affect children of any age, but where vaccine coverage is low, up to 30% of 15-month olds can be found to have had one of these three illnesses already. Studies looking at the optimal timing of the MMR vaccine have demonstrated that immunogenicity does occur if administered before 1 year of age, but maternal antibodies may still be present, and therefore there may be a reduced response to the vaccine.

Further Reading

Ma SJ, Li X, Xiong YQ, Yao AL, Chen Q. Combination measles-mumps-rubella-varicella vaccine in healthy children: a systematic review and meta-analysis of immunogenicity and safety. *Medicine*. 2015;94(44):e1721.

A8.7   Answer D: *Vibrio cholerae*

A killed whole-cell vaccine is available for *V. cholerae* which contains four strains; O1 (subtypes Inaba and Ogawa) and biotypes El Tor and classical. Two doses of the vaccine provide effective protection against cholera for at least 3 years, while a single dose provides short-term protection sufficient for some circumstances such as travel or acute natural disaster recovery programmes. The vaccine is administered orally and is indicated in travellers (2 years and older) who are travelling to an area at risk of cholera. Specifically, it is often used for aid workers and those with itineraries covering areas where cholera epidemics are occurring.

There are currently no effective vaccines against *C. jejuni*, *Shigella* spp. or *Giardia lamblia*. While there is a vaccine available against typhoid fever, there is no effective human vaccine against the other *Salmonella* spp.

Further Reading

Bi Q, Ferreras E, Pezzoli L, Legros D, Ivers LC, Date K, Qadri F, Digilio L, Sack DA, Ali M, Lessler J, Luquero FJ, Azman AS. Protection against cholera from killed whole-cell oral cholera vaccines: a systematic review and meta-analysis. *Lancet Infect Dis*. 2017;17(10):1080–1088.

A8.8   Answer D: Yellow fever vaccination should be given and early re-vaccination considered

Yellow fever is a flavivirus infection transmitted by day biting *Aedes* spp. mosquitos and is prevalent across 13 countries in Latin America and 31 countries in sub-Saharan Africa, including Nigeria, as relevant in this case. There is an effective (protective levels achieved in 99% by 28 days) vaccine available, but this is a live-attenuated vaccine and as such is contraindicated in several patient cohorts. Notably, it must not be given to those who: are aged less than 6 months, have had an anaphylactic reaction to a previous dose of YF vaccine/ any components of the vaccine or egg, have thymus dysfunction or who are immunocompromised (including previous bone marrow or solid organ transplant, ongoing immunosuppressive agents, severe primary immunodeficiency or HIV infection with low CD4 counts). There are further precautions associated in several other groups, including HIV infection with high CD4 counts, infants aged 6–9 months, those aged over 60 years and pregnant and breastfeeding women.

Specifically for pregnant women, as in this case, there is a theoretical risk of foetal infection. However, the benefits from vaccination of those travelling to yellow fever endemic areas are thought to outweigh the risks, and the vaccine should be advocated after providing counselling to the expectant mother around the potential risks and benefits. However, lower seroconversion rates (39%) have been observed in pregnant women compared to controls in prospective studies. Therefore, while vaccination might be considered to confer at least 35 years of protection to the majority of those who are vaccinated (i.e. those who are immunocompetent, over 2 years of age and are not pregnant at the time of vaccination), vaccination of pregnant women may warrant early re-vaccination.

Further Reading

The WHO Strategic Advisory Group of Experts (SAGE) on Immunization Documents on Yellow Fever. 2013. Available at: www.who.int/immunization/diseases/yellow_fever/en/

A8.9 **Answer C: He is not protected from yellow fever and should be re-vaccinated**
Yellow Fever Certificate requirements for travel must be considered for those undertaking international travel, and this varies on a country-by-country basis. In this specific case, Brazil is a country where there is endemic yellow fever in several parts, particularly in the interior of the country including the Amazonian basin. As such, travellers to these regions are at risk of acquiring yellow fever, and there is a clear clinical indication to vaccinate accordingly. The patient in this scenario has no contraindications to administration of this live vaccine, and as such it should be given. Separate to the assessment of whether there is a clinical need for the Yellow Fever vaccine, there must be an assessment of Yellow Fever Certificate requirements. In this case the cruise up the Amazon overrides this concern, but if the patient had only been sailing to areas without clear risk of yellow fever disease, yet where there were travel requirements for Yellow Fever Certification, then a decision has to be made. The alternatives are (i) whether he should have an exemption issued (preferable and is taken into legal consideration at border control) or (ii) whether he should have the vaccine purely to meet travel regulations (within the license of the vaccine but as his age puts him at increased risk of vaccine-associated viscerotropic disease).

Where exemptions are given, it must be made clear that a medical exemption does not confer protection to yellow fever. Therefore, for those who are travelling to yellow fever endemic areas, but who have an absolute contraindication to the live vaccine, careful discussion of whether travel is wise at all should be had. Finally, best practice is for a discussion to also be had around the validity of medical exemption certificates, and how although the World Health Organisation says they should be taken into consideration at border control, each country retains sovereign right to decide upon entry of travellers.

Yellow Fever Certificates of vaccination (and exemptions) are given on a specific yellow booklet in accordance to the International Health Regulations (2005). They should only be re-issued where the clinician re-issuing has clear unambiguous evidence of prior vaccination.

Further Reading

The International Health Regulations. 2005. Available at: http://apps.who.int/iris/bitstream/10665/ 43883/1/9789241580410_eng.pdf (in particular Annex 7).

Chapter

9 The Management of HIV Infection, Opportunistic Infections and Complications of Other Causes of Immunocompromise

Patients living with human immunodeficiency virus (HIV) have particular health needs relating to their diagnosis, the opportunistic infections which can affect them, and the chronic disease management of their condition which is impacted by the disease process itself and the medication used to control it. Practitioners working with patients living with human immunodeficiency virus must hold knowledge of the pathophysiology and natural history of the disease, the therapeutic options available for virological control and the likely complication from HIV and the medications. Practitioners must be able to safely monitor and interpret the test results of patients living with human immunodeficiency virus. They must also be able to advise on strategies to decrease onwards transmission of HIV, including pre-and post-exposure prophylaxis. Practitioners managing patients living with human immunodeficiency virus must be able to identify and treat the opportunistic infections which may arise.

Questions

Q9.1 A 24-year-old male presents with fever, rash and arthralgia. He reports multiple unprotected sexual exposures a few months ago. Investigations reveal:

White cell count: 6.9×10^9/L

Lymphocytes: 2.6×10^9/L

Rapid point of care HIV test: reactive

CD4 count: 950 cells/μL

Which of the following statements is most correct in this case?
A. This represents seroconversion illness
B. He is manifesting an AIDS-defining illness
C. This is a false positive
D. He is not infectious for HIV
E. Treatment with antiretrovirals should commence when CD4 count is <350 cells/μL

Q9.2 A 51-year-old male who is HIV positive attends clinic for review. He has been on antiretroviral therapy for 6 months and now has an undetectable viral load and a CD4 count of 615 cells/μL. However, he spent a long period off therapy, but with a high viral load, when younger. What end-organ disease does HIV virus directly cause?
A. Nephropathy
B. Enteritis

    C. Hepatitis

    D. Retinitis

    E. Arthropathy

Q9.3 A 32-year-old female presents with breathlessness and is diagnosed with *Pneumocystis carinii* pneumonia. A HIV test returns positive. Which laboratory test is useful for prognostic purposes in new diagnoses of HIV?

    A. HIV envelope antibody

    B. HIV p24 antigen

    C. HIV viral load

    D. CD4 count

    E. HIV plasma RNA

Q9.4 A 55-year-old, HIV-positive Kenyan male presented with weakness and numbness of his left arm and leg. He was diagnosed with HIV 5 years previously and has struggled with adherence to medication. His last CD4 count was 60 cells/μL. On examination, he had hemiparesis of the left side with hemi-sensory loss. MRI scan shows a focal mass lesion in the right hemisphere. What is the most likely cause of this presentation?

    A. *Toxoplasma gondii*

    B. Progressive multifocal leukoencephalopathy

    C. Primary CNS lymphoma

    D. *Cryptococcus neoformans*

    E. *Mycobacterium tuberculosis*

Q9.5 A 40-year-old female who is HIV-positive presents with confusion, seizures and an altered level of consciousness. She is originally from France and known IgG positive to *Toxoplasma gondii*. MRI did not show any focal lesions and a lumbar puncture was undertaken due to no evidence of raised intracranial pressure. CSF examination revealed a positive PCR for *T. gondii*. Her previous CD4 count was <200 cells/μL in outpatients 8 months ago and was started on PCP prophylaxis with co-trimoxazole, but developed a rash and medication was changed to dapsone. What treatment regime would be recommended?

    A. Liposomal amphotericin

    B. Sulphadiazine with pyrimethamine

    C. Clindamycin with pyrimethamine

    D. Atovaquone with pyrimethamine

    E. Azithromycin with pyrimethamine

Q9.6 A 35-year-old, HIV-positive male presents with fever, weight loss and decreased appetite. On examination, he has widespread lymphadenopathy. Computerised tomography of his chest and abdomen is undertaken (Figure 9.1).

    His blood tests show:

        CD4 count of 114 cells/μL

        Plasma HIV viral load of 65,000 copies/ml

        HHV8 viral load of 10,000 copies/mL

Lymph node biopsy shows an onion-skin appearance on histopathology with interfollicular plasmablasts expressing HHV8 latent nuclear antigen.

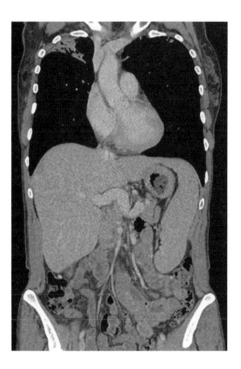

Figure 9.1 Thoracoabdominal computerised tomograph, coronal plane.

What is the likely diagnosis?
A. Primary effusion lymphoma (PEL)
B. Kaposi's sarcoma
C. Multicentric Castleman's disease
D. Hodgkin's lymphoma
E. Non-Hodgkins's lymphoma

Q9.7 A 35-year-old male presents to his local general practitioner (GP) with multiple purple raised lesions on his trunk and arms. He had seen his GP for dry skin over the face last year when he was prescribed emollients. He is homosexual and works as a dancer. His male partner has been recently diagnosed HIV positive and he is concerned this may be Kaposi's sarcoma (KS). He has pulmonary or gastrointestinal symptoms. Which of the following treatments are not established for Kaposi's sarcoma?
A. Introduction of antiretroviral therapy
B. Intralesional vinblastine
C. Liposomal anthracyclines
D. Ganciclovir
E. Paclitaxel chemotherapy

Q9.8 A 60-year-old female from Cambodia was visiting family in the United Kingdom when she felt unwell and attended the emergency department. She was complaining of weight loss, fever and cough. On examination, it was noted that she had cervical and inguinal lymphadenopathy with hepatosplenomegaly. She had multiple papular skin lesions with central necrotic umbilication mainly on the trunk and upper limbs. Her rapid HIV test was reactive and blood showed anaemia and mild thrombocytopenia. What would be the initial treatment regime?

A. Commence antiretroviral therapy
B. Liposomal amphotericin B
C. Antituberculous therapy
D. Itraconazole
E. Paclitaxel chemotherapy

Q9.9 A 29-year-old male presented with pneumococcal pneumonia 2 weeks previously. His HIV test was positive and further results reviewed at his follow-up HIV outpatient appointment showed a CD4 count of 651 cells/μL and a viral load of 352,000 copies/mL. He is self-employed and explains that he wants to start treatment as soon as possible due to concerns of being unwell, which will have a financial implication to his family. When would you recommend he starts antiretroviral therapy?

A. Immediately
B. When his CD4 count falls below 350 cells/μL
C. When his CD4 count falls below 250 cells/μL
D. When his CD4 count is between 350 and 500 cells/μL
E. When he develops signs and symptoms of an opportunistic infection

Q9.10 A 24-year-old male known to be HIV positive on treatment denies problems with adherence to his medication. He was diagnosed after partner notification and has not suffered from an opportunistic infection. He has maintained a reasonable CD4 count but his last viral load was 354 copies/mL 6 months ago and in clinic his viral load is 460 copies/mL. He has never reached an undetectable viral load of <50 copies/mL. What is the definition of his current viral response to treatment?

A. Virological failure
B. Incomplete virological response
C. Virological rebound
D. Low-level viraemia
E. Virological blip

Q9.11 A 23-year-old female was recently diagnosed with HIV disease. She was diagnosed with oesophageal candidiasis, *Mycobacterium tuberculosis* and pneumocystis pneumonia during a recent admission to hospital. She has started antiretroviral therapy. She comes to clinic and her pregnancy test is positive. Based on her menstrual cycle, she is in the first trimester of pregnancy. Which of the following medications would be safe to continue to treat her illnesses?
A. Co-trimoxazole
B. Efavirenz
C. Moxifloxacin
D. Itraconazole
E. None of the above

Q9.12 An HIV-positive patient attended the outpatient clinic after commencing a new therapy regime 3 month previously complaining of nightmares. He had started an ART containing regime of tenofovir-DF, emtricitabine and efavirenz. His HIV viral load was undetectable. The patient does not want to continue the current regime and wants to change therapy. Based on the likely drug to be switched, which of the following medications will need a dose increase for the first week?
A. Raltegravir
B. Maraviroc
C. Dolutegravir
D. Rilpivirine
E. Elvitegravir/cobicistat

Q9.13 A 55-year-old patient from West Africa was referred to the HIV outpatient department following a positive test for HIV-2 disease. After basic genotypic resistance testing, no significant mutations were found. HIV-2 shows innate resistance to which class of antiretrovirals?
A. Non-nucleoside reverse transcriptase inhibitors (NNRTI)
B. Nucleoside reverse transcriptase inhibitor (NRTI)
C. Protease inhibitors
D. Integrase inhibitors
E. Chemokine (C-C motif) receptor 5 (CCR5) antagonists

Q9.14 A 22-year-old, HIV-negative patient presents after a weekend which involved sexual activity at a sex party. He is a man who has sex with men (MSM). He recalls having unprotected receptive anal intercourse while under the influence of alcohol and recreational drugs 48 hours earlier. He knows the individual is HIV positive and he accompanies him to the clinic appointment. The sexual partner is known to the clinic and consents to disclose his latest results. He was diagnosed 1 year previously and is currently on antiretroviral therapy, with his last HIV plasma viral load undetectable (<50 copies/mL). Four months previously he had a viral load of 350 copies/mL. There was no significant resistance on genotypic testing.

The patient is concerned about contracting HIV and wonders if there is anything to do. How would you treat this individual?
A. Reassure that transmission is low risk and no treatment needed
B. Offer post-exposure prophylaxis with truvada and raltegravir for 14 days

C. Offer post-exposure prophylaxis with truvada and raltegravir for 28 days
D. Offer post-exposure prophylaxis with truvada and efavirenz for 14 days
E. Offer post-exposure prophylaxis with truvada and efavirenz for 28 days

Q9.15 A 37-year-old female with known HIV was admitted with fever and shortness of breath with a dry cough. She had stopped taking her antiretroviral medication 3 years previously due to social circumstances. She was diagnosed with PCP when the broncho-alveolar lavage tested positive for *Pneumocystis* PCR. She was treated with high-dose co-trimoxazole (septrin) and made a full recovery. She was counselled on the importance of compliance with long-term therapy and agreed to take her medication. She was seen in clinic 6 months later and her CD4 count was 230 cells/μL, and she remained on oral septrin. Which of the following statements is true regarding PCP prophylaxis?

A. Dapsone is first-line therapy for PCP prophylaxis
B. Once CD4 counts drop below 200 cells/μL, PCP prophylaxis should continue for life
C. Following treatment of PCP, if the CD4 counts rise above 200 cells/μL for 3 months, PCP prophylaxis can be stopped
D. Co-trimoxazole is first-line prophylaxis for PCP before dapsone because of toxicity issues rather than increased efficacy
E. G6PD status needs to be established prior to therapy with pentamidine

Q9.16 A 44-year-old female with known advanced HIV disease was admitted with fever, reduced consciousness and a history of 3 weeks of headache. On examination, she was confused with a Glasgow Coma Scale of 13. A lumbar puncture was performed showing a markedly raised opening pressure. On microbiological examination, India ink staining showing encapsulated organisms and the cryptococcal antigen test in both blood and cerebrospinal fluid was positive. A diagnosis was made and the patient was started on caspofungin (an echinocandin). She continued to deteriorate and was changed to liposomal amphotericin and flucytosine.

Which of the following reasons would make choosing an echinocandin for this indication inappropriate?

A. *Cryptococcus neoformans* is resistant to echinocandins as it does not contain $(1,3)\beta$-glucan synthase
B. Echinocandins have poor penetration into the central nervous system
C. Echinocandins have no in-vitro activity against Cryptococcal species
D. Echinocandins are prohibitively expensive given the prolonged therapy needed for *Cryptococcal meningitis*
E. Echinocandins have multiple drug interactions with HIV antiviral regimes and may complicate therapy if needed to be changed

Q9.17 A 56-year-old female in induction-phase chemotherapy for acute myeloid leukaemia develops a fever and breathlessness. High-resolution computerised tomography of the chest indicates a pneumonitis. Samples from broncho-alveolar lavage are sent.

Microscopy: no organisms seen

Bacterial culture: scanty *Streptococcus oralis*

Fungal culture: no growth

Viral PCR: adenovirus detected.

Which other clinical syndrome does the pathogen in this case commonly cause?

A. Genital cancer
B. Kerato-conjunctivitis
C. Genital ulcers
D. Hand, foot and mouth ulcers
E. Aseptic meningitis

Q9.18 A 34-year-old male who is on tacrolimus having received a kidney transplant 5 years previously presents with fever, fatigue and cervical adenopathy. His blood tests demonstrate:

CMV PCR: negative

EBV PCR: negative

HHV6 PCR: positive

Which disease is HHV6 is associated with?

A. Fifth's disease
B. Roseola infantum
C. Kaposi's sarcoma
D. Castleman's disease
E. Oral hairy leukoplakia

Q9.19 A 7-year-old female was treated for relapsed acute lymphoblastic leukaemia with methotrexate, cytarabine and cyclophosphamide. Chemotherapy was given by central venous access via a Hickmann® line. She attended the emergency department with neutropenic fever. No localising symptoms or signs were identified. She was commenced on piperacillin-tazobactam and vancomycin with resolution of the fever. Seventy-two hours after admission, blood cultures flagged positive. Gram stain from blood culture showed fungal hyphae without chlamydospores (Figure 9.2). She was commenced on liposomal amphotericin but remained febrile at day 7 post admission. Her fever settled on removal of the central venous catheter and changing her antifungal therapy to voriconazole.

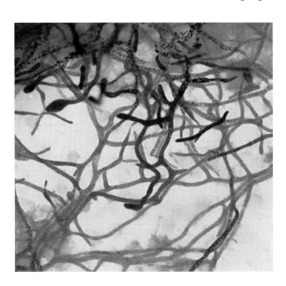

Figure 9.2 Gram stain from a positive blood culture. (A black and white version of this figure will appear in some formats. For the colour version, please refer to the plate section.)

Which is the most likely organism identified?
A. *Fusarium solani*
B. *Malassezia furfur*
C. *Candida auris*
D. *Paecilomyces lilacinus*
E. *Aspergillus fumigatus*

Q9.20 A 50-year-old male was undergoing an autologous stem cell transplantation for acute myeloid leukaemia when he developed a febrile illness 10 days after receiving the stem cells. He was neutropenic and broad-spectrum antibiotics where commenced with meropenem and amikacin. He continued to spike fevers despite introduction of antifungal therapy. He had developed lesions on his skin and parenchymal changes in the chest radiograph. A high-resolution chest CT showed widespread changes consistent with fungal aetiology. Blood cultures flagged positive after 3 days with filamentous fungi growing on subsequent sub-culture (Figure 9.3).

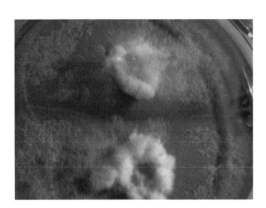

Figure 9.3 Appearance of isolate after 5 days aerobic sub-culture on Sabouraud Dextrose Agar at 25°C. (A black and white version of this figure will appear in some formats. For the colour version, please refer to the plate section.)

Which is the most likely fungal pathogen causing the above presentation?
A. *Fusarium solani*
B. *Aspergillus fumigatus*
C. *Paecilomyces* spp.
D. *Penicillium* spp.
E. *Scopulariopsis* spp.

Q9.21 A 33-year-old male was undergoing a haemopoietic stem cell transplantation for acute myeloid leukaemia. He was 7 days into the transplantation following return of stem cells and was neutropenic. He was tachycardic and febrile. He complained of some oral and abdominal pain with some associated diarrhoea. On examination, he was pale and lethargic with a temperature of 38.5°C. There was a Hickmann® line in situ which was non-tender with a clean exit site. The abdomen had some mild generalised tenderness. Per rectal examination was not performed but no blood was seen on stool examination. He was commenced on piperacillin-tazobactam and amikacin as per local protocol for the management of febrile neutropenia.

Investigations revealed:

- Haemoglobin: 80 g/L
- Platelet count: 30×10^9/L
- Total white cell count: 0.2×10^9/L
- Total neutrophil count: 0.0×10^9/L
- Creatinine: 110 μmol/L
- Blood culture: no growth after 48 hours incubation

The patient was reviewed 72 hours later on the consultant ward round where he was afebrile.

What would be your next management plan regarding the antimicrobials?
A. No bacterial cause found so add an antifungal
B. Continue both piperacillin-tazobactam and gentamicin until neutrophil count $>0.5 \times 10^9/L$
C. Stop gentamicin and continue piperacillin-tazobactam until neutrophil count $>0.5 \times 10^9/L$
D. Stop all antimicrobials at 72 hours
E. Change to second line antibiotic therapy with meropenem

Q9.22 A 44-year-old male was admitted with fever and persistent cough. He had undergone a renal transplantation for polycystic kidney disease 5 years ago. He took tacrolimus as anti-rejection medication. He had no significant travel history, no pets and lived in a two-bed maisonette which had recently been renovated. On examination, he was pyrexial and tachypnoeic. Chest radiograph revealed non-specific changes in both lung fields. CT imaging of the chest showed small nodular changes with surrounding ground glass changes.

A bronchoscopy was performed and the microbiology laboratory subsequently reported growth of a mould (Figure 9.4).

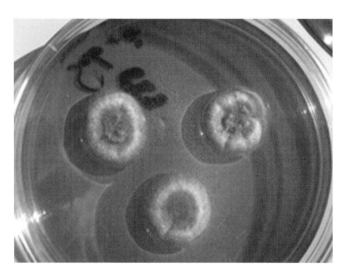

Figure 9.4 Appearance of isolate after 5 days aerobic sub-culture on Sabouraud Dextrose Agar at 30°C. (A black and white version of this figure will appear in some formats. For the colour version, please refer to the plate section.)

What would be the most appropriate first-line therapy?
A. Liposomal amphotericin B alone
B. Micafungin and liposomal amphotericin B
C. Voriconazole and liposomal amphotericin B
D. Voriconazole alone
E. Caspofungin

Q9.23 A 35-year-old male presents with a dry cough and feeling short of breath on minimal exertion. He works as a scaffolder and has a long-term male partner. On examination, he is comfortable at rest, with some mild bi-basal crepitations on auscultation. Chest radiograph shows bilateral haziness. Computed tomography of the chest shows bilateral widespread ground glass shadowing with sub-pleural margin sparing.

Point of care HIV test: reactive

Which is the likely pathogen causing this presentation?

A. Cytomegalovirus
B. *Mycobacterium tuberculosis*
C. *Pneumocystis jirovecii*
D. *Mycobacterium avium complex*
E. *Streptococcus pneumoniae*

Q9.24 A male with recurrent staphylococcal infections is investigated for a possible immune system disorder. On laboratory investigation, it is noted that his neutrophils fail to stain with nitroblue-tetrazolium dye. What is the most likely cause of his immunodeficiency?

A. Myeloperoxidase deficiency
B. Chronic granulomatous disease
C. IgA deficiency
D. Familial Mediterranean fever
E. Alpha-1-antitrypsin deficiency

Q9.25 A 55-year-old male renal transplant patient attended a summer wedding where the reception was held in the garden of the couple's home. The couple own two snakes and a lizard which were on display for the guests. There was a buffet dinner which included oysters and vegetarian sandwiches.

Which scenario is the least likely to be a risk to the individual?

A. Pet reptiles in the home
B. Eating sprouts in a sandwich
C. Eating raw oysters
D. Drinking pasteurised juices
E. Eating from a buffet at a summer wedding

Q9.26 A 14-year-old male patient with hypogammaglobulinaemia develops persistent diarrhoea. He had previously been treated for *Campylobacter* infection. He was clinically well with non-bloody diarrhoea. The microbiology laboratory isolates *Campylobacter jejuni* in stool culture. His blood cultures did not grow any organism after 5 days of incubation. What is the therapy of choice?

A. Fosfomycin
B. Colistin
C. Erythromycin
D. Ciprofloxacin
E. Amoxicillin

Q9.27 A 55-year-old male patient with bowel cancer is receiving chemotherapy via a central venous catheter. He is bought in by ambulance after collapsing at home. On arrival he is hypotensive, tachycardic and febrile. Examination does not reveal an obvious source of the infection. He was given piperacillin-tazobactam and gentamicin as per local policy for treatment of suspected neutropenic sepsis. The blood culture grows an organism and Gram stain demonstrates a Gram negative rod.

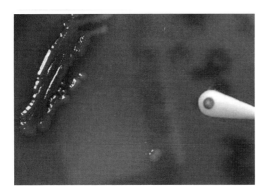

Figure 9.5 Growth on blood agar incubated in an aerobic environment at 37°C for 24 hours, with result of oxidase test.

What is the likely organism?
A. *Escherichia coli*
B. *Citrobacter freundii*
C. *Salmonella enteritidis*
D. *Pseudomonas aeruginosa*
E. *Proteus mirabilis*

Answers

A9.1 **Answer A: This represents seroconversion illness**
The pre-test probability of the HIV test being positive was high due to the history and risk exposure, thus making a false-positive test unlikely. He is early in the infection and, therefore, the long-term effect on CD4 count is not apparent. The START study was published in 2015 and enrolled 4,685 adults with CD4 cell counts above 500 cells/µL in 35 countries, and randomised them to start ART immediately or to defer ART until the CD4 count fell below 350 cells/µL. The risk of developing AIDS, a serious non-AIDS event or of death was reduced by 57% in those who were randomised to start earlier, after a median follow-up period of 3 years. The results were similar in high-income when compared to low- and middle-income countries, and driven mainly by a difference in rates of AIDS events, particularly TB and cancers.

Further Reading

INSIGHT START study Group, Lundgren JD, Babiker AG, Gordin F, Emery S, Grund B, Sharma S, Avihingsanon A, Cooper DA, Fätkenheuer G, Llibre JM, Molina JM, Munderi P, Schechter M, Wood R, Klingman KL, Collins S, Lane HC, Phillips AN, Neaton JD. Initiation of antiretroviral therapy in early asymptomatic HIV infection. *N Engl J Med.* 2015;373(9):795–807.

A9.2 Answer A: Nephropathy

HIV-associated nephropathy (HIVAN) is a form of focal segmental glomerulosclerosis (FSGS) with associated interstitial inflammation. It is caused by direct invasion of kidney epithelial cells by HIV virus. Other types of chronic kidney diseases are seen in association with HIV, but these are immune complex-mediated and include IgA nephropathy, membrano-proliferative glomerulonephritis and a glomerulonephritis that resembles that of lupus. Instigating antiretroviral therapy can improve HIVAN. Additional steroids and angiotensin-converting enzyme inhibitors have been suggested to have a beneficial effect, but the evidence is not strong. Enteritis and retinitis in HIV is typically caused by opportunistic infections rather than the HIV virus itself. Hepatitis can occur for several reasons in HIV-positive patients, including co-infection with hepatitis B or C or as a result of antiretroviral therapy (particularly the non-nucleotide reverse transcriptase inhibitors). Arthritides occur frequently in HIV-positive individuals, with Reiter syndrome and reactive arthritis representing the most common causes. Non-inflammatory arthralgia is also common in HIV-positive individuals (up to 45%), but the pathophysiology behind this is uncertain, and may involve transient bone ischaemia.

Other main end-organ diseases caused directly by HIV virus are the HIV-associated neurocognitive disorders (HAND), including the AIDS dementia complex (ADC). ADC typically occurs in those who have prolonged periods of high viral loads and low CD4 counts. Antiretroviral therapy may delay (data is less clear on whether it is preventative) ADC.

Further Reading

Kalayjian RC. The treatment of HIV-associated nephropathy. *Adv Chronic Kidney Dis.* 2010;17(1):59–71.

A9.3 Answer D: CD4 count

The CD4 count is the strongest laboratory prognostic indicator for patients newly diagnosed with HIV. For those diagnosed with HIV who did not present with an opportunistic infection (i.e. those presenting for sexual health or occupational screening or after an exposure event), data from the Strategic Timing of Antiretroviral Treatment study group has now indicated net benefits for initiation of antiretroviral therapy in HIV-positive adults with a CD4+ > 500 cells/µL compared to the previous suggested starting range of 350 cells/µL.

Initial HIV viral load (i.e. HIV plasma RNA) can be used as a diagnostic test for the presence of HIV, but is more frequently used to influence which antiretroviral regime should be commenced (some regimes are associated with higher rates of virological failure in those with high pre-treatment HIV RNA). Once antiretroviral therapy has been commenced, HIV viral load is used to monitor response to therapy and detect virological failure. The p24 antigen can be used as an early diagnostic test (i.e. before HIV serology becomes positive) for those who have been exposed to HIV virus. HIV envelope antibodies may be neutralising or (more frequently) non-neutralising. These have obvious diagnostic value in serological tests, but are also an area of ongoing interest to aid development of prophylactic and therapeutic interventions for people living with HIV.

Further Reading

Burton DR, Mascola JR. Antibody responses to envelope glycoproteins in HIV-1 infection. *Nat Immunol.* 2015;16:571–576.

The INSIGHT START Study Group. Initiation of antiretroviral therapy in early asymptomatic HIV infection. *N Engl J Med.* 2015;373:795–807.

A9.4 Answer A: *Toxoplasma gondii*

Toxoplasma abscesses are the most common cause of mass lesions among immunocompromised individuals worldwide, including sub-Saharan Africa. The primary infection in immunocompetent patients is often asymptomatic but can be a mononucleosis presentation similar to EBV. Seropositivity for toxoplasma varies worldwide and depends on age, dietary habits and proximity to cats. In France, rates approach 90%; in the United Kingdom and United States, rates are 10–40%. The lifetime risk of an untreated HIV-positive IgG seropositive for *T. gondii* patient for toxoplasma encephalitis is 25%. It is now a standard practice to treat any HIV patient with a CD4 count of <200 cells/µL and a brain mass lesion with anti-toxoplasma therapy unless an alternative diagnosis has been made.

Further Reading

Nelson M, Dockrell D, Edwards S; BHIVA guidelines subcommittee. British HIV Association and British Infection Association guidelines for the treatment of opportunistic infection in HIV-seropositive individuals 2011. *HIV Med.* 2011;12(S2):1–140.

A9.5 Answer C: Clindamycin with pyrimethamine

First-line therapy for toxoplasma encephalitis is sulphadiazine with pyrimethamine. Patient should be screened for G6PDH deficiency prior to starting therapy due to the risk of haemolysis with sulphur-containing drugs. Second-line therapy for patients who cannot take sulphur drugs is clindamycin with pyrimethamine. Folinic acid should be given with pyrimethamine-containing regimes. Clindamycin-containing regimes show slightly less efficacy but sulphadiazine regimes have significantly more side-effects. Other regimes including azithromycin, doxycycline or dapsone are not as effective.

Further Reading

Nelson M, Dockrell D, Edwards S; BHIVA Guidelines Subcommittee. British HIV Association and British Infection Association guidelines for the treatment of opportunistic infection in HIV-seropositive individuals 2011. *HIV Med.* 2011;12(S2):1–140.

A9.6 Answer C: Multicentric Castleman's disease

Castleman's disease is classified into localised (LCD) and multicentric (MCD) forms. The localised form usually presents in young adults with isolated masses in the mediastinum or neck. In contrast, MCD is associated with multiple organ involvement, typically with adenopathy and extensive hepato-splenomegally, as in this case, and has a more aggressive course. MCD is an HHV8-driven disease similar to PEL and Kaposi's sarcoma. PEL can develop in the presence of MCD demonstrating the association between the diseases. It is recommended that histological confirmation requires immunocytochemical staining for HHV8 and IgM lambda, and all patients should have blood levels for HHV8 to support the diagnosis. Rituximab should be first-line treatment with MCD and chemotherapy added for aggressive disease.

Further Reading

Bower M, Palfreeman A, Alfa-Wali M, Bunker C, Burns F, Churchill D, Collins S, Cwynarski K, Edwards S, Fields P, Fife K, Gallop-Evans E, Kassam S, Kulasegaram R, Lacey C, Marcus R, Montoto S, Nelson M, Newsom-Davis T, Orkin C, Shaw K, Tenant-Flowers M, Webb A, Westwell S, Williams M. British HIV association guidelines for HIV-associated malignancies 2014. *HIV Med.* 2014;15(S2):1–92.

A9.7   Answer D: Ganciclovir

Kaposi's sarcoma (KS) is the most common tumour in HIV-positive individuals and is an AIDS-defining illness. It is caused by the Kaposi sarcoma herpesvirus (KSHV). It is characterised by cutaneous or mucosal lesions which are graded into patch, plaque or nodular disease. Visceral disease is uncommon and affects 14% of patients with KS. Current recommendations state that Kaposi's should be confirmed histologically, and further investigations outside of dermatology should be guided by symptoms, such as endoscopy or CT scans. HAART should be started on all patients with KS. Local radiotherapy or intralesional vinblastine can be used for early stage TO KS for symptomatic or cosmetic improvement. Advanced KS should receive chemotherapy with liposomal anthracyclines as first line. Paclitaxel chemotherapy is second-line treatment for refractory disease. Aciclovir, ganciclovir and valganciclovir have been looked at for preventative therapy but results are poor, and although frequency of KS can be reduced, the risk can return to baseline on stopping treatment.

Further Reading

Bower M, Palfreeman A, Alfa-Wali M, Bunker C, Burns F, Churchill D, Collins S, Cwynarski K, Edwards S, Fields P, Fife K, Gallop-Evans E, Kassam S, Kulasegaram R, Lacey C, Marcus R, Montoto S, Nelson M, Newsom-Davis T, Orkin C, Shaw K, Tenant-Flowers M, Webb A, Westwell S, Williams M. British HIV association guidelines for HIV-associated malignancies 2014. *HIV Med.* 2014;15(S2):1–92.

A9.8   Answer B: Liposomal amphotericin B

The most likely diagnosis in an HIV-positive patient from South-east Asia with lesions that are umbilicated (similar to molluscum) would be penicilliosis. The fact that she has systemic signs and symptoms suggests a disseminated disease, and histoplasmosis and *Cryptococcus* can have similar presentations. Liposomal amphotericin is first-line treatment for penicilliosis, histoplasmosis and cryptococcosis, and therefore the most appropriate treatment choice. Penicilliosis is caused by *Penicillium marneffei* which is a dimorphic fungus common in SEA. Biopsy with fungal culture should be sought in these cases. Patients should be treated with amphotericin B induction for 2 weeks followed by itraconazole maintenance.

Further Reading

Nelson M, Dockrell D, Edwards S. British HIV Association and British Infection Association guidelines for the treatment of opportunistic infection in HIV-seropositive individuals 2011. *HIV Med.* 2011;12(S2):1–140.

A9.9   Answer A: Immediately

Previous BHIVA recommendations stated that individuals with chronic infection should start ART when their count falls below 350 cells/μL. The START study enrolled 4,685 adults with CD4 cell counts above 500 cells/μL (median 651 cells/μL) in 35 countries to either starting immediately or deferring until <350 cells/μL. There was a 57% reduction in risk of developing AIDS, a serious non-AIDS event or of death if therapy was started earlier. Therefore, the recommendations are that if a patient is committed to taking ART, then it should be started irrespective of CD4 count.

Further Reading

Churchill D, Waters L, Ahmed N, Angus B, Boffito M, Bower M, Dunn D, Edwards S, Emerson C, Fidler S, Fisher M, Horne R, Khoo S, Leen C, Mackie N, Marshall N, Monteiro F, Nelson M, Orkin C, Palfreeman A, Pett S, Phillips A, Post F, Pozniak A, Reeves I, Sabin C, Trevelion R, Walsh J, Wilkins E, Williams I, Winston A. British HIV association guidelines for the treatment of HIV-1-positive adults with antiretroviral therapy 2015. *HIV Med.* 2016;17(S4): S2–S104.

A9.10   Answer B: Incomplete virological response

The following definitions are used to characterise a patient's virological response to treatment:

- *Virological suppression*: achieving and maintaining a VL level <50 copies/mL
- *Virological failure:* incomplete virological response after commencing treatment or evidence of virological rebound to >200 copies/mL
- *Incomplete virological response*: two consecutive VL >200 copies/mL after 24 weeks without ever achieving VL <50 copies/mL
- *Virological rebound*: failure to maintain a VL below the limit of detection (<50 copies/mL) on two or more consecutive occasions.
- *Low-level viraemia*: a persistent VL between 50 and 200 copies/mL
- *Virological blip:* after virological suppression a single VL between 50 and 200 copies/mL followed by an undetectable result.

Current recommendations state that a virological blip is usually not of clinical concern and should necessitate clinical vigilance and adherence reinforcement. A single result of >200 copies/mL should have a rapid retest and genotypic resistance test as it may be indicative of virological failure. If there is low-level viraemia or repeated viral blips, then resistance testing should be done.

Further Reading

Churchill D, Waters L, Ahmed N, Angus B, Boffito M, Bower M, Dunn D, Edwards S, Emerson C, Fidler S, Fisher M, Horne R, Khoo S, Leen C, Mackie N, Marshall N, Monteiro F, Nelson M, Orkin C, Palfreeman A, Pett S, Phillips A, Post F, Pozniak A, Reeves I, Sabin C, Trevelion R, Walsh J, Wilkins E, Williams I, Winston A. British HIV association guidelines for the treatment of HIV-1-positive adults with antiretroviral therapy 2015. *HIV Med.* 2016;17(S4):S2–S104.

A9.11   Answer B: Efavirenz

No ARV has a licence for use in the first trimester of pregnancy. Only zidovudine has a licence in the third trimester. The most robust data on teratogenicity and first-trimester

ART exposure are from the Antiretroviral Pregnancy Registry (APR), which reports rates of birth defects during ART. It needs >200 reports before the APR report, and now there are over 200 prospective reports in the APR of first-trimester exposure for abacavir, atazanavir, darunavir, efavirenz, emtricitabine, lamivudine, lopinavir, nevirapine, ritonavir, tenofovir and zidovudine. No signal of increased risk has been demonstrated. There were concerns over the safety of efavirenz based on pre-clinical animal studies, but a systematic review and meta-analysis in 2014 did not reveal increased risk. Current recommendation is efavirenz which can be initiated in women of childbearing potential, can be continued in women who conceive and commenced in pregnancy, but the data should be discussed with the patient. Co-trimoxazole, moxifloxacin and itraconazole are contraindicated in pregnancy and alternative therapy should be introduced.

Further Reading

De Ruiter A, Taylor GP, Clayden P, Dhar J, Gandhi K, Gilleece Y, Harding K, Hay P, Kennedy J, Low-Beer N, Lyall H, Palfreeman A, O'Shea S, Tookey P, Tosswill J, Welch S, Wilkins E. British HIV Association guidelines for the management of HIV infection in pregnant women 2012 (2014 interim review). *HIV Med.* 2014;15(S4):1–77.

Ford N, Mofenson L, Shubber Z, Calmy A, Andrieux-Meyer I, Vitoria M, Shaffer N, Renaud F. Safety of efavirenz in the first trimester of pregnancy: an updated systematic review and meta-analysis. *AIDS.* 2014;28(S2):S123–S131.

A9.12 Answer B: Maraviroc

Induction of drug-metabolising enzymes by efavirenz persists upon cessation. No high-quality data exists on how to switch away from efavirenz to an alternative, and if the patient has an undetectable viral load, then it is unlikely to be clinically significant.
A pharmacokinetic study in HIV-positive individuals showed that the induction effect necessitated an increase in maraviroc dose to 600 mg twice daily from 300 mg twice daily (standard dose) for 1 week.

Further Reading

Churchill D, Waters L, Ahmed N, Angus B, Boffito M, Bower M, Dunn D, Edwards S, Emerson C, Fidler S, Fisher M, Horne R, Khoo S, Leen C, Mackie N, Marshall N, Monteiro F, Nelson M, Orkin C, Palfreeman A, Pett S, Phillips A, Post F, Pozniak A, Reeves I, Sabin C, Trevelion R, Walsh J, Wilkins E, Williams I, Winston A. British HIV association guidelines for the treatment of HIV-1-positive adults with antiretroviral therapy 2015. *HIV Med.* 2016;17(S4):S2–S104.

Waters L, Jackson A, Else L, Rockwood N, Newell S, Back D, Nelson M, Gazzard B, Boffito M. Switching safely: pharmacokinetics, efficacy and safety of switching efavirenz to maraviroc twice daily I patients on suppressive antiretroviral therapy. *Antivir Ther.* 2015;20:157–163.

A9.13 Answer A: Non-nucleoside reverse transcriptase inhibitors (NNRTI)

HIV-2 predominates in West Africa with a much lower prevalence than HIV-1 disease. HIV-2 shows genetic diversity with at least eight different groupings (A-H) from a primate reservoir. Like HIV-1, HIV-2 exhibits mutations which are either baseline or secondary response to antiretroviral therapy. The structure of the NNRTI-binding pocket of HIV-2 differs from HIV-1 conferring innate resistance; therefore, it is recommended not to use this class. The current preferred first-line therapy is tenofovir, emtricitabine and lopinavir/ritonavir.

Further Reading

Gilleece Y, Chadwick DR, Breuer J, Hawkins D, Smit E, McCrae LX, Pillay D, Smith N, Anderson J. British HIV association guidelines for antiretroviral treatment of HIV-2 positive individuals 2010. *HIV Med.* 2010;11:611–619.

A9.14 Answer C: Offer post-exposure prophylaxis with truvada and raltegravir for 28 days

The current guidance for post-exposure prophylaxis following sexual exposure (PEPSE) recommends that if the source's HIV status is unknown, then proactive attempts should be made to establish HIV status. If the source individual is known to be HIV positive then treatment history, viral load and resistance profile should be determined. PEPSE is not recommended if the source is on antiretrovirals with confirmed and sustained (>6 months) undetectable plasma HIV viral load (<200 copies/mL). If there are doubts, then PEP should be given following unprotected receptive anal intercourse. Truvada and raltegravir for 28 days are the first-line treatments and should be initiated as soon as possible after exposure, preferably within 24 hours but can be up to 72 hours. Follow-up HIV testing at 8–12 weeks after exposure should be undertaken.

Further Reading

Cresswell F, Waters L, Briggs E, Fox J, Harbottle J, Hawkins D, Murchie M, Radcliffe K, Rafferty P, Rodger A, Fisher M. UK guideline for the use of HIV post-exposure prophylaxis following sexual exposure, 2015. *Int J STD AIDS.* 2016;27(9):713–738.

A9.15 Answer C: Following treatment of PCP, if the CD4 counts rise above 200 cells/μL for 3 months, PCP prophylaxis can be stopped

Systematic reviews found that co-trimoxazole reduced the incidence of PCP compared with placebo or pentamidine. One systematic review and one randomised controlled trial found no significant difference between high- and low-dose co-trimoxazole for PCP prophylaxis, although adverse effects were more common with the higher dose.
A randomised controlled trial showed that primary and secondary prophylaxis against PCP can be safely discontinued after the CD4 cell count has increased to 200 cells/μL for more than 3 months.

Further Reading

Lopez Bernaldo de Quiros JC, Miro JM, Peña JM, Podzamczer D, Alberdi JC, Martínez E, Cosin J, Claramonte X, Gonzalez J, Domingo P, Casado JL, Ribera E. A randomized trial of the discontinuation of primary and secondary prophylaxis against *Pneumocystis carinii* pneumonia after highly active antiretroviral therapy in patients with HIV infection. Grupo de Estudio del SIDA 04/98. *N Engl J Med.* 2001;344(3):159.

A9.16 Answer B: Echinocandins have poor penetration into the central nervous system

Echinocandins work by inhibiting $\beta(1,3)$-D-glucan synthase and thereby disturbing the integrity of the fungal cell wall. *C. neoformans* is resistant to echinocandins by a mechanism unrelated to $(1,3)\beta$-glucan synthase resistance. It is thought that echinocandin resistance is due to the high content of other sugar polymers (β-1,6 glucans) since their biosynthesis is not affected by echinocandins. Echinocandins do have in-vitro activity. Current guidance recommends liposomal amphotericin B and flucytosine for the induction phase followed by fluconazole as the maintenance phase. The addition of flucytosine speeds up sterilisation of the CSF and reduces the chance of relapse.

Further Reading

Nelson M, Dockrell D, Edwards S. British HIV Association and British Infection Association guidelines for the treatment of opportunistic infection in HIV-seropositive individuals 2011. *HIV Med.* 2011;12(S2):1–140.

A9.17 Answer B: Kerato-conjunctivitis

Adenovirus most commonly causes illness of the respiratory system (pneumonia, croup and bronchitis); however, depending on the infecting serotype, they may also cause various other illnesses, such as gastroenteritis (40 and 41), kerato-conjunctivitis (8, 19 and 37), cystitis and rash illness. Anogenital cancers are associated with specific serotypes of human papilloma virus (HPV). Genital ulcers can be caused by several pathogens, but the most common cause is herpes simplex 1 and 2. Hand, foot and mouth disease is caused by an enterovirus, and enteroviridae are also the most common cause of aseptic meningitis in the United Kingdom.

Further Reading

Lenaerts L, De Clercq E, Naesens L. Clinical features and treatment of adenovirus infections. *Rev Med Virol.* 2008;18(6):357–374.

A9.18 Answer B: Roseola infantum

Human herpes virus 6 (HHV6) is a DNA virus, of which there are two subtypes of HHV-6 termed HHV-6A and HHV-6B (the latter the most common). Infection is nearly ubiquitous in early childhood where the virus usually causes a mild self-limiting fever, with exanthem subitum (Roseola infantum) only being observed in 10% of cases. Following infection, subsequent latency is established in myeloid progenitors. The virus periodically re-activates, particularly in the immunocompromised, and can lead to an infectious mononucleosis-like syndrome. This is more serious in post-transplant recipients and in HIV-positive individuals. HHV6 is frequently incorporated into human genome, however, and diagnosis of active disease is complex. There is some evidence that while qualitative and real-time quantitative PCR cannot distinguish active from latent/integrated HHV6, reverse transcriptase PCR may be more useful. Parvovirus B19 causes Fifth disease (also known as erythema infectiousum), HHV-8 causes Kaposi's sarcoma and is associated with Castleman's disease. EBV is associated with oral hairy leukoplakia.

Further Reading

Caserta MT, Hall CB, Schnabel K, Lofthus G, Marino A, Shelley L, Yoo C, Carnahan J, Anderson L, Wang H. Diagnostic assays for active infection with human herpesvirus 6 (HHV-6). *J Clin Virol.* 2010;48(1):55–57.

A9.19 Answer D: *Paecilomyces lilacinus*

Paecilomyces spp. and *Fusarium* spp. both cause hyalohyphomycosis. *Paecilomyces* spp. are found ubiquitously within the environment. These are uncommon pathogens, with *P. lilacinus* and *P. variotii* the two species most frequently associated with human illness. Ocular and cutaneous disease are the most common presentations, however, fungaemia is reported and associated with haematological malignancies and indwelling prosthetic material. *Fusarium* spp. are the most common cause of fungal keratitis worldwide. In patients with immunodeficiency, *Fusarium* spp. can cause disseminated disease and is second only to *Aspergillus* spp. within this population. Cutaneous manifestations of fusariosis can precede fungaemia, and blood cultures may be positive in up to 40% of cases.

Further Reading

Pastor FJ, Guarro J. Clinical manifestations, treatment and outcome of *Paecilomyces lilacinus* infections. *Clin Microbiol Infect*. 2006 Oct;12(10):948–960.

A9.20 Answer A: *Fusarium solani*

Invasive fusariosis is an important cause of fungal infection in immunocompromised individuals and is an important condition due to high mortality. The most common fungal infection in this case would be *Aspergillus* spp., however, this is rarely seen in blood cultures or skin lesions. Disseminated fusariosis classically has skin lesions and haematogenous spread. Most infections are caused by *F. solani* spp. complex and *Fusarium oxysporum* spp. complex. Most species show high MICs to antifungal therapy, including voriconazole and posaconazole. The use of corticosteroids or prolonged neutropenia is associated with a worse outcome. Optimum therapy is not known but the introduction of liposomal amphotericin (rather than amphotericin deoxycholate), voriconazole or combination therapy has increased survival rates.

Further Reading

Nucci M, Marr KA, Bvehreschild MJ, de Souza CA, Velasco E, Cappellano P, Carlesse F, Queiroz-Telles F, Sheppard DC, Kindo A, Cesaro S, Hamerschlak N, Solza C, Heinz WJ, Schaller M, Atalla A, Arikan-Akdagli S, Bertz H, Galvão Castro C Jr, Herbrecht R, Hoenigl M, Härter G, Hermansen NE, Josting A, Pagano L, Salles MJ, Mossad SB, Ogunc D, Pasqualotto AC, Araujo V, Troke PF, Lortholary O, Cornely OA, Anaissie E. Improvement in the outcome of invasive fusariosis in the last decade. *Clin Microbiol Infect*. 2014;20(6):580–585.

A9.21 Answer D: Stop all antimicrobials

This patient has no identifiable microbiological cause of the fever. The fever has settled over the last 48 hours with negative blood cultures. Examination did not reveal a localising source. Therefore, antimicrobials should be stopped, irrespective of the neutrophil count. There is conflicting advice from current international guidance as the 2011 US guidance (re-approved in 2013) recommends that in patients with unexplained fever the initial regimen should be continued until clear signs of marrow recovery; the traditional endpoint is an increasing neutrophil count exceeding 500 cells/mm^3. The opposing view from European and British guidelines would support stopping antibiotics. The ECIL 2011 guidance recommend discontinuation of antimicrobials after 72 hours if the patient is stable and afebrile for 48 hours. The NICE guidance also supports discontinuation of empiric antibiotic therapy in patients who have responded to treatment, irrespective of neutrophil count. A randomised controlled trial published in 2017 showed no significant difference in mortality or adverse events in patients who had antimicrobials stopped after 72 hours of apyrexia. The conclusion was in support of the ECIL recommendations.

Further Reading

Aguilar-Guisado M, Espigado I, Martin-Pena A, Gudiol C, Royo-Cebrecos C, Falantes J, Vázquez-López L, Montero MI, Rosso-Fernández C, de la Luz Martino M, Parody R, González-Campos J, Garzón-López S, Calderón-Cabrera C, Barba P, Rodríguez N, Rovira M, Montero-Mateos E, Carratalá J, Pérez-Simón JA, Cisneros JM. Optimisation of empirical antimicrobial therapy in patients with haematological malignancies and febrile neutropenia (How Long study): an open-label, randomised, controlled phase 4 trial. *Lancet Haematol.* 2017;4(12):e573–e583.

Averbuch D, Orasch C, Cordonnier C, Livermore DM, Mikulska M, Viscoli C, Gyssens IC, Kern WV, Klyasova G, Marchetti O, Engelhard D, Akova M. European guidelines for empirical antibacterial therapy for neutropenic patients in the era of growing resistance: summary of the 2011 4th European Conference on Infections in Leukaemia. *Haematologica.* 2013;98 (12):1826–1835.

National Institute for Health and Care Excellence. Neutropenic sepsis: prevention and management in people with cancer. NICE guideline (CG151). 2012. Available at: www.nice.org.uk/guidance/cg151

A9.22 Answer D: Voriconazole alone

The choice of antifungal agent depends on whether prophylactic antifungal therapy has been given, which may influence the choice of empiric or definitive treatment. If the patient has been on triazole prophylaxis, then an alternative class should be used such as liposomal amphotericin. This patient has not been on prophylaxis. The organism shown is Aspergillus flavus, and therefore voriconazole is strongly recommended as the initial choice of therapy. Alternatives include liposomal amphotericin and isavuconazole. Combination therapy is not recommended routinely. Invasive pulmonary aspergillosis should be treated for a minimum 6–12 weeks depending on the degree and duration of immunosuppression, site of disease and evidence of disease improvement.

Further Reading

Patterson TF, Thompson GR 3rd, Denning DW, Fishman JA, Hadley S, Herbrecht R, Kontoyiannis DP, Marr KA, Morrison VA, Nguyen MH, Segal BH, Steinbach WJ, Stevens DA, Walsh TJ, Wingard JR, Young JA, Bennett JE. Practice guidelines for the diagnosis and management of *Aspergillosis*: 2016 Update by the Infectious Diseases Society of America. *Clin Infect Dis.* 2016;63(4):e1–e60.

A9.23 Answer C: *Pneumocystis jirovecii*

The common term for *P. jirovecii* infection is PCP, which is due to the previous species name of *Pneumocystis carinii*. This was changed considering the fact *P. carinii* was a rat pathogen. PCP is still commonly used and referred to as "pneumocystis pneumonia." Symptoms of PCP include fever, non-productive cough (sputum hyperviscosity), dyspnoea (especially on exertion), weight loss and night sweats. There is a characteristic appearance on chest X-ray of widespread pulmonary infiltrates with an associated arterial oxygen level markedly lower than would be expected from symptoms. The diagnosis can be definitively confirmed by histological identification of the causative organism in sputum or BAL. Staining with toluidine blue, silver stain, periodic-acid Schiff (PAS) or immunofluorescence assay will show characteristic cysts. The most common diagnostic technique is PCR, and serum β-D-glucan will also be raised.

Further Reading
Stringer J, Beard C, Miller R, Wakefield A. A new name (*Pneumocystis jirovecii*) for pneumocystis from humans. *Emerg Infect Dis*. 2002;8(9):891–896.

A9.24   **Answer B: Chronic granulomatous disease**
Functional disorders of neutrophils are often hereditary. They are disorders of phagocytosis or deficiencies in the respiratory burst (including chronic granulomatous disease and myeloperoxidase deficiency). Phagocytes produce reactive oxygen species to destroy bacteria following phagocytosis called the respiratory burst (NADPH oxidase). Individuals with these deficiencies are vulnerable to infections with catalase-positive organisms such as *Staphylococcus aureus*. The nitroblue-tetrazolium (NBT) test is the original and most widely-known test for chronic granulomatous disease; this test is negative in CGD and positive in normal individuals. A similar test uses dihydrorhodamine (DHR). In MPO deficiency, the majority of individuals show no signs of immunodeficiency but can present particularly with *Candida albicans* infections. Patients with MPO deficiency have a respiratory burst with a normal NBT dye test, as opposed to CGD of childhood, but do not form bleach due to their lack of peroxide.

Further Reading
Mauch L, Lun A, O'Gorman MR, Harris JS, Schulze I, Zychlinsky A, Fuchs T, Oelschlägel U, Brenner S, Kutter D, Rösen-Wolff A, Roesler J. Chronic granulomatous disease (CGD) and complete myeloperoxidase deficiency both yield strongly reduced dihydrorhodamine 123 test signals but can be easily discerned in routine testing for CGD. *Clin Chem*. 2007;53(5):890.

A9.25   **Answer D: Drinking pasteurised juices**
Unlike the limited species tropism exhibited by *Salmonella* Typhi, non-typhoidal *Salmonella* species are widely distributed among pets, particularly reptiles, and have also been documented to cause outbreaks associated with bean sprouts and non-pasteurised juice. In relation to food-borne Salmonellosis, infection is caused by ingestion of viable bacteria. The infectious dose is usually quite large. *Campylobacter* is the most common cause of bacterial gastrointestinal infections in the United Kingdom. *Campylobacter* is thermotolerant and needs a lower infecting dose. Cross-contamination of ready-to-eat foods in the food preparation environment is an important route of transmission. *Vibrio parahaemolyticus* is associated with shellfish and can cause a marked disease in immunocompromised individuals. *V. parahaemolyticus* is a marine bacterium fond in coastal and estuarine waters. It is rare but associated with imported seafood. Growth is reported between 14°C and 40°C, and therefore does not occur if stored at proper refrigeration temperatures; freezing does not kill *V. parahaemolyticus*.

Further Reading

Health Protection Agency. Guidelines for Assessing the Microbiological Safety of Ready-to-Eat Foods. London: Health Protection Agency. 2009. Available at: www.gov.uk/government/publications/ ready-to-eat-foods-microbiological-safety-assessment-guidelines

A9.26 Answer C: Erythromycin

Patients with primary hypogammaglobulinaemia, such as X-linked agammaglobulinaemia and common variable immunodeficiency, have recurrent infections, predominantly of the respiratory and intestinal tract. Recurrent *Giardia lamblia* infections may result in chronic diarrhoea, whereas chronic *C. jejuni* infections may cause recurrent bacteraemia and cellulitis. In X-linked agammaglobulinaemia, persistent enterovirus infections (notably echovirus) are associated with chronic meningoencephalitis. Studies in children with *C. jejuni* dysentery have shown benefit from early treatment with erythromycin. Individuals with hypogammaglobulinaemia who have recurrent *C. jejuni* bacteremia may require fresh-frozen plasma or HNIG/IgM concentrates in addition. A placebo-controlled study showed erythromycin promptly eradicates *C. jejuni* from the faeces but does not alter the natural course of uncomplicated enteritis when therapy begins four or more days after the onset of symptoms.

Further Reading

Anders BJ, Lauer BA, Paisley JW, Reller LB. Double-blind placebo controlled trial of erythromycin for treatment of *Campylobacter enteritis. Lancet.* 1982;1(8264):131–132.

Janssen R, Krogfelt KA, Cawthraw S, van Pelt W, Wagenaar JA, Owen RJ. Host-pathogen interactions in *Campylobacter* infections: the host perspective. *Clin Microbiol Rev.* 2008;21(3):505–518.

A9.27 Answer D: *Pseudomonas aeruginosa*

Pseudomonas spp. are Gram-negative, aerobic, non-sporing rods with one or more polar flagella providing motility, and are also oxidase and catalase positive. They are beta haemolytic, indole negative, methyl red negative, Voges Proskauer test negative and citrate positive. They produce a sweet grape like odour and can produce a green pigment. They are a common pathogen in the healthcare setting and can cause severe sepsis in patients with neutropenia. Empirical choice of antibiotics for patients with neutropenic fever most commonly include an anti-pseudomonal beta-lactam.

Further Reading

Heinz WJ, Buchheidt D, Chistopeit M, von Lilienfeld-Toal M, Cornely OA, Einsele H, Karthaus M, Link H, Mahlberg R, Neumann S, Ostermann H, Penack O, Ruhnke M, Sandherr M, Schiel X, Vehreschild JJ, Weissinger F, Maschmeyer G. Diagnosis and empirical treatment of fever of unknown origin (FUO) in adult neutropenic patients: guidelines of the Infectious Diseases Working Party (AGIHO) of the German Society of Haematology and Medical Oncology (DGHO). *Ann Hematol.* 2017;96(11):1775–1792.

National Institute for Health and Care Excellence. Neutropenic sepsis: prevention and management in people with cancer. NICE guideline (CG151). 2012. Available at: www.nice.org.uk/guidance/cg151

Chapter 10

Travel and Geographical Health; Imported Infection and the Provision of Pre-travel Health Advice

The nature of infectious diseases means that they are not bound by political or social boundaries. Practitioners in infectious diseases, microbiology and virology must, therefore, be competent in the recognition and management of imported infections and be aware of mechanisms to identify prevalent infections in different geographical areas. Practitioners must also be able to recognise problems of non-communicable diseases among immigrants from low- and middle-income settings. Practitioners in infectious diseases must also be competent in giving pre-travel medical advice including vaccination against communicable diseases and prophylaxis (both physical and chemical).

Questions

Q10.1 A 34-year-old male presents after extensive travel to South-east and South Asia over the preceding 6 months with tiredness. His blood tests demonstrate:

Haemoglobin: 91 g/L
White cell count: 7.9×10^9/L
Neutrophils: 3.1×10^9/L
Lymphocytes: 2.3×10^9/L
Eosinophils: 2.0×10^9/L
Platelets: 370×10^9/L
Folate: 5 µg/L
B_{12} 90 pmol/L

Which enteric pathogen is most likely to be associated with this presentation?
A. *Schistosomiasis mekongi*
B. *Taenia solium*
C. *Strongyloides stercoralis*
D. *Taenia saginata*
E. *Diphyllobothrium latum*

Q10.2 A 32-year-old male presents with a fever after staying in a rural farm in West Africa. Which of the following viruses has no known animal reservoir?
A. Rabies virus
B. Coronavirus
C. Cytomegalovirus
D. Hantavirus
E. Lassa fever virus

Q10.3 A 40-year-old female returns from a holiday visiting friends in New England, United States. She had spent 3 weeks travelling around the state and enjoyed long walks in the forests. She describes being bitten on multiple occasions. She complains of a headache and rash. On examination, there is a localised annular lesion on her left lower limb which has a pale centre suspicious of an insect bite. There is no evidence of meningism and no focal neurological signs. She is concerned about Lyme's disease as she has a friend who has been diagnosed with this in the United States and has chronic fatigue. What would be your next management steps?

A. Perform an enzyme-linked immunoassay (EIA) and treat with doxycycline immediately

B. Commence intravenous ceftriaxone

C. Perform two-tiered testing and await results before giving treatment

D. Do not perform any tests and give treatment with doxycycline

E. Perform two-tiered testing and treat with doxycycline immediately

Q10.4 A 45-year-old female presents with fever, headache, myalgia and diarrhoea. She had returned from a 2-week vacation to the United States 10 days ago. She enjoys walking and visited rural areas in the upper mid-State of Wisconsin and Lake Michigan. Physical examination was unremarkable. She describes noticing multiple insect bites.

Investigations revealed:
- Haemoglobin: 95 g/L
- Platelet count: 78×10^9/L
- Total white cell count: 2.3×10^9/L
- Total neutrophil count: 1.8×10^9/L
- Total lymphocyte count: 0.4×10^9/L
- Peripheral blood film showed morulae in the cytoplasm of granulocytes.

Based on the history above what is the most likely vector of the disease?

A. Black legged tick – *Ixodes scapularis*

B. Lone star tick – *Amblyomma americanum*

C. American dog tick – *Dermacentor variabilis*

D. Rocky mountain wood tick – *Dermacentor andersoni*

E. Soft tick – *Ornithodoros* spp.

Q10.5 A 20-year-old male presented with complaints of fever, joint pains, headache and dark urine. He had travelled to the upper Midwestern United States with friends enjoying rural activities, including water sports, hiking and rock climbing. He denies any bites, didn't notice many animals on his walks and did not have direct contact. His friends are all well with no similar symptoms. He had a splenectomy 2 years previously secondary to a motorcycle accident and takes prophylactic penicillin. On examination, he looked pale with an abdominal scar evident but no other relevant features.

Investigations revealed:
- Haemoglobin: 80 g/L
- Platelet count: 60×10^9/L
- Total white cell count: 6.5×10^9/L
- Total neutrophil count: 4.8×10^9/L

- Creatinine: 210 μmol/L
- ALT: 330 U/L
- Peripheral blood film showed intra-erythrocytic parasites.

What is the likely diagnosis for his presentation?
A. Ehrlichiosis
B. Lyme disease
C. Babesiosis
D. Rocky mountain spotted fever
E. Tuleraemia

Q10.6 Three days after returning from the United States a 24-year-old female presents unwell to the local emergency department. She complains of fever, headache, anorexia, sore throat and abdominal pain. She enjoys walking and spent a long weekend camping. On examination, she was meningitic with photophobia. She was excessively lacrimating and crying in pain. Bilateral conjunctivitis and pre-auricular lymphadenopathy were noted.
  Investigations revealed:
- Haemoglobin: 95 g/L
- Platelet count: 44×10^9/L
- Sodium: 128 mmol/L
- Total white cell count: 8.5×10^9/L
- Total neutrophil count: 6.8×10^9/L
- Creatinine: 310 μmol/L
- ALT: 550 U/L
- Creatine kinase: 15,000 U/L

What is your recommended antibiotic treatment regimen to instigate based on the likely infective cause?
A. Meropenem
B. Ceftriaxone
C. Streptomycin and chloramphenicol
D. Doxycycline and gentamicin
E. Ciprofloxacin and doxycycline

Q10.7 During a routine antenatal anomaly ultrasound scan, a 25-year-old female was informed that the foetus has a reduced head circumference. A male child was born at 35 weeks, and microcephaly confirmed with other congenital abnormalities. The mother had gone on a holiday with her husband to Brazil at 12 weeks of pregnancy. She did not seek travel advice prior to departure. During her 2-week holiday she describes a short illness of headache, muscle pain and swelling in her small joints of her hands. She did not seek medical attention as she presumed it to be related to pregnancy. The illness self-resolved. Which pathogen is the most likely cause?
A. Zika virus
B. Chikungunya virus
C. Malaria
D. Dengue virus
E. Cytomegalovirus

Q10.8 A 32-year-old male returns from Sierra Leone and presents with fever, cough and flu-like symptoms. What is the essential next step in managing this patient?
  A. Isolate at a containment level 4 facility
  B. Send a malaria blood film
  C. Start on chloroquine
  D. Wait for blood culture results
  E. Send stool for MC&S and ova, cysts, and parasites

Q10.9 A 37-year-old male returns from celebrations in Hanoi where he drank duck blood. He presents with cough, malaise and a flu-like illness. What management step should be taken next?
  A. Admit to ward and start oral amantadine
  B. Isolate the patient with respiratory precautions
  C. Discharge to the community with oral erythromycin
  D. Admit to ward and commence ceftriaxone
  E. Admit and start intravenous aciclovir

Q10.10 A 45-year-old female with a history of recent travel to Spain presents with confusion, severe pneumonia and diarrhoea. What antimicrobial regime should be initiated for this patient?
  A. Ciprofloxacin and metronidazole
  B. Amoxicillin and clarithromycin
  C. Levofloxacin
  D. Co-amoxiclav and clarithromycin
  E. Ciprofloxacin and clarithromycin

Q10.11 A 28-year-old female with recent travel to Africa and the Middle East presents with a 3-week history of fever, night sweats, an enlarged spleen and a tender spine. A blood culture becomes positive (Figure 10.1).

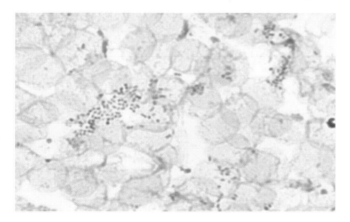

Figure 10.1 Gram stain from a positive blood culture. (A black and white version of this figure will appear in some formats. For the colour version, please refer to the plate section.)

What is the most likely diagnosis in this patient?
  A. Tuberculosis
  B. Visceral leishmaniasis
  C. Hydatid disease
  D. Brucellosis
  E. Malaria

Q10.12 A 32-year-old male presents with haematuria. He has just returned from a round-the-world tour, which included East Africa, South Asia and South-east Asia. He described swimming in fresh water lakes 3 months ago. Microscopy of a terminal urine sample is conducted (Figure 10.2).

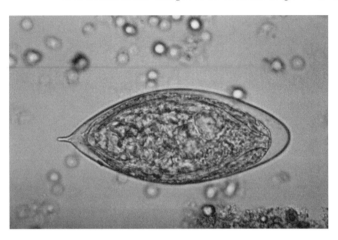

Figure 10.2 Light microscopy of urine sample prepared in 10% (v/v) formalin in water.

Which of the following is the most likely organism?
A. *Schistosoma mekongi*
B. *Schistosoma japonicum*
C. *Schistosoma intercalatum*
D. *Schistosoma haematobium*
E. *Schistosoma mansoni*

Q10.13 A 24-year-old female presents with acute abdominal pain and vomiting. She is flushed and hypotensive and urticarial wheals are noted. She reports eating raw fish. What is the most likely diagnosis?
A. Chlonorchiasis
B. Diphyllobothrium
C. Anisakiasis
D. Gnathostomiasis
E. Strongyloidiasis

Q10.14 A 26-year-old male presents with abdominal pain and diarrhoea immediately on return from India. He reported eating street food on his way to the airport. What is the most common bacterial cause of traveller's diarrhoea?
A. *Campylobacter jejuni*
B. Enterotoxigenic *Escherichia coli*
C. *Salmonella* spp.
D. *Shigella* spp.
E. Astrovirus

Q10.15 A 54-year-old female presents with a diarrhoeal illness 24 hours after consumption of seafood from a street vender in the Caribbean. Which investigation is needed?
A. Stool culture for *Vibrio* spp.
B. Stool microscopy for *Cyclospora cayetanensis*

    C. Stool culture for *Escherichia coli* O157 H:7

    D. Stool culture for *Campylobacter jejuni*

    E. Stool culture for *Bacillus cereus*

Q10.16 A 28-year-old backpacker has recently returned from a 1-month trip to Peru. He seeks medical advice for a long-standing (3-week) volumous watery diarrhoea. Stool culture is negative, as is stool viral PCR. Which of the following is the most likely cause?

    A. *Giardia intestinalis*

    B. *Cryptosporidium parvum*

    C. *Necator americanus*

    D. *Cyclospora cayetanensis*

    E. *Shigella sonnei*

Q10.17 A 25-year-old male with a previous gastrectomy visits his family in a small village in Bangladesh. Two weeks after his return he develops fever and malaise without diarrhoea. Which pathogen is the most likely cause?

    A. *Campylobacter jejuni*

    B. *Salmonella* Paratyphi

    C. *Vibrio cholerae*

    D. *Citrobacter freundii*

    E. *Shigella sonnei*

Q10.18 A 25-year-old male with a previous gastrectomy visits his family in a small village in Bangladesh. Two weeks after his return he develops fever and malaise without diarrhoea. What is the optimal empiric antimicrobial therapy?

    A. Ampicillin

    B. Co-trimoxazole

    C. Chloramphenicol

    D. Ceftriaxone

    E. Nalidixic acid

Q10.19 A 22-year-old male presents to his local general practitioner with groin pain. He discloses having unprotected intercourse with a sex worker while on a business trip to Nigeria a few weeks ago. On examination, he has a painful ulcer on the glans of his penis which bleeds easily on light touch and painful inguinal lymphadenopathy. What is the most likely cause of his symptoms?

    A. Chancroid

    B. Syphilis

    C. Herpes simplex

    D. Human immunodeficiency virus

    E. Gonorrhoea

Q10.20 A 50-year-old male attended the emergency department with watery diarrhoea and dehydration. He lives in Delhi, India, and works as a business man for an international bank. He landed in the United Kingdom 6 hours prior to the onset of symptoms, which included acute-onset watery diarrhoea, vomiting, abdominal cramps and fever. He is opening his bowels every 2 hours with an estimated 500 mL in volume. He has not travelled outside Delhi recently, and lives with two children who remain well. He visited a Chinese style restaurant in Delhi the evening before travel and ate vegetarian food. He travelled business class and ate fish for main course on the aeroplane. On admission, he was clinically dehydrated, tachycardic with mild diffuse abdominal tenderness but no distension. Per rectum examination showed a small amount of faeces on the glove and no blood.

Investigations revealed:
- Haemoglobin: 120 g/L
- Total white cell count: 12.1×10^9/L
- Creatinine: 250 μmol/L
- Potassium: 6.4 mmol/L

Macroscopic appearance of the stool was liquid taking the form of the stool pot (Figure 10.3a), and culture in the enterics laboratory demonstrated an oxidase-negative organism (Figure 10.3b).

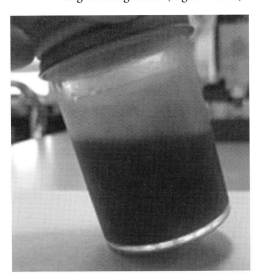

Figure 10.3a Stool specimen.

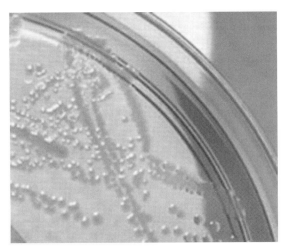

Figure 10.3b Growth on thiosulfate citrate bile salts sucrose incubated in an aerobic environment at 37°C for 24 hours. (A black and white version of this figure will appear in some formats. For the colour version, please refer to the plate section.)

Which is the most likely organism to cause this presentation?
A. *Plesiomonas shigelloides*
B. *Vibrio cholerae*
C. *Campylobacter jejuni*
D. *Vibrio parahaemolyticus*
E. *Shigella* spp.

Q10.21 A 55-year-old female returns from a trip to Kenya with a large travelling party. She was travelling around rural Kenya including game reserves. She developed abdominal pain, fever and constipation 5 days after returning to the United Kingdom. On examination, she had mild abdominal tenderness but no distension or guarding. She was pyrexial and tachycardic. The day after admission her blood cultures flag positive and grow *Salmonella* Typhi. She was treated with 10 days of intravenous ceftriaxone and her fever settled.

She recovers completely from the enteric fever, but 1 year later *S.* Typhi is isolated from a stool sample. Which of the following is the most likely condition?
A. Dumper's illness
B. Presumptive carriage
C. Chronic carriage
D. Anasarca
E. Cary–Blair syndrome

Q10.22 A 37-year-old engineer who works abroad returns from the Philippines with dysuria and epididymitis with a rash on his body and hands and is investigated for sexually transmitted infections. Prior to moving to the Philippines he underwent a full sexual health screen 6 months previously. The screen consisted of HIV, syphilis, chlamydia and gonorrhoea testing which was normal.
   Investigations revealed the following:
- Syphilis screening EIA: positive
- Treponemal pallidum haemagglutination (TPHA): positive
- Venereal Disease Reference Laboratory (VDRL) test: negative

What is the most likely diagnosis?
A. Primary syphilis
B. Secondary syphilis
C. Symptomatic tertiary syphilis
D. Past treated disease
E. HIV co-infection

Q10.23 A 22-year-old man developed a painful penile ulcer on return from a trip to Thailand. On examination, there was an ulcer on the coronal sulcus which had a ragged edge with a grey base which bled easily on palpation. He was otherwise systemically well.

A sample was taken of the ulcer for microscopy which revealed Gram-negative coccobacilli. Which is the most likely organism?
A. *Haemophilus paraphrophilus*
B. *Burkholderia pseudomallei*

    C. *Haemophilus ducreyi*
    D. *Haemophilus influenzae*
    E. *Treponema pallidum*

Q10.24 A 32-year-old man gets repatriated from Vietnam to Australia with severe pneumonia. He was trekking in Vietnam with a group of friends for a 2-month period. Half way during his trip he developed shortness of breath and high fever. He had recently been on a 10-day expedition in deep jungle and had suffered a minor machete injury which healed well. He was admitted to a local hospital in Vietnam and rapidly deteriorated needing intensive care support. His chest CT showed bilateral pneumonia with an abscess noted in his liver.
    Broncho-alveolar lavage culture demonstrated:
- Microscopy: Gram-negative bacilli
- Culture: Oxidase-positive colonies resistant to gentamicin and colistin on disc diffusion methodology

He was treated with a combination of ceftazidime and co-trimoxazole where he made a reasonable clinical recovery but suffered from acute respiratory distress syndrome requiring a long tracheostomy wean and repatriation to his home country of Australia. Which is the most likely organism causing the illness?
    A. *Haemophilus influenzae*
    B. *Burkholderia pseudomallei*
    C. *Chlamydophila psittaci*
    D. *Pseudomonas aeruginosa*
    E. *Stenotrophomonas maltophilia*

Q10.25 A 20-year-old returns from Africa and develops scaly lesion on his scalp with loss of hair. There are other lesions on the upper arms which are hypopigmented, scaly and macular.

Microscopy of skin scrapings demonstrates yeasts with short hyphae. Which is the most likely causative organism?
    A. *Malassezia furfur*
    B. *Candida tropicalis*
    C. *Microsporum* spp.
    D. *Trichophyton rubrum*
    E. *Trichophyton mentagrophytes*

Q10.26 A 29-year-old female patient presents for pre-travel advice. She is travelling to Kenya, including towns and safari parks. She reports a past medical history of depression, although she is currently only medicated with an oral contraceptive pill. Which malaria prophylaxis is most appropriate for this patient?
    A. Mefloquine
    B. Atovaquone-proguanil
    C. Chloroquine
    D. Artemisinin
    E. Doxycycline

Q10.27 A 27-year-old female patient presents for pre-travel advice. She is travelling to the Gambia, including trekking in the National Park. She is 16 weeks pregnant. Which malaria prophylaxis is most appropriate for this patient?
A. Mefloquine
B. Atovaquone-proguanil
C. Chloroquine
D. Artemisinin
E. Doxycycline

Q10.28 A 64-year-old male presents for pre-travel advice. He has ischaemic heart disease and atrial fibrillation and is on bisoprolol, atorvastatin and warfarin. Which malaria prophylaxis is most appropriate for this patient?
A. Mefloquine starting 2 weeks prior to entering the malaria endemic region
B. Atovaquone-proguanil starting 2 days prior to entering the malaria endemic region
C. Mefloquine starting 2 days prior to entering the malaria endemic region
D. Atovaquone-proguanil starting 2 weeks prior to entering the malaria endemic region
E. Doxycycline starting 2 days prior to entering the malaria endemic region

Q10.29 An 18-year-old male returns from an extended trip staying with relatives in rural Nigeria. He reports 3 weeks of being intensely itchy, affecting his entire body. Examination reveals a faint popular rash on some extensor surfaces and numerous excoriations over his entire body. What is the most likely cause?
A. *Malassezia furfur*
B. *Onchocerca volvulus*
C. *Coccidiodes immitis*
D. *Brugia malayi*
E. *Wucheria bancrofti*

Q10.30 A 22-year-old female medical student recently returned from Tanzania and presents with a history of haematuria. On investigation, schistosomal serology is shown to be positive. Which of the following is the treatment of choice?
A. Albendazole
B. Ivermectin
C. Mebendazole
D. Praziquantel
E. Suramin

Q10.31 A 27-year-old female returns from climbing Mount Kilimanjaro and presents with a fever. Her blood results demonstrate:

Heamoglobin: 79 g/L
White cell count: 11.3×10^9/L
Platelet count: 27×10^9/L
Blood film: *Plasmodium falciparum* seen, 2.5% parasitaemia

Which treatment should be initiated?
A. Oral chloroquine
B. Intravenous quinine

C. Oral atovaquone-proguanil
D. Oral mefloquine
E. Intravenous chloroquine

Q10.32 A 19-year-old gap year student recently returned from a 1-year trip around the world, which included Egypt, The Gambia, Uganda, Tanzania and Brazil. She paid privately for an asymptomatic health screen for the returning traveller. Stool concentration demonstrated the causative organism (Figure 10.4).

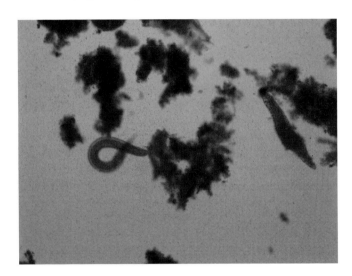

Figure 10.4 Light microscopy of stool sample prepared in 10% (v/v) formalin in water.

Which of the following drugs is most efficacious?
A. Mebendazole
B. Ivermectin
C. Praziquantel
D. Albendazole
E. Suramin

Q10.33 A 22-year-old male returned from Saudi Arabia 10 days ago and presents with a history of fever, cough and shortness of breath. His uncle works in a local slaughterhouse. On examination, he looks unwell, with a respiratory rate of 30 and crepitations widespread on auscultation. Chest radiograph shows widespread infiltrates. He is hypoxic in type 1 respiratory failure. He is intubated and admitted to the intensive care department.

What is the most likely diagnosis?
A. Middle East respiratory syndrome (MERS)
B. Avian influenza
C. Influenza A
D. Severe Acute Respiratory Syndrome (SARS)
E. Human metapneumovirus

Answers

A10.1 Answer E: *Diphyllobothrium latum*

Other intestinal worms cause a variety of pathological changes to enteric mucosa either through direct physical or chemical tissue damage or through inducement of specific immunological response. The hookworms *Ancylostoma duodenale* and *Necator americanus* can, on occasion, lead to anaemia through direct blood loss from their attachment and injection of anticoagulants into mucosal capillaries; however, symptomatic anaemia from this cause alone is unusual. Infestation with other intestinal worms can lead to a protein-losing enteropathy. Direct nutritional deficiencies from helminths are unusual and is unlikely to be symptomatic without other factors influencing diet and nutrition. Exceptions include *A. duodenale* and *N. americanus*, which can cause a vitamin A deficiency, and *D. latum* which can cause a specific vitamin B_{12} deficiency through direct absorption of this factor before the host can absorb and utilise it. B_{12} deficiency can similarly occur with *Giardia lamblia* infection.

Further Reading

Webb C, Cabada MM. Intestinal cestodes. *Curr Opin Infect Dis.* 2017;30(5):504–510.

A10.2 Answer C: Cytomegalovirus

Cytomegalovirus (CMV) isolated from animals (specifically monkeys) differs from that which infects humans in terms of genomic structure, and there have so far been no reported cases of cross-transmission to humans from other hosts. The rabies virus may infect any warm-blooded animal, including humans, though natural transmission has only been documented among mammals. Viruses in the genus Hantavirus are unique in that they are transmitted by aerosolised rodent excreta or rodent bites, whereas all other genera in the Bunyaviridae family (i.e. Orthobunyavirus, Nairovirus, Phlebovirus and Tospovirus) are arthropod-borne viruses. The primary animal host of Lassa virus is the Natal multimammate Mouse (indigenous to most of Sub-Saharan Africa), with viral transmission to humans likely to occur through contact with urine or faeces of infected animals. Coronaviruses have been associated with civets (severe acute respiratory syndrome - SARS) and camels (Middle East respiratory syndrome – MERS), with increased incidence of disease in humans among those in close proximity to these animals, although the primary host species is unclear and bats have been implicated.

Further Reading

Brook CE, Dobson AP. Bats as 'special' reservoirs for emerging zoonotic pathogens. *Trends Microbiol.* 2015;23(3):172–180.

A10.3 Answer D: Do not perform any tests and give treatment with doxycycline

There are three stages of *Borrelia burgdorferi* infection: early localised, early disseminated and late disseminated. The classic sign of localised disease is erythema migrans (EM), a gradually expanding annular lesion >5 cm in diameter. In America, approximately 70–80% of patients with Lyme disease have EM, which may have accompanying fever, lymphadenopathy and myalgia. If untreated, it can spread haematogenously causing early disseminated disease with multiple lesions, meningitis, facial palsy or carditis. In the United States, late disseminated disease is often recurrent joint infection whereas neurological disease is uncommon. Patients who have a lesion consistent with EM such as our patient and travelled to Lyme-endemic areas can be given a diagnosis without lab testing. All other manifestations need serological confirmation, which should be a two-tiered serologic test comprising EIA/ELISA followed by Western immunoblot.

Further Reading

Moore A, Nelson C, Molins C, Mead P, Schriefer M. Current guidelines, common clinical pitfalls, and future directions for laboratory diagnosis of Lyme disease, United States. *Emerg Infect Dis.* 2016;22(7):1169–1177.

A10.4 **Answer A: Black-legged tick – *Ixodes scapularis***
The most likely diagnosis for this patient is anaplasmosis, which is suggested by visualisation of morulae in the cytoplasm of granulocytes. The epidemiology is important due to the overlapping geographical distribution of Lyme disease and anaplasmosis, which is prevalent in the upper mid-west and north-eastern United States. The black-legged tick transmits both Lyme and anaplasma.

Lone star tick transmits *Ehrlichia chaffeensis* and *Ehrlichia ewingii* (causes ehrlichiosis), tularemia and STARI (Southern Tick-Associated Rash Illness). American dog tick and rocky mountain wood tick transmits tularaemia and rocky mountain spotted fever. The soft tick transmits tick-borne relapsing fever (*Borrelia hermsii, Borrelia parkerii* or *Borrelia turicatae).*

Further Reading

U.S. Department of Health and Human Services. CDC. Tick-borne Diseases of the United States: A reference manual for healthcare providers. Third Edition, 2015. Available at: https://stacks.cdc.gov/view/cdc/46358/cdc_46358_DS1.pdf

A10.5 **Answer C: Babesiosis**
Babesiosis is a tick-borne illness caused by parasites that infect red blood cells. Most cases in the United States are caused by *Babesia microti* transmitted by *Ixodes scapularis.* Transfusion- and congenital-related infections can occur. Infection can range from asymptomatic to life threatening, but particular risk factors include asplenia, advanced age and immunosuppression. Presentation is similar to malaria. Diagnosis can be made by identification of intra-erythrocytic *Babesia* parasites on peripheral blood smear or positive PCR. Treatment for significant illness is combination of either atovaquone and azithromycin or clindamycin and quinine for 7–10 days.

Further Reading

U.S. Department of Health and Human Services. CDC. Tick-borne Diseases of the United States: A reference manual for healthcare providers. Third Edition, 2015. Available at: https://stacks.cdc.gov/view/cdc/46358/cdc_46358_DS1.pdf

A10.6 **Answer C: Streptomycin and chloramphenicol**
The most likely pathogen in this case is *Francisella tularensis* which causes tularaemia. Naturally occurring disease has been reported across the United States, except Hawaii. It is a tick-borne illness primarily from ticks including dog tick (*Dermacentor variabilis*), the wood tick (*Dermacentor andersoni*) and the lone star tick (*Amblyomma americanum*). It can be spread via inhalation and direct inoculation and has been identified as a potential bioterrorism pathogen. Clinical presentation can be vague, however, specific presentations can occur depending on factors such as portal of entry, (ulcero)glandular, oropharyngeal, pneumonic,

typhoidal (no localising symptoms) and in this particular case, oculoglandular. Treatment regimens include ciprofloxacin, gentamicin, streptomycin and doxycycline, but if meningitis is suspected, then it is recommended that chloramphenicol is added to streptomycin.

Further Reading

Tarnvik A. WHO Guidelines on Tularaemia. Vol. WHO/CDS/EPR/2007.7. Geneva: World Health Organization, 2007. Available at: www.who.int/csr/resources/publications/deliberate/WHO_CDS_EPR_2007_7/en/

U.S. Department of Health and Human Services. CDC. Tick-borne Diseases of the United States: A reference manual for healthcare providers. Third Edition, 2015. Available at: https://stacks.cdc.gov/view/cdc/46358/cdc_46358_DS1.pdf

A10.7   Answer A: Zika virus

Zika virus (ZIKV) is a member of the genus flavivirus. It was first isolated from a monkey in the Zika forest in Uganda in 1947. Symptoms of ZIKV are similar to dengue and chikungunya. Most cases are asymptomatic but fever, joint pain (predominance of smaller joints), rash, conjunctivitis, headache and muscle/eye pain can occur. ZIKV is transmitted by the infected Aedes mosquito. Usual incubation period is 3–12 days. In October 2015, the Brazil International Health Regulations detected an unusual increase in cases of congenital microcephaly. This was followed by the detection of ZIKV from blood and tissue of a baby who died after birth with microcephaly and other congenital abnormalities. There has also been an increase in reporting of Guillain–Barre syndrome and other neurological syndromes, as well as autoimmune syndromes in areas where ZIKV outbreaks have been reported. ZIKV has spread from Africa and now autochthonous transmission has been reported in multiple countries in South America. There is no current antiviral treatment or vaccination. Avoidance of mosquito bites is advised, especially to pregnant travellers.

Further Reading

Public Health England. Zika virus (ZIKV): clinical and travel guidance, 2018. Available at: www.gov.uk/guidance/zika-virus

A10.8   Answer B: Send a malaria blood film

Returned travellers from some areas of the world (Figure 10.5), particularly some areas of Africa, are at risk of viral haemorrhagic fever and pose a risk to healthcare professionals and other patients.

UK national guidelines state it is essential that tests for malaria are undertaken during the clinical assessment of suspected cases of viral haemorrhagic fever (VHF), along with other essential tests, which may influence the immediate management of the patient. In addition to a malaria blood film this includes full blood count, urea and electrolytes, liver function tests, C-reactive protein, glucose, clotting and blood cultures. A stool culture should not be sent. The local laboratory that processes the malaria film should be made aware that the sample is coming and that the patient is at risk of having a VHF, so that they can process it appropriately. The sample should be taken using aseptic non-touch techniques, and placed in a suitable receptacle as soon as it is taken. This will depend upon local availability, but at a minimum this should involve double bagging of the specimen and placement in a hardened plastic receptacle which is then taken by hand to the laboratory – i.e. not in a pneumatic tube delivery system. Risk stratification of the patient to high, moderate or low risk can then be made, enabling subsequent decisions about patient movement from negative pressure side rooms onwards to Category 4 facilities.

If the case is identified as malaria, chloroquine should not be used for treatment given the prevalence of chloroquine resistance. Instead, quinine or artesunate-based therapy should be used.

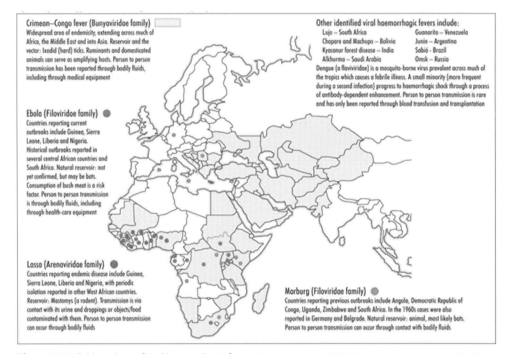

Crimean–Congo fever (Bunyaviridae family)
Widespread area of endemicity, extending across much of Africa, the Middle East and into Asia. Reservoir and the vector: Ixodid (hard) ticks. Ruminants and domesticated animals can serve as amplifying hosts. Person to person transmission has been reported through bodily fluids, including through medical equipment

Ebola (Filoviridae family)
Countries reporting current outbreaks include Guinea, Sierra Leone, Liberia and Nigeria. Historical outbreaks reported in several central African countries and South Africa. Natural reservoir: not yet confirmed, but may be bats. Consumption of bush meat is a risk factor. Person to person transmission is through bodily fluids, including through health-care equipment

Lassa (Arenaviridae family)
Countries reporting endemic disease include Guinea, Sierra Leone, Liberia and Nigeria, with periodic isolation reported in other West African countries. Reservoir: Mastomys (a rodent). Transmission is via contact with its urine and droppings or objects/food contaminated with them. Person to person transmission can occur through bodily fluids

Other identified viral haemorrhagic fevers include:
Lujo – South Africa   Guanarito – Venezuela
Chapare and Machupo – Bolivia   Junin – Argentina
Kyasanur forest disease – India Sabiá - Brazil
Alkhurma – Saudi Arabia   Omsk – Russia
Dengue (a flaviviridae) is a mosquito-borne virus prevalent across much of the tropics which causes a febrile illness. A small minority (more frequent during a second infection) progress to haemorrhagic shock through a process of antibody-dependent enhancement. Person to person transmission is rare and has only been reported through blood transfusion and transplantation

Marburg (Filoviridae family)
Countries reporting previous outbreaks include Angola, Democratic Republic of Congo, Uganda, Zimbabwe and South Africa. In the 1960s cases were also reported in Germany and Belgrade. Natural reservoir: animal, most likely bats. Person to person transmission can occur through contact with bodily fluids

Figure 10.5 Epidemiology of viral haemorrhagic fevers (from Moore et al., 2014). (A black and white version of this figure will appear in some formats. For the colour version, please refer to the plate section.)

Further Reading
Moore LSP, Moore M, Sriskandan S. Ebola and other viral haemorrhagic fevers: a local operational approach. *Br J Hosp Med.* 2014;75(9):515–522.

A10.9 Answer B: Isolate the patient with respiratory precautions
Poultry and fowl have been associated most significantly with human outbreaks of novel influenza virus, and to a lesser extent, implicated in the spread of some coronaviruses. Specific public health concerns arise over the transmission of "avian" influenza strains (influenza A H5N1) to humans who come in close contact with poultry and fowl, as well as in the context of tourist travel to Vietnam, particularly around those who partake of the local "Tiết canh", or (fresh) duck-blood pudding.

Patients who present on return from trips abroad with symptoms and signs consistent with severe influenza should be placed in respiratory isolation to minimise the risk of potential onward transmission of the virus. Healthcare workers and other visitors to the room should wear an FFP3 mask. Suitable tests should be sent (usually including a viral swab for multi-plex PCR), and if there is clinical concern that this is influenza, then oseltamivir started. Bacterial infections, particularly bacterial pneumonia, do sometimes follow or even present concurrently with influenza, and should be considered and treated where found with appropriate antibacterial agents.

Further Reading

Investigation and management of possible human cases of avian influenza A/H7N9, in travellers returning to the UK. Public Health England. Available at: www.gov.uk/government/uploads/system/uploads/attachment_data/file/358673/Investigation_and_management_of_possible_human_cases_of_avian_influenza_A_H7N9__flow_diagram_July_new.pdf

A10.10 Answer D: Co-amoxiclav and clarithromycin

In the United Kingdom, the most common cause of community-acquired pneumonia (CAP) is *Streptococcus pneumoniae*, with less common causes including *Haemophilus influenza*, *Staphylococcus aureus* and *Mycoplasma pneumoniae*. Rarer causes in the United Kingdom are *Chlamydophilia* spp. and *Legionella pneumophilia*, the latter usually being associated with institutional outbreaks. Outside the United Kingdom, and particularly in countries with a higher average temperature, *Legionella* spp. pneumonia is more frequent, and several cases have been reported among travellers returning from Spain. Yet, at the same time *S. pneumoniae* remains a common cause, although antimicrobial resistance prevalence differs between the United Kingdom and Spain, in particular, with Spain having higher rates of penicillin-resistance among pneumococcal isolates. To that end, empiric treatment for patients with moderate to severe, community-acquired pneumonia, such as the current patient, should follow the national guidelines. In the United Kingdom the national pneumonia guidelines were published by the British Thoracic Society (BTS) in 2009, but the National Institute for Health and Care Excellence (NICE) published updated guidelines, with some overlap and some variations, in 2014. Both sets of guidance state that dual antibiotic therapy with amoxicillin and a macrolide should be considered for patients with moderate severity community-acquired pneumonia, and for those with high severity, this should be a beta-lactamase stable beta-lactam (such as co-amoxiclav) and a macrolide.

Microbiological samples should be sent in this case, including a blood culture and a sputum culture, but urinary antigen tests for *S. pneumoniae* and *L. pneumophilia* should also be sent. A confirmed case of *Legionella pneumoniae* should be treated with clarithromycin and rifampicin.

Further Reading

2015 Annotated BTS Guideline for the management of CAP in adults: Summary of recommendations. Available at: www.brit-thoracic.org.uk/document-library/clinical-information/pneumonia/adult-pneumonia/annotated-bts-cap-guideline-summary-of-recommendations/ (This document integrates the 2009 BTS guidelines on CAP with those published in 2014 by NICE)

Phin N, Parry-Ford F, Harrison T, Stagg HR, Zhang N, Kumar K, Lortholary O, Zumla A, Abubakar I. Epidemiology and clinical management of Legionnaires' disease. *Lancet Infect Dis.* 2014;14(10):1011–1021.

A10.11 Answer D: Brucellosis

Brucella abortus (cattle) and *B. melitensis* (goats and sheep) are the two most commonly encountered species causing human brucellosis. Acquisition is typically through contact with unpasteurised milk of infected animals, either through diet or from working with livestock. Brucella typically presents in an indolent fashion, often with fever, sweating and arthralgia and myalgia. Local disease most commonly occurs in bones and joints (particularly lumbar spine spondylodiscitis and sacroilitis), in the testis as orchitis or as pneumonia, with less common manifestations including endocarditis and neurobrucellosis. Diagnosis is through culture (blood cultures, bone marrow aspirate or tissue/pus specimens) where organisms are small Gram-negative cocco-bacilli, which grow on blood agar and are oxidase positive), or through serology. Treatment is based on doxycycline, either given with gentamicin or with rifampicin.

Tuberculosis is the most likely differential in this case, but the explicit dietary history in the context of travel to Africa and the Middle East make Brucella more likely. While visceral leishmaniasis frequently gives rise to splenomegaly, spinal tenderness would be uncommon. Hydatid disease caused by *Echinococcus granulosus* causes cystic disease, which most commonly affects the liver or the lung. Malaria frequently gives rise to splenomegaly, a malaria film should be sent in this case, but again the history suggests brucellosis more strongly.

Further Reading

Dean AS, Crump L, Greter H, Hattendorf J, Schelling E, Zinsstag J. Clinical manifestations of human brucellosis: systematic review and meta-analysis. *PLoS Negl Trop Dis.* 2012;6(12):e1929.

A10.12   Answer D: *Schistosoma haematobium*

Schistosomiasis occurs after cercariae, released from their fresh water snail hosts, penetrate the skin of swimmers and waders in infested water bodies. They then migrate through the vascular system, through several organs including the lungs, before ending in the venous beds of either the intestine (*S. mansoni, S. intercalatum, S. japonicum* and *S. mekongi*) or the bladder (*S. haematobium*) and cause disease in these areas, respectively. Although several of the *Schistosoma* species have geographic specific sounding names, the global distribution of schistosomiasis is broad. Specifically for *S. haematobium*, the helminth can be found in all freshwater in southern and sub-Saharan Africa (as well as the Nile River valley), the Middle East, parts of South America (including Brazil, Suriname and Venezuela) and the Caribbean (Dominican Republic, Martinique, Guadeloupe and St Lucia) and Asia (southern China, Laos and the Philippines). The three major *Schistosoma* species can be differentiated on microscopy; *S. haematobium* has a prominent terminal spine (as in this case), *S. mansoni* as a large lateral spine and *S. japonicum* has only a small vestigial lateral spine. Alternatively, diagnosis can be made serologically. Treatment for schistosomiasis is with praziquantel, although this should be given once the adult schistomal worms are mature (at least 6–8 weeks after exposure).

Further Reading

Gray DJ, Ross AG, Li YS, McManus DP. Diagnosis and management of schistosomiasis. *BMJ.* 2011;342:d2651.

A10.13   Answer C: Aniskiasis

Anisakiasis is caused by infection with *Anisakis simplex*, a nematode which usually infests fish in a crustacean-fish-marine mammal life cycle. Human disease arises when infested raw fish is eaten; freezing prevents disease but salting and light pickling does not. It is most prevalent in Scandinavia, the Netherlands, Japan and along the Pacific coast of South America. Three types of presentation predominate: (i) acute abdominal symptoms including pain and vomiting (occurring several hours after ingestion); (ii) an allergic response with urticarial and on occasion anaphylaxis (this may overlap with the abdominal symptoms and again occur several hours after ingestion); or (iii) obstructive abdominal symptoms occurring later, 1–2 weeks after ingestion (which may mimic an acute Crohn's presentation). Within hours of ingestion of infective larvae, violent abdominal pain, nausea and vomiting may occur. Occasionally, the larvae are coughed up. If the larvae pass into the bowel, a severe eosinophilic granulomatous response may also occur 1–2 weeks following infection, causing symptoms mimicking Crohn's disease. Treatment is largely supportive, and the nematodes die without specific therapy.

Chlonorchiasis typically presents with symptoms related to liver disease, including an enlarged tender liver or jaundice, although abdominal symptoms can manifest. Diphyllobothrium infection usually results in mild abdominal symptoms or weight loss, although in some cases disrupted B_{12} absorption can lead to a megaloblastic anaemia. Gnathostomiasis can lead to intestinal symptoms, but these occur several days after ingestion. Further migration of this nematode under the skin can lead to an erythema chronicum migrans-type rash, and visceral or neurological migration of the worm can cause organ-specific disease. Strongyloidiasis can present with gastrointestinal symptoms or a Löffler's syndrome during the pulmonary migratory phase. Dissemination of the worm to other organs can cause specific complications. Hyperinfection (classically in the context of HTLV-1 infection, but also seen with some other immunocompromised conditions) can eventually lead to catastrophic disease, including shock, meningitis, renal impairment and respiratory failure.

Further Reading
Audicana MT, Kennedy MW. Anisakis simplex: from obscure infectious worm to inducer of immune hypersensitivity. *Clin Microbiol Rev.* 2008;21(2):360–379.

A10.14 Answer B: Enterotoxigenic *Escherichia coli*
Travellers' diarrhoea has been defined as three or more loose stools in 24 hours with or without at least one symptom of cramps, nausea, fever or vomiting. The most common causes are bacterial (60–85% of cases) and the most important bacterial pathogen is *E. coli* (predominantly ETEC). Parasites account for about 10% and viruses for 5%. *E. coli* will usually cause mild self-limiting diarrhoea for less than 72 hours. Diarrhoea lasting longer than 14 days suggests more unusual organisms, including *Giardia* spp., *Entamoeba* spp., *Cyclospora* spp. and *Cryptosporidium* spp. Dysentery occurs more commonly with some pathogens *(Salmonella* spp., *Shigella* spp. and *Campylobacter* spp.). In children under 5 years, rotavirus is a common pathogen.

Further Reading
Steffen R, Hill DR, DuPont HL. Traveller's diarrhoea: a clinical review. *JAMA.* 2015;313(1):71–80.

A10.15 Answer A: Stool culture for *Vibrio* spp.
The genera *Vibrio* has many species, of which three are the most commonly encountered; *Vibrio cholera, V. parahaemolyticus* and *V. vulnificans*. While *V. cholera* is typically transmitted through contaminated water, *V. parahaemolyticus* and *V. vulnificans* are typically acquired from eating contaminated seafood. *V. vulnificans* can also be acquired through open wounds exposed to contaminated water when swimming or wading. *V. parahaemolyticus* can be isolated from stool. Routine blood cultures should be performed

when *V. vulnificus* is suspected, and bullae, ecchymoses and abscesses are often productive sites to aspirate material for Gram stain and culture. Additional cultures are guided by clinical symptoms and may include ocular, peritoneal, sputum, cervical and stool cultures. Stool cultures require a thiosulfate citrate bile (TCBA) salts sucrose agar for isolation.

C. cayetanensis causes gastroenteritis, with symptoms including watery diarrhoea, loss of appetite, weight loss, abdominal bloating and cramping, increased flatulence, nausea, fatigue and low-grade fever. Typically, patients present with a persistent watery diarrhoea lasting several days. *E. coli* O157 H:7 causes haemolytic-uraemic syndrome. *C. jejuni* is typically associated with undercooked chicken and causes enteritis, where bloating and abdominal cramps, in particular, predominate. *B. cereus* can cause an acute toxin-mediated enteritis, but stool cannot be cultured to determine this; primary samples of the infected food source is needed.

Further Reading

Butt AA, Aldridge KE, Sanders CV. Infections related to the ingestion of seafood Part I: viral and bacterial infections. *Lancet Infect Dis*. 2004 Apr;4(4):201–212.

A10.16 Answer B: *Cryptosporidium parvum*

Cryptosporidium spp. are well recognised as causes of diarrhoeal disease in immunocompromised hosts but can also cause prolonged diarrhoea in immunocompetent hosts on occasion. Symptoms typically appear from 2 to 10 days after the infection and last for up to 2 weeks, or in some cases, up to 1 month. The disease can be asymptomatic. Diarrhoea is usually watery with mucus and haematochezia is rare. In addition to watery diarrhoea, there are often stomach cramps and a low fever. Individuals who are asymptomatic are nevertheless infective, and even after symptoms have finally subsided, an individual is still infective for some weeks. Severe diseases, including pancreatitis, can occur.

Giardiasis is characterised by prolonged abdominal discomfort, sometimes diarrhoea, and commonly eructation and flatulence. *S. sonnei* typically presents with an acute cramping abdominal pain with diarrhoea, but on the whole is self-limiting. *N. americanus*, a human hookworm, typically causes no abdominal symptoms, but in high worm burdens can cause an iron-deficiency anaemia.

Further Reading

Checkley W, White AC Jr, Jaganath D, Arrowood MJ, Chalmers RM, Chen XM, Fayer R, Griffiths JK, Guerrant RL, Hedstrom L, Huston CD, Kotloff KL, Kang G, Mead JR, Miller M, Petri WA J9, Priest JW, Roos DS, Striepen B, Thompson RC, Ward HD, Van Voorhis WA, Xiao L, Zhu G, Houpt ER. A review of the global burden, novel diagnostics, therapeutics, and vaccine targets for cryptosporidium. *Lancet Infect Dis*. 2015;15(1):85–94.

A10.17 Answer B: *Salmonella* Paratyphi

Enteric fever (or typhoid fever) can be caused by *S*. Typhi or *S*. Paratyphi. Gastric acid presents a significant barrier to infection, and the inoculated dose required to cause disease is reduced where there is a relative reduction in gastric acidity (i.e. those on proton pump inhibitors and the elderly). The bacteria invade the intestinal mucosa and can then haematogenously disseminate. The incubation period for enteric fever ranges from 7 to 14 days, but longer periods of up to 8 weeks have been reported. Diagnosis is through culture, either from stool samples or from blood cultures. Serology is available, but is highly unreliable and should not routinely be requested.

Further Reading

Wain J, Hendriksen RS, Mikoleit WL, Keddy KH, Ochiai RL. Typhoid fever. *Lancet*. 2015;385 (9973):1136–1145.

A10.18 Answer D: Ceftriaxone

In much of South-east Asia, *Salmonella* Typhi and *Salmonella* Paratyphi strains display a high resistance to ampicillin, chloramphenicol and co-trimoxazole, above 50%, and ciprofloxacin resistance is also very high to trust empiric therapy with this agent. Resistance to quinolones is first indicated in vitro through laboratory disc susceptibility testing looking for decreased zone sizes to nalidixic acid. Treatment must be guided by antimicrobial susceptibility testing, although on the whole initial empiric therapy with a third-generation cephalosporin is indicated while cultures are awaited. Some *Salmonella* spp. displaying extended-spectrum beta-lactamase phenotypes, resistant to cephalosporins, have been seen, and therapy with other agents, including azithromycin or carbapenems, may be indicated on occasion.

Further Reading

Crump JA, Sjölund-Karlsson M, Gordon MA, Parry CM. Epidemiology, clinical presentation, laboratory diagnosis, antimicrobial resistance, and antimicrobial management of invasive *Salmonella* infections. *Clin Microbiol Rev*. 2015;28(4):901–937.

A10.19 Answer A: Chancroid

Chancroid is a sexually transmitted bacterial infection caused by *Haemophilus ducreyi* and causes painful genital ulceration. It used to be a common cause of genital ulceration but is now much less common due to the widespread use of effective antibiotics, increased condom usage in sex workers and use of syndrome management algorithms. It can cause painful inguinal lymphadenopathy, which can develop into buboes needing aspiration of incision and drainage. The genital ulcers are painful, found on the prepuce, frenulum and glans in men and labia minora and fourchette in women. Ulcers have a ragged undermined edge with a grey or yellow base that bleeds on touch. Ulcers can be single or multiple. PCR-based diagnostic technique are most sensitive. Single-dose oral azithromycin or intra-muscular ceftriaxone are first-line therapies.

Further Reading

O'Farrell N, Lazaro N. UK National Guideline for the management of chancroid 2014. *Int J STD AIDS*. 2014;25(14):975–983.

A10.20 Answer B: *Vibrio cholerae*

The key to the diagnosis of cholera in this case is the degree of watery diarrhoea, travel history and appearance on TCBS plate. India has outbreaks of cholera and should always be considered in the differential, irrespective of the patient demographic. TCBS plate should be set up based on risk assessment, and yellow colonies are classic. Oxidase test is positive in cholera but should never be performed directly from the TCBS plate as this will give false results, as in this case. The patient responded well to oral ciprofloxacin and aggressive rehydration.

Further Reading

Public Health England. UK Standards for Microbiology Investigations. B 30: Investigation of faecal specimens for enteric pathogens, 2014. Available at: www.gov.uk/government/publications/smi-b-30-investigation-of-faecal-specimens-for-enteric-pathogens

A10.21 Answer C: Chronic carriage

Relapse of enteric fever can occur in immunocompetent individuals and typically occurs 2–3 weeks following resolution of fever. The chronic carriage of salmonellae is defined as the shedding of a *Salmonella* spp. for more than 12 months following acute infection. Post illness, screening for *S.* Typhi is not routinely performed. The optimal approach to eradication is not known, but if the known isolate was fluoroquinolone-sensitive, then the use of a 4-week course is recommended by some. The gallbladder is a classic site of persistence, and therefore cholecystectomy is still an option, but performed infrequently. Cary–Blair is the type of transport medium used for clinical specimens suspected to contain enteric pathogens. Anasarca is the name given to massive and excessive fluid accumulation usually associated with heart failure, cirrhosis and nephrotic syndrome.

Further Reading

Date KA, Newton AE, Medalla F, Blackstock A, Richardson L, McCullough A, Mintz ED, Mahon BE. Changing patterns in enteric fever incidence and increasing antibiotic resistance of enteric fever isolates in the United States, 2008-2012. *Clin Infect Dis.* 2016;63(3):322–329.

A10.22 Answer E: HIV co-infection

Unless the patient has previously been treated, the most likely diagnosis is HIV co-infection. Clinically, the presence of the rash does not fit with primary syphilis and would most likely be secondary syphilis. Secondary syphilis should have a positive VDRL/RPR test but is not shown in this case. A false-negative RPR/VDRL test may occur in secondary or early latent syphilis due to the prozone phenomenon when testing undiluted serum. This may be more likely to occur in HIV-infected individuals. When clinical findings are suggestive of syphilis but serological tests are non-reactive, alternative tests (e.g. biopsy of a lesion, dark ground microscopy) may be useful for diagnosis.

Further Reading

Kingston M, French P, Higgins S, McQuillan O, Sukthankar A, Stott C, McBrien B, Tipple C, Turner A, Sullivan AK. UK national guidelines on the management of syphilis 2015. *Int J STD AIDS.* 2016;27(6):421–446.

A10.23 Answer C: *Haemophilus ducreyi*

In order to make a diagnosis of chancroid (*H. ducreyi*), there are two main methods: PCR- and culture-based methods. To obtain culture material superficial pus should be removed, and then material at the base of the lesion should be taken. *H. ducreyi* is a fastidious organism that is difficult to grow, and therefore should be plated immediately or within 4 hours of the sample being taken. GC agar supplemented with 1–2% bovine haemoglobin, 5% foetal calf serum or Mueller–Hinton agar enriched with 5% chocolatised horse blood are recommended. However, culture sensitivity is still low <80%, and PCR-based technologies increase the sensitivity of testing to >95%.

Further Reading

O'Farrell N, Lazaro N. UK National Guideline for the management of chancroid 2014. *Int J STD AIDS*. 2014;25(14):975–983.

A10.24 Answer B: *Burkholderia pseudomallei*

Melioidosis is endemic in parts of South-east Asia and northern Australia, where *B. pseudomallei* is found in soil and surface water. *B. pseudomallei* grows on a large variety of culture media and cultures typically become positive in 24–48 hours, colonies are wrinkled, have a metallic appearance and possess an earthy odour. On Gram staining, the organism is a Gram-negative bacillus with a characteristic "safety pin" appearance (bipolar staining). On sensitivity testing, the organism appears highly resistant and that differentiates it from *Burkholderia mallei*, which is, in contrast, sensitive to a large number of antibiotics. Ceftazidime or meropenem should be the initial antibiotics of choice as they have a low level of naturally occurring resistance. The addition of septrin is not routinely recommended and does not decrease either mortality or relapse rate. The initial antibiotic choice (ceftazidime or meropenem) should be continued for at least 2 weeks depending on the clinical scenario. It may be extended in case of a deep focus such as osteomyelitis. This should be followed by a 12-week course of eradication phase treatment. The relapse rate after full eradication is 10%, but rises to 30% if a course of oral therapy is >8 weeks. Co-trimoxazole is the first-line oral treatment for eradication therapy.

Further Reading

Lipsitz R, Garges S, Aurigemma R, Baccam P, Blaney DD, Cheng AC, Currie BJ, Dance D, Gee JE, Larsen J, Limmathurotsakul D, Morrow MG, Norton R, O'Mara E, Peacock SJ, Pesik N, Rogers LP, Schweizer HP, Steinmetz I, Tan G, Tan P, Wiersinga WJ, Wuthiekanun V, Smith TL. Workshop on treatment of and postexposure prophylaxis for *Burkholderia pseudomallei* and *B. mallei* infection, 2010. *Emerg Infect Dis*. 2012;18(12):e2.

A10.25 Answer A: *Malassezia furfur*

Tinea capitis can be caused by any one of the several dermatophytes (filamentous fungi) belonging to the genera *Trichophyton* and *Microsporum*; the genus *Epidermophyton* is not known to invade the hair. Three types of in vivo hair invasion are recognised: Ectothrix (exterior of the hair shaft – *Microsporum canis*, *Microsporum gypseum*, *T. mentagrophytes*, *Trichophyton equinum* and *Trichophyton verrucosum*), Endothrix (within the hair shaft only – anthropophilic fungi only e.g. *Trichophyton tonsurans*, *T. violaceum*) and Favus (usually caused by *Trichopyton schoenleinii* produces favuslike crusts or scutula and corresponding hair loss). In the United Kingdom, *T. tonsurans* accounts for greater than 90% of cases of Tinea Capitis. Malassezia species are basidiomycetous yeasts and part of our normal skin microbiota. It causes tinea versicolor (Pityriasis versicolor) which is a common superficial fungal infection, and unlike other tinea infections, this is not a dermatophyte. Topical ketoconazole shampoo to affected areas has shown good efficacy.

Further Reading

Hald M, Arendrup MC, Svejgaard EL, Lindskov R, Foged EK, Saunte DM. Evidence-based Danish guidelines for the treatment of Malassezia-related skin diseases. *Acta Derm Venereol*. 2015;95 (1):12–19.

A10.26 Answer B: Atovaquone-proguanil

Atovaquone-proguanil is the agent of choice in this patient given her co-morbidities. Mefloquine, while safe and side-effect-free for the majority of users, may have severe and permanent adverse side-effects in a minority of patients and can cause severe depression, anxiety, paranoia, aggression, nightmares, insomnia and seizures. It should be avoided in those with a past medical history of psychiatric disease. Chloroquine should be avoided in most areas of the world as chloroquine-resistant *Plasmodium falciparum* is widespread. Artemisinin and quinine are used for treatment of falciparum malaria. Doxycycline would be an alternative choice for this patient, and additional contraceptive precautions are not required when using non-enzyme-inducing antimicrobials such as doxycycline.

Further Reading

Public Health England. Guidelines for malaria prevention in travellers from the UK, 2015. Available at: www.gov.uk/government/uploads/system/uploads/attachment_data/file/461295/2015.09.16_ACMP_guidelines_FINAL.pdf

A10.27 Answer A: Mefloquine

Pregnant travellers should be advised about the risks associated with malaria in pregnancy; pregnant women who acquire malaria are more likely to develop severe sequelae (including hypoglycaemia, jaundice, pulmonary oedema, severe anaemia and renal failure), and have a higher mortality. Miscarriage, premature delivery and neonatal death may occur, as may congenital malaria, which is rare and occurs with *Plasmodium vivax* most commonly. Furthermore, diagnosing *P. falciparum* malaria in pregnancy can be more difficult as parasites sequester in the placenta and false-negative blood films may occur.

Pre-travel advice for pregnant travellers should focus on bite avoidance, advising topical application of 50% DEET (which has a good safety record in children and pregnancy, although care must be taken to avoid ingestion if breast feeding) and remaining indoors between dusk and dawn. The main chemotherapeutic agent advised is mefloquine, which should be used with caution in first trimester, but where benefit outweighs risk, it can be used in all trimesters. There is no evidence of harm to pregnant mothers or foetuses when mefloquine is used, either from increased still births, miscarriages or teratogenicity. For atovaquone-proguanil, there is a lack of evidence on safety in pregnancy, although neither is there any evidence of teratogenicity; currently, the advice is to avoid use of atovaquone-proguanil for antimalarial chemoprophylaxis in pregnancy unless there are no other options, when a risk-benefit analysis should be undertaken as to whether it is indicated in the second and third trimesters.

Doxycycline should be avoided as it is teratogenic. Chloroquine resistance is too high for its effective use in chemoprophylaxis. Artemisinin is used for treatment, not prophylaxis.

Further Reading

Public Health England. Guidelines for malaria prevention in travellers from the UK, 2015. Available at: www.gov.uk/government/uploads/system/uploads/attachment_data/file/461295/2015.09.16_ACMP_guidelines_FINAL.pdf

A10.28 Answer A: Mefloquine starting 2 weeks prior to entering the malaria endemic region

Travellers to malaria endemic regions who have pre-existing medical conditions must be counselled carefully, including taking appropriate travel insurance. For patients on coumarins, including warfarin, consideration must be given to potential disturbance of the international normalised ratio (INR) from chemotherapeutic agents. Mefloquine is not considered to adversely affect the INR for those taking warfarin and should be started 2 weeks before entering a malaria endemic region; this is not only in line with achieving full malarial protection from this agent but also to enable an INR to be measured after the traveller has started the mefloquine, yet before their departure, in case warfarin dose adjustment is required. Atovaquone-proguanil has, rarely, been reported to cause an enhanced effect of warfarin; where mefloquine is contraindicated atovaquone-proguanil can be used, but rather than being started 2 days prior to travel as normal, should instead be commenced 2 weeks prior to entering a malaria endemic region to enable the INR to be checked. Doxycycline may enhance the anticoagulant effect of warfarin and should be avoided.

Careful consideration around choice of antimalarial prophylaxis must also be given to to those paitents with a history of epilepsy. Mefloquine and chloroquine are contraindicated in epilepsy, and for doxycycline the half-life may be reduced by phenytoin, carbamazepine and barbituates. Atovaquone-proguanil can be used safely in epilepsy.

Further Reading

Public Health England. Guidelines for malaria prevention in travellers from the UK, 2015. Available at: www.gov.uk/government/uploads/system/uploads/attachment_data/file/461295/2015.09.16_ACMP_guidelines_FINAL.pdf

A10.29   Answer B: *Onchocerca volvulus*

O. volvulus is found mainly in West and Central Africa, but intermittent cases are reported in the Caribbean, some regions of South America and Yemen. This nematode is transmitted by the *Simuliam* spp. Black Fly which inhabits rivers and has a bacterial endosymbiont thought to cause most aspects of human disease – *Wolbachia* spp. Although mortality from this disease is extremely rare, the attributable morbidity is high, with three main clinical manifestations recognised: (i) acute onchodermatitis, presenting as in this case with intense pruritis, papules and sometimes vesicles and pustules; (ii) 9–24 months after inoculation, chronic dermatitis may occur with subcutaneous nodules, lichenification and skin atrophy and depigmentation; (iii) ocular onchocerciasis, characterised by itchy eyes, photophobia and eventually punctate keratitis and corneal fibrosis. A less common manifestation of onchocerciasis is nodding disease, presenting as seizures. Diagnosis is through skin snip biopsies, either placed in saline for microscopy to look for microfilariae emerging from the sample, or through PCR where available. Alternatively, a patch test, using topical application of diethylcarbamazine, will elicit localised pruritis and oedema in those infected, but false positive reactions may occur in those with other filarial diseases. Classically, treatment was with ivermectin, active against the microfilaria, but not against the adult worms, so repeated dosing is usually needed. For ocular onchocerciasis, concomitant steroids may be indicated. Alternatively, doxycycline, active against the endosymbiont *Wolbachia* spp. may be given.

M. furfur is a yeast which causes Pityriasis versicolour, dandruff and seborrheic dermatitis.

C. immitis is an environmental yeast that can cause a pneumonia, associated with headaches, rash and myalgia. *B. malayi* and *W. bancrofti* are the two nematodes which cause lymphatic filariasis. They display nocturnal periodicity, meaning blood films for diagnosis are best obtained between midnight and 2 a.m.; in contrast, blood films for loa loa should be taken at midday.

Further Reading

Moore LSP, Chiodini PL. Tropical helminths. *Medicine*. 2010;38(1):47–51.

A10.30 Answer D: Praziquantel

Schistosomiasis is a parasitic disease caused by blood flukes with a highest prevalence in sub-Saharan Africa. The life cycle requires an intermediate host (snails) and definitive host (humans) to complete the life cycle. Schistosomiasis is acquired from fresh water such as lakes, with Lake Malawi a classic example. The infectious cercariae penetrates the human host and initial infection can cause a local "swimmers itch." Acute schistosomiasis can follow, known as Katayama fever, but most patients do not realise they are infected. Chronic infection depends on the infecting species but will often progress in non-treated individuals. Praziquantel is the drug of choice. The mechanism of Praziquantel is postulated to increase permeability of the membranes of parasite cells to calcium ions, which alters the tegument structure. Mass population treatment can reduce the prevalence and morbidity of the condition. Treatment for *Schistosoma haematobium*, *S. mansoni* or *S. intercalatum* is 40 mg/kg in one or two divided doses, but a higher dose of 60 mg/kg is recommended for treatment of *S. japonicum* or *S. mekongi*.

Further Reading

Cioli D, Pica-Mattoccia L, Basso A, Guidi A. Schistosomiasis control: praziquantel forever?
  Mol Biochem Parasitol. 2014;195:23.

A10.31 Answer B: Intravenous quinine

A diagnosis of *P. falciparum* malaria is a medical emergency and necessitates immediate assessment and therapy. Symptoms ranging from isolated fever to more complex presentations with diarrhoea, cough, myalgia and headache may manifest between 6 days and 3 months after inoculation (by the night biting *Anopheles* spp. mosquito). Diagnosis is through blood film (thick film for detection, thin film for speciation and to determine parasitaemia) or rapid diagnostic lateral flow tests. PCR is available in some centres. Treatment is dependent upon whether features of severity are present or not. Uncomplicated *P. falciparum* should be treated with an artemisinin combination therapy (ACT) with oral artemether-lumefantrine (Riamet®) as the drug of choice. Atovaquone-proguanil (Malarone®) can be used if an ACT is not available. Current UK guidelines for severe or complicated malaria indicate intravenous artesunate as the drug of choice, but intravenous quinine should be used if artesunate is unavailable. Indicators for severe disease include:

- Evidence of cerebral malaria (impaired consciousness or seizures)
- Evidence of acute respiratory distress or pulmonary oedema
- Evidence of renal impairment (oliguria or creatinine >265 μmol/L))
- Evidence of anaemia (Hb < 80 g/L)
- Shock (BP <90/60 mmHg)
- Disseminated intravascular coagulation
- Hypoglycaemia (<2.2 mmol/L)
- Acidosis (pH < 7.3)
- Parasitaemia > 10%

For non-falciparum malaria (*P. ovale, P. vivax P. knowlesi,* or *P. malariae*) oral chloroquine is the treatment of choice. To clear liver stage hypnozoites, *P. vivax* and *P. ovale* require additional treatment with primaquine. Primaquine is contraindicated in patients with glucose-6-phosphate dehydrogenase deficiency (G6PD), where it may cause severe haemolysis.

Further Reading
Lalloo DG, Shingadia D, Bell DJ, Whitty CJ, Beeching NJ. Chiodini PL; PHE Advisory Committee on Malaria Prevention in UK Travellers. *J Infect.* 2016;72(6):635–649.

A10.32 Answer B: Ivermectin
Strongyloidiasis is caused by *Strongyloides stercoralis*, which is often asymptomatic in immunocompetent patients but can cause disseminated disease in the immunosuppressed. Eosinophilia may be the only biochemical abnormality, which should prompt serological testing of individuals from endemic countries. Thiabendazole and albendazole have activity against Strongyloides but have lower cure rates. Albendazole has a reported 50–60% cure rate compared to 90–100% cure rate for two doses of ivermectin.

Further Reading
Muennig P, Pallin D, Challah C, Khan K. The cost-effectiveness of ivermectin vs. albendazole in the presumptive treatment of strongyloidiasis in immigrants to the United States. *Epidemiol Infect.* 2004;132(6):1055.

A10.33 Answer A: Middle East respiratory syndrome (MERS)
MERS is a viral infection caused by MERS coronavirus (MERS-CoV), which was first identified in a 2012 in a patient from Saudi Arabia with severe respiratory failure with multi-organ involvement. MERS-CoV is the first beta-coronavirus of the C phylogenetic lineage known to infect humans. Dromedary camels are considered to be the likely source of animal-to-human transmission with subsequent human-to-human transmission. In 2015, an outbreak of imported MERS-CoV in South Korea led to 186 cases and 36 deaths across multiple healthcare facilities. The rate of MERS-CoV seropositivity is 23 times higher in slaughterhouse workers than the general population. Incubation time is 2–14 days and frequently results in severe disease, however, asymptomatic and mild infections have been reported. Diagnosis is made by real-time PCR of respiratory samples. No antiviral treatment is available and management is predominantly supportive but mortality rates are high.

Further Reading
Arabi YM, Balkhy HH, Hayden FG. Middle east respiratory syndrome. *N Engl J Med.* 2017;376 (6):584–594.

Index